Traditional He
Medicines

Lakshman Karalliedde *dedicates this book to Kanthi, Janaka, Dhammika and Sidantha for their love and affection and above all for their courage, determination and resolve to overcome adversity;*

My teachers, particularly A. Sinnatamby, Bertie Dias, Ivan Jansze, Leslie Handunge, R L Kannangara, Rev Clarence Peiris, Charles de Silva, Drs Francis de Silva, Thistle Jayawardena, L C 'Chokka' Fernando, P A P Joseph, Chris Uragoda, Upali Weerackody, Professors Tony Adams, Stanley Feldman, H S Keerthisinghe, C Barr Kumarakulasinghe, Senaka Bibile; and

My friends, particularly Palitha Abeykoon, Roger Abeyaratne, Lakshman Attygalle, Y C Chang, Ranjit and Anura Eriyagama, Anton Fernando, Wimal Jayaratnam, N Ganeshananthan, Tissa Kappagoda, Sarath Kapuwatte, Indra and Lalitha Katugaha, Dayantha and Sunil Liyanage, Keerthi Makuloluwa, Bernie Peiris, Aldo Pereira, N Poopalasingham, Nimal Senanayake, Syed Ahmed, Harendra Rasiah, A H Sheriff Deen, Mahes de Silva, Naomal Soysa, R Swaminathan, Bertram Tittawella, Nahil Wijesuriya, John Henry, Timothy Marrs, Bob Maynard, Virginia Murray, Ray Radford, Guy Rathcliffe, John Restall, Trevor Thomas, Glyn Volans, and Brian Widdop, who have all done so much to teach, guide, help and support me in innumerable ways during good times and especially during rough times.

Indika Gawarammana *dedicates this book to Rukmali, Radhini, Raje Thiruini and his parents Ranaweera and Leela.*

Traditional Herbal Medicines

a guide to their safer use

Dr Lakshman Karalliedde MB BS DA FRCA
Consultant, Chemical Hazards and Poisons Division (London)
Health Protection Agency, UK;
Visiting Senior Lecturer, King's College Medical School, London, UK

Dr Indika Gawarammana MB BS MD MRCP
Senior Lecturer in Medicine and Consultant Physician
Department of Medicine, Faculty of Medicine, Peradeniya, Sri Lanka;
Director of Clinical Research, South Asian Toxicology Research Collaboration,
Faculty of Medicine, Sri Lanka;
Conjoint Lecturer in Clinical Toxicology, University of Newcastle, Australia

EDITORIAL ADVISOR:
Debbie Shaw
Medical Toxicology Unit
Guy's & St Thomas' NHS Foundation Trust, London, UK

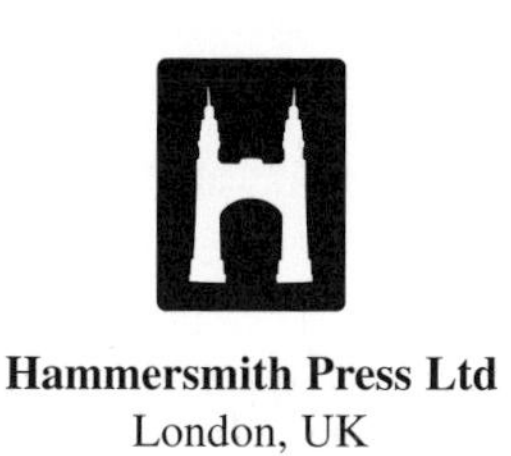

Hammersmith Press Ltd
London, UK

First published in 2008 by Hammersmith Press Limited
496 Fulham Palace Road, London SW6 6JD, UK
www.hammersmithpress.co.uk

Disclaimer
Whilst the advice and information in this book are believed to be true and accurate at the date of going to press, neither the author nor the publisher can accept any legal responsibility or liability for any errors or omissions that may be made. In particular (but without limiting the generality of the preceding disclaimer) while every effort has been made to ensure that the contents of this book are accurate, it must not be treated as a substitute for qualified medical advice. Neither the Author nor the Publisher can be held responsible for any loss or claim arising out of the use, or misuse, of the suggestions made or failure to take medical advice.

The Authors and Publisher have made every endeavour to ensure all sources of information are acknowledged. Any omissions are the result of oversight and can be rectified if brought to our attention.

British Library Cataloguing in Publication Data: A CIP record of this book is available from the British Library.

ISBN 978-1-905140-04-6

Commissioning editor: Georgina Bentliff
Designed by Julie Bennett
Copyediting by Carolyn Holleyman
Proof reading by Carrie Walker
Typesetting by Phoenix Photosetting, Chatham, Kent
Production by Helen Whitehorn, Pathmedia
Printed and bound by TJ International Ltd, Padstow, Cornwall, UK
Cover images: *Top* © Corbis
Left © Roy Morsch/CORBIS
Middle © Image Source/Corbis
Right © David Aubrey/CORBIS

Contents

Chapter 2 Commonly Used Herb

About the Authors, Editors and Contributors

THE AUTHORS/EDITORS

Dr Lakshman Karalliedde (MB BS, DA, FRCA) and **Dr Indika Gawarammana** (MB BS, MD, MRCP) grew up in the central hills of Sri Lanka amidst strong beliefs in and heritage of Ayurvedic Medicine. They both studied allopathic medicine, first at the medical schools in Sri Lanka and then, for their post-graduate training and examinations, in the UK. Both worked at the Medical Toxicology Unit of Guy's & St Thomas NHS Trust for seven and two years respectively. The Medical Toxicology Unit developed an interest in the toxicology of traditional medicines in the 1990s. Lakshman Karalliedde and Indika Gawarammana have considerable respect for the Traditional Medical Systems despite being aware of the paucity of sound scientific evidence as regards efficacy and safety, and they and their families continue to use both traditional and allopathic medicines. Lakshman Karalliedde, after retirement from the Medical Toxicology Unit, is now Consultant Toxicologist at the Chemical Hazards and Poisons Division (London) of the Health Protection Agency, UK and Visiting Senior Lecturer at King's College School of Medicine. Indika Gawarammana is Senior Lecturer in Medicine and Consultant Physician at the Faculty of Medicine, University of Peradeniya, Sri Lanka and Director of Clinical Research at the South Asian Clinical Toxicology Research Collaboration (SACTRC) based in Sri Lanka. (He is also a Conjoint Lecturer in Clinical Toxicology at the University of Newcastle, Australia.) Lakshman Karalliedde is also closely associated with the collaboration to develop toxicology in Sri Lanka and in South East Asia.

THE EDITORIAL ADVISOR

Debbie Shaw heads the herbals work at the Chinese Medicine Advisory Service, Medical Toxicology Unit (MTU), Guy's & St Thomas's NHS Foundation Trust, London, UK. She has been actively involved in reviewing and investigating suspected adverse reactions to herbal and traditional medicines for the past 11 years. She works closely with the Royal Botanic Gardens Kew, and has participated in the development of the Chinese Medicinal Plants Centre. She is a member of the Herbal Signals Review Panel for the Uppsala Monitoring Centre (WHO Collaborating Centre for International Drug Monitoring), and an advisor to the American Herbal Pharmacopoeia.

THE AUTHOR OF THE FOREWORD

Professor Virginia Murray, FFPH, FRCP, FFOM, FRCPath
Consultant Medical Toxicologist

Virginia Murray trained in medicine before joining the Guy's Poisons Unit, London in 1980. In 1986 she was appointed as a consultant medical toxicologist. In 1989 she started the Chemical Incident Research Programme and was the Director of the Chemical Incident Response Service from 1996. Since April 2003 she has worked for the Health Protection Agency's Chemical Hazards and Poisons Division. She is the Visiting Professor in Health Protection at King's College, London.

ASSISTANT EDITORS

Heather Wiseman BSc, MSc
Senior Scientist
Guy's & St Thomas' NHS Foundation Trust, London, UK

Dr Anomi Panditharatne MB BS, MD (Ophthal), FRCS (Ophthal) (Glasgow)
University College London Hospital, London, UK

Rita Fitzpatrick BSc
Senior Scientist
Guy's & St Thomas' Poisons Unit,
Guy's & St Thomas' NHS Foundation Trust, London, UK

CONTRIBUTIONS BY

Edwin Chandraharan MB BS, MS (Obs & Gyn), DFFP, MRCOG
Consultant Obstetrician & Gynaecologist,
St George's Healthcare NHS Trust, London, UK

Narlaka Jayasekera MB BS, MRCS
Specialist Registrar in Trauma and Orthopaedic Surgery,
West Midlands (Oswestry) Training Scheme,
Princess Royal Hospital, Telford, UK

INDEX AND GLOSSARY COMPILED BY

Thusharika Gooneratne-Karalliedde BSc, MSc

Foreword

Many people around the world use traditional or herbal remedies as their treatment of choice and many consider that, because 'they are natural', these remedies are intrinsically safe. In my experience as a medical toxicologist this is not necessarily true.

Traditional remedies are of increasing interest to many people, not only patients but also western (allopathic) medicine practitioners. Data show that usage in developed countries is increasing significantly. But the knowledge of potential adverse effects is not taught routinely to the practitioners or patients who use these remedies. Information on adverse health effects is not easily available to those members of the public who decide to seek traditional remedies, often without telling their western (allopathic) doctors.

Why do patients not discuss the use of traditional remedies with their western (allopathic) doctors? Possibly because they are concerned that their wish for medicine other than that prescribed by their western doctor may undermine their doctor-patient relationship. Equally, western doctors may not seek to know what other remedies their patients may be taking, because they do not know what risks these might present. Risks of adverse health effects therefore exist – sometimes just because of poor communication and insufficient knowledge.

In the old days traditional remedy practitioners would have had knowledge of the adverse effects associated with their remedies. However, this information was rarely recorded and is not readily available in scientific literature.

As a practitioner of western medicine, I have not been involved in efficacy studies of these remedies but as a medical toxicologist (specialist in poisons) I am cautious about the use of traditional remedies. I have been involved in responding to adverse health effects associated with the use of these remedies for some years. The reported effects have been due to innate toxicity of the remedy, to interactions with allopathic medicines, or even to misidentification, to inappropriate use and/or poor quality of plant materials.

I have led a five year project to assess and document adverse health effects from traditional remedies seen at the Guy's Poisons Unit. Although a series of scientific papers has been published from this work, it has become increasingly apparent that up until now there has been no clear, easily accessible source of information for western medical practitioners, traditional remedy practitioners or members of the public. This book, *Traditional Herbal Medicines – a guide to their safer use*, goes a long way to providing this information.

This book highlights the care that needs to be exercised in the use of traditional remedies. It is not a guide to the primary use of traditional remedies. It is more a book summarising the effects and potential hazards from their use. It is not a 'pharmacopoeia'. *Traditional Herbal Medicines* is for the public and for the professionals (allopathic and traditional) who may not be aware of what other systems of medical practice may prescribe.

The book, in its Introduction, covers data for the public and for medial professionals:

- The public are guided through the increase in use, particularly in developed countries, of traditional remedies and the nature of diseases for which they are used (e.g. diseases where there are no specific 'cures' or remedies in allopathic medicine such as childhood eczema, sickle cell disease, malignancies, obesity and problems associated with sexual dysfunction – impotence and subfertility).
- Medical professionals are guided through the widespread use of traditional remedies. Information on why certain communities (e.g. immigrant population groups) tend to use the herbal medicines more frequently is included and an indication of the potentially harmful constituents that these preparations may contain. Information about toxic effects or interactions which cause major difficulties in diagnosis and treatment is summarised. Information is also provided on aspects of assessments of efficacy- more objective in allopathic medicine and more subjective in traditional medicines- the need for each group of clinicians to learn from each other.

This book provides summary details on the types of diseases where members of the public seek to use traditional remedies and the types of remedies that they may be given. Chapter 1 describes some common medical disorders from an allopathic (western) perspective and the treatments used in allopathic medicine and a list, in alphabetical order, of some of the herbs that have been used for such disorders. No attempt is made at any stage to compare efficacy for any particular disease state.

Some 300 pen pictures of herbs commonly used in herbal and traditional remedies are provided in Chapter 2 indicating plant components, usual uses, and other uses, probable mode of action, adverse effects and precautions. The readers are referred to other more comprehensive texts for detailed reviews.

Chapter 3 summarise data on the known harmful constituents of herbal medicines. Heavy metals (usually referred to as contaminants), allopathic medications (usually referred to as adulterants), animal and human body parts, toxic plant alkaloids and pesticides are described. Reports from the scientific literature illustrating adverse health effects are included. The toxic effects of harmful contaminants are indicated at the end of the chapter along with a list of the herbal medicines that have been found to contain such toxic constituents.

Precautions that should be followed during pregnancy, breast feeding, old age, infancy, heart disease, liver disease, allergies and other diseases are addressed in Chapter 4. Information on herbal and traditional remedies that may act as hallucinogens or stimulants with the probability of causing dependence /addiction is provided.

Finally chapter 5 provides a summary of the known and possible interactions between western (allopathic) medicine and herbal and traditional remedies. It also provides summary data on known herbal and traditional remedy to herbal and traditional remedy interactions, known as herb-herb interactions.

So where to in the future? More information is needed on the risks from adverse health effects. Please remember to report any effects on the 'Reporting suspected adverse drug reactions' page of the Medicines and Healthcare products Regulatory Agency (MHRA): http://www.mhra.gov.uk/home/idcplg?IdcService=SS_GET_PAGE&nodeId=287. Healthcare professionals and patients, parents or carers can make a report.

Virginia Murray

Introduction

Despite the benefits of conventional Western (allopathic) medicine, more and more of us are using traditional medicines. Estimates suggest that over 50% of the population use some form of traditional medical practice at least once during their life time, either in addition to or instead of conventional medicine.

In the US, approximately 160 million adults are believed to use traditional medicines and over 1500 herbal medicines are sold annually for a total of nearly US$ 5 billion. This constitutes the fastest growing sector of the US pharmaceutical market, according to the US President's Commission on Dietary Supplements.

The *Archives of Internal Medicine* in October 2006 reported that in the US 21% of adult prescription medication users admitted to using non-vitamin dietary supplements (which includes herbal medicines) and that 69% of those did not discuss this use with a conventional medical practitioner.

In the UK, a study of Scottish prescription data for 1,891,669 patients in 2003–2004 revealed that 49% of general medical practices prescribed homeopathic remedies and 32% of practices prescribed herbal remedies.

A recent publication in the *British Medical Journal* (25 November 2006) estimated 'that up to 80% of all patients with cancer take a complementary treatment or follow a dietary programme to help treat their cancer'. The *NHS Directory of Complementary and Alternative Practitioners* lists 29 directories. The article stated that alternative medicine is big business with a market value in the UK alone of £250 million in the year 2005 and that the current prediction is that sales will increase by 7% per annum.

Worldwide, WHO estimates that 50% of the population of Canada and 75% of the population of France have tried complementary or alternative medicine, which often includes herbal remedies. In Japan, 85% of doctors prescribe not only allopathic medicine but also traditional herbal medicine (called kampo) which is covered by health insurance. If patients suffering from a single specific disease state, e.g. HIV/AIDS, are considered, some form of traditional medicine, predominantly of plant origin, is likely to be used by 75% of them, an estimate that is similar for patients in San Francisco, London and South Africa.

The global market for medicines of herbal origin was worth US$ 60 billion in 2003, and the consensus is that this market is continuing to increase. Herbal remedies continue to be the first choice of healthcare in many developing countries. In Africa for example, up to 80% of the population depend on herbal medicines, according to WHO estimates. A recent study by Roll Back Malaria Initiative found that in Ghana, Mali, Nigeria and Zambia, herbal medicine is the first choice for home treatment of nearly two-thirds of children with high fever. In India, where the traditional Ayurvedic medicine uses over 1200 different herbs, herbal medicine is regularly used by about 65% of the approximately one billion population.

One of the key reasons for increased use in developed countries is the generally accepted perception that 'natural' products are safe: they have stood the test of time and do not carry the risks inherent in newly developed conventional medicines. There is insufficient awareness that the ingredients that make traditional medicines effective may also be capable of causing serious illness such as allergy, liver or kidney malfunction, blindness, cancer or even death. Herbal medicines should be used with the same degree of caution as conventional medicines, but this is difficult given the lack of information available about effectiveness, optimum dose or adverse effects.

Acknowledging that much of the evidence remains anecdotal, we have brought together what is currently known about the safe use of traditional medicines in what we hope will prove a user-friendly guide, highlighting the key safety issues:

- poisons intrinsic to herbal and mineral ingredients
- potential interactions with conventional medicines and medical procedures
- possible adulterants and contaminants
- problems for vulnerable groups, including pregnant mothers and infants
- the importance of not delaying seeking conventional medical help.

We have written this guide not only for users of traditional medicines, but also for those who prescribe them, and for practitioners of conventional medicine. Depending on the group to which you belong, you may find there are some sections that you will want to skip over, so we have used a highly structured format to help you to find the information you need to use these potentially powerful medicines safely.

Note for health professionals

If you are a practitioner of allopathic medicine it is essential that you are aware of the significant increase in the use of traditional medicines, particularly by migrant population groups. You should take time to document traditional medicine use by your patients, remembering that many people who use herbal remedies are reluctant to reveal this even to members of their family.

Safety and efficacy are major issues associated with any form of medical practice, and it is important for you to be familiar with the issues discussed in this book that influence the safety of traditional medicines, particularly herbal medicines. These are:

1. The presence of intrinsically toxic constituents to which a patient may be exposed while using herbal medicines.
2. The potential for adulteration and contamination of herbal products and possible adverse health effects that may result.
3. The disadvantages or dangers of delays in seeking allopathic medical care that may be caused by using herbal medicines that may be of doubtful efficacy.
4. The vulnerability of some specific population groups to adverse effects of herbal medicines. Pregnant women, breastfeeding mothers, infants and older people and people suffering from some medical conditions that are well defined in the allopathic medical literature should avoid using herbal preparations or take them only under close supervision.
5. The dangers to patients of not revealing their use of herbal medicines to allopathic practitioners who may prescribe allopathic medicine prior to surgical interventions and investigations or to treat disease. The interaction of allopathic medicine with herbal medicine could render the allopathic medicine ineffective or could cause life-threatening adverse effects.

Conventional allopathic Western medical practice has evolved during centuries of scientific study and critical review. In developed or industrialized countries where literacy, accessibility to healthcare, effective communication links and the availability and affordability of medications have all facilitated the development and utilization of this form of medical practice, allopathic medicine is now familiar and acceptable to most population groups.

Traditional medicines have an even longer history, during which the medicines and their method of use have been developed by communities to provide readily available remedies to their population groups.

Herbal medicines have maintained their popularity in all regions of the developing world especially where the availability and cost of allopathic medicines and of allopathic medical practitioners are dominant considerations in the provision and delivery of healthcare. Literate, affluent people in developed countries use herbal medicines because they believe that natural products are safe and must be beneficial to health, or because they are suspicious of synthetic chemical products. Others turn to herbal medicines when they believe allopathic medicine offers little or no hope or comfort. This is particularly the case for people suffering from chronic disorders or diseases of uncertain causation or pathology which cannot be cured, only controlled, by allopathic medicine (e.g. skin disorders, chronic fatigue, HIV, obesity), or terminal illnesses (e.g. malignant disease).

The rapidly increasing use and growing popularity of traditional medicines in developed countries is intriguing and is to some extent being stimulated by increasing scientific interest in herbal medicine. WHO estimates that of the 35,000–70,000 species of plants that are used for medicinal purposes around the world, some 5000 have been submitted to biomedical scrutiny. Scientific evidence of efficacy is beginning to emerge from randomized controlled trials in which herbs compare favourably with placebo. Evidence is emerging for herbs such as St John's wort, used for mild depression; ginkgo biloba, used for some forms of dementia; saw palmetto, used for benign prostatic hyperplasia; and horse chestnut, used for chronic venous insufficiency. Of course, a number of commonly used pharmaceuticals are of botanical origin – aspirin, digoxin and quinine being three well-known examples.

Other issues of concern relating to traditional herbal medicines are:

1. The therapeutic/toxic constituent/s of the plant may vary in amount due to geographical variations, stage of maturity of the plant or plant component and/or improper storage.
2. Contamination with toxic or harmful elements such as heavy metals may occur during preparation.
3. There may be huge variations in the concentrations of ingredients used in medicines prepared by different manufacturers or at different times, and in the potency of those ingredients.
4. Practitioners or manufacturers may deliberately incorporate allopathic medications which may be banned in some countries or are only available on prescription from an allopathic practitioner in other countries.
5. The labelling of some herbal medicines may be inaccurate, in indicating both the constituents and the amounts of the constituents used, which may be compounded by the fact that the labelling may be in a language not familiar to users.
6. Sociocultural, religious and other factors may result in different therapeutic regimens or dosages of very similar herbal medicines for a particular disease state.
7. There is seldom any biochemical or physiological evidence for the efficacy of a herbal medicine on a disease state.
8. Although many countries have systems for monitoring adverse reactions to herbal medicines, for example the yellow card system in the UK, nevertheless adverse effects of many herbs are poorly documented. Manufacturers of unlicensed products may not comply with normal safety monitoring requirements. Health professionals do not always report adverse effects with herbal medicines. In addition adverse effects may not be associated with the herbal medicine responsible, because the

patient has not told their doctor that they are using the medicine. Even when an adverse symptom is correctly attributed to use of a herbal product the identity of the constituents may be uncertain.

9. There is less stringent regulation of herbal medicine practitioners when compared with allopathic practitioners. Although schemes for the training and assessment of competence and knowledge for the practice of herbal or traditional medicine are being introduced or are already in use in many countries, there are no internationally accepted standards.

The preparation, distribution and marketing of traditional medicines are largely unregulated (though this is changing in some countries). Although many of the issues listed above make it difficult to regulate herbal medicines and practitioners, it is disappointing that there has been so little progress in implementing regulation in those countries which have had well-developed systems for regulating allopathic medicines and practitioners in place for decades, particularly when one considers the increasing popularity of traditional medicine in such countries. Health authorities need to develop guidelines and analytical facilities to ensure the safety of imported herbal medicines and to develop mechanisms to monitor and assess the practice of traditional medicines. The publication in the *British Medical Journal* quoted earlier (November 2006) suggests 'that the alternative medicines industry should be subject to the level of scrutiny that defines pharmaceuticals'.

The author, Dr Waxman, suggests reclassifying these agents as drugs – for this is after all how they are marketed – and that in this context, the current EU initiative to bring forward legislation on this matter is welcomed. The yellow card system which enables practitioners, pharmacists, nurses and patients to report adverse effects of allopathic medicines should be encouraged for herbal medicines.

The Uppsala Monitoring Centre runs the WHO Programme for International Drug Monitoring, taking adverse reaction reports (ADRs) from over 80 countries around the world. Their ADR database has over 3.7 million reports collected since 1968, with only 16,154 reports on adverse effects of herbal medicine.

It is not the intent of this introduction to seek explanations for the infinitely small number of reports of adverse drug reactions of traditional medicines when compared with allopathic medicines. However, the reporting of adverse effects by all associated with the use of herbal traditional medicines needs to be encouraged and publicized.

As with allopathic medicines, the manufacturers have a responsibility to ensure the production of herbal medicines according to Good Manufacturing Practice (GMP) prior to distribution of their products in a country. It is likely that herbal medicines will be subjected to GMP scrutiny by the end of this decade in many developed countries. The manufacturers should also consider their responsibility to ensure that labelling is accurate and legible, and should carry out testing of the products in a manner similar to the manufacturers of allopathic medications.

If the results of a recent survey in Scotland provide an accurate picture of the extent of homeopathic and herbal prescribing throughout the UK, it 'raises questions about homeopathic/herbal provision in the National Health Service which should prompt critical review'.

REFERENCES

Gardiner P, Graham RE, Legedza TR, Eisenberg DM, Phillips RS. Factors associated with dietary supplement use among prescription medication users. *Archives of Internal Medicine* 2006:166:1968–1974.

Ross S, Simpson CR, McLay JS. Homeopathic and herbal prescribing in general practice in Scotland. *British Journal of Clinical Pharmacology* 2006:23, published online 23 June 2006.

Waxman J. Shark cartilage in the water. Personal view. *British Medical Journal* 2006:333:1129.

www.who-umc.org

1

Common Medical Disorders

with Treatment Options in Allopathic Medicine and Herbal Medicine

This chapter explores the possibilities of providing optimal safe care by utilizing the resources of both allopathic and herbal medicine.

Traditional systems of medicine such as Unani, Ayurveda or Chinese medicine each have their own understanding and interpretation of disease and a different approach to its medical management. Their explanations of disorders of body function and causes of disease may be difficult for Western, or 'allopathic,' physicians and patients educated in the Western tradition to understand.

This chapter:

1. Describes some common medical disorders from an allopathic viewpoint, providing basic information on signs and symptoms and the treatment used by allopathic physicians.
2. Lists herbal medicines used for the medical disorders, discussed in alphabetical order. (Please note these lists cannot be exhaustive.) It is not intended to be a recommendation for use, but an indication of the varied herbal medicines that have been known/reported to be used for the medical disorders discussed. Some of these herbs, though used in the past, are now considered to be toxic (e.g. aconite) and are no longer recommended for use. It is also important that some of these herbs, particularly essential oils, should not be used systemically (taken by mouth) and hence it is mandatory that patients seek information from

Ayurvedic, Unani or Chinese herbal practitioners as to which of these herbs should be used only as external applications.
3. Makes no attempt to compare efficacy of herbal medicines and allopathic medicines for medical disorders.
4. Discusses some of the dangers which we believe could result from delays in seeking appropriate allopathic medical care.
5. Emphasizes the need to study and document information on herbal medicines using criteria that would make both users and those prescribing more comfortable with the safe use of herbal medicines in medical practice, either on their own or as adjuncts to allopathic medications.

The following are among the several reasons for the increasing popularity of herbal medicines:

1. For some disease states which are protracted or chronic, allopathic medicine offers unsatisfactory relief to the individual and/or the family, e.g. childhood asthma, childhood eczema, psoriasis, depression, insomnia, arthritis, irritable bowel syndrome, malignancies and disorders such as sickle cell disease.
2. There may be doubts or suspicion about the safety of allopathic medications that have been prescribed, e.g. corticosteroids, drugs used in chemotherapy, antidepressants or anti-inflammatory agents.
3. Individuals who have experienced adverse effects from allopathic medications may be reluctant to continue using them.
4. There may be no over-the-counter allopathic medications available to treat those conditions for which some people would prefer to obtain their own medication without consulting a physician, e.g. menstrual abnormalities, concerns regarding fertility, slimming and some skin disorders.

In allopathic medicine, efficacy tends to be assessed in a more objective manner than in therapy with herbal medicines. Allopathic medicine uses measurements of physiological parameters (temperature, blood sugar, blood pressure) and sophisticated investigations (e.g. CAT scans, MRI scans, biomarkers) to assess efficacy. In contrast herbal practitioners rely on patient interviews and subjective responses from recipients to assess efficacy.

It would be useful for each to learn from the other: for herbal practitioners to make better use of investigative facilities and for allopathic practitioners to pay greater attention to the patient's subjective responses. This is already happening to some extent, for patient satisfaction has become an increasingly important aspect of allopathic medical practice in the past decade.

All medical practitioners need to be aware of the socioeconomic and cultural factors that influence their patients, including their preferences for, and frequency of use of, different types of medications. It is also necessary to be aware that patients may use several medications at the same time, sometimes using both allopathic and herbal preparations. When patients present with disorders which cannot be easily diagnosed, it is particularly important to consider the possibility that this could be due to an interaction between allopathic and herbal medicines, or to an adverse effect from either a herbal or allopathic medication. The simultaneous use of more than one kind of medicine also makes it difficult to attribute efficacy to any one of them.

The lack of information on long-term or subtle effects of herbal medicines such as carcinogenicity, mutagenicity and teratogenicity is considered a serious drawback at present. Such information would give medical practitioners more confidence in prescribing herbal medicines either alone or in addition to allopathic products.

SOURCES

The following sources were used in the compilation of this chapter:

Barnes J, Anderson LA, Phillipson JD (Eds). *Herbal Medicines*, 2nd edn. London: Pharmaceutical Press, 2002.

Boon NA, Chilvers E, Colledge N et al. (Eds). *Davidson's Principles and Practice of Medicine*, 20th edn. Edinburgh: Elsevier Churchill-Livingstone, 2006.

Fetrow CW, Avila JR. *Professionals' Handbook of Complementary and Alternative Medicines*, 2nd edn. Philadelphia: Springhouse, 2001.

Gruenwald J, Brendler T, Jaenicke C. *PDR for Herbal Medicines*, 2nd edn. Montvale, New Jersey: Medical Economics Co, 2000.

Haslett C, Chilvers E, Boon NA. *Davidson's Principles and Practice of Medicine*, 19th edn. Edinburgh: Elsevier Churchill-Livingstone, 2002.

McIntyre A. *The Top 100 Herbal Remedies*. London: Duncan Baird Publishers, 2006.

Peters D (Ed). *New Medicine*. London: Dorling Kindersley, 2005.

Scott G, Springfield EP. *Pharmaceutical Monographs for 60 South African Plant Species used as Traditional Medicines*. South African National Biodiversity Institute (SANBI) Plant Information, 2004.

Vries J de. *The Pharmacy Guide to Herbal Remedies*. Edinburgh: Mainstream Publishing, 2001.

Weatherall DJ, Ledingham JGG, Warrell DA. *Oxford Textbook of Medicine*, 3rd edn. Oxford: Oxford University Press, 1996.

CLINICAL PROBLEMS DISCUSSED IN THIS CHAPTER

CHAPTER CONTENTS LIST

The above disorders are discussed according to the systems/structures in which they occur as follows:

Skin disorders
- Acne
- Eczema
- Fungal infections of the skin – ringworm, athlete's foot
- Warts – veruccas
- Scabies
- Lice
- Psoriasis

General disorders or symptoms
- Obesity
- Asthma – bronchial asthma
- Headache
- Pain

Growths – Tumours – Cancers
Diabetes – Diabetes mellitus
Acute sore throat
Raised blood cholesterol
Bleeding
Fever
Mouth ulcers
Vitiligo
Goitre
Hypertension (high blood pressure)
Ischaemic heart disease – Angina – Heart attacks
Gout
Cystitis
Hives or urticaria (nettle rash)

Liver and gallbladder disease
Jaundice
Viral hepatitis
Cirrhosis
Gallstones

Disorders of blood
Anaemia
Leukaemia

Abdominal (gastrointestinal) disorders
Constipation
Diarrhoea
Abdominal pain
Severe acute pain/discomfort in the abdomen
Chronic or recurrent abdominal pain
Weight loss
Malabsorption
Haematemesis (vomiting of blood)
Bleeding per rectum
Gastritis and peptic ulcer disease
Irritable bowel syndrome

Musculoskeletal system disorders
Joint pains
Arthritis
Fibromyalgia
Osteoporosis
Backache

Sexually transmitted diseases
AIDS/HIV
Gonorrhoea
Syphilis

Gynaecological disorders
Amenorrhoea
Infertility
Dysmenorrhoea (painful menstruation or pain with periods)
Endometriosis
Menorrhagia (heavy periods)
Menopause
Premenstrual syndrome (PMS)

Nervous system and mental function
Depression
Anxiety
Fits – epilepsy
Impairment of memory and dementia

Male and female sexual dysfunction
Erectile dysfunction and impotence
Female sexual dysfunction

Eye disorders
Conjunctivitis
Glaucoma
Diabetic retinopathy

Ear, nose and throat disorders
Earache and ear infections
Catarrh and sinusitis
Tinnitus

Tiredness all the time (TATT)

***NOTE*:** Do bear in mind that, of the herbs listed for each condition below, some, e.g. some herbs used in the treatment of HIV/AIDS, are known to interact with allopathic medications, either increasing or decreasing their effect (see chapter 5, on Interactions).

SKIN DISORDERS

ACNE

Acne is a common skin condition characterized by red pimples on the skin. It particularly affects women and teenagers, and may continue into the third decade of life, but only rarely beyond that. Acne occurs when sebaceous glands below the surface of the skin secrete excessive amounts of sebum. The sebum builds up under the surface of the skin because the skin's pores have become blocked by dead skin cells, and causes blackheads or comedones to form. Sometimes the inflammation is made worse by excessive growth of a bacterium, *Propionibacterium acnes*, which normally lives in the sebaceous glands without causing harm.

Secretion of sebum is stimulated mainly by male hormones (androgens) and by the female hormone progesterone, but is reduced by other female hormones, such as oestrogens, which thus tend to reduce acne. Applications of tars, and other agents, such as chlorinated hydrocarbons and oily cosmetics, to the skin of the face can make acne worse.

Comedones can be treated with topical application of benzoyl peroxide or tretinoin. Washes, soaps or antiseptics are of little or no benefit. If antibiotic treatment is contemplated, it is mandatory that treatment be continued for three months before concluding that there is no response to the antibiotic. Oxytetracycline is the antibiotic of choice and minocycline is an alternative. Isotretinoin therapy for four months is effective in moderate to severe acne unresponsive to antibiotics. Scarring is best treated by excision or carbon dioxide laser treatment.

Rosacea is a persistent eruption on the face of unknown cause characterized by redness and papules which respond to oxytetracycline. It may sometimes be associated with inflammation of the eyes (blepharitis, conjunctivitis).

ACNE:

Some herbs used in treatment

Acidophilus	Hawthorn
Aloe	Jojoba
Burdock	Marigold
Chamomile (washes)	Milk thistle (tea)
Chickweed	Oregon grape
Cleavers (tea)	Nettle (tea)
Coriander	Red clover (tea)
Dandelion (tea)	Rose water (washes)
Echinacea	Tea tree (topical)
Elderflower (washes)	

Some herbal medicines considered to cause or worsen acne

Fucus (kelp). The association between halogen salts and acneiform eruptions is well established. Ingestion of kelp products has been associated with the worsening of pre-existing acne and the development of acnei-form eruptions.

ECZEMA

The terms eczema and dermatitis are synonymous and refer to distinctive changes in the skin characterized by redness and swelling with ill-defined margins, papules, vesicles, exudates (fluid that seeps out – weeping) and cracking. The onset can be acute or chronic.

These skin eruptions are caused by a number of factors which can be grouped as follows:

Atopic eczema. This is caused by a genetic predisposition to common substances found in the environment, like pollen and house dust mite. It is seen usually during the first two years of life and generally affects 1 in 10 school children. The main features are itching, scratching and dryness of skin. During infancy, the onset is often acute and involves the face and the trunk. The nappy areas are usually spared. In childhood, the rashes appear on the back of the knees, front of the elbows, wrists and ankles. In adults, the face and trunk are more likely to be affected. Children with atopic eczema have an increased incidence of food allergies (e.g. eggs, cow's milk, fish, wheat and soya) which can cause an immediate urticarial reaction with little or no worsening of the eczema. When eczematous lesions persist for long periods it will cause difficulty in sleeping, loss of schooling and behavioural abnormalities.

Allopathic treatment consists of moisturizers, 'wet wraps', tar and ichthammol paste bandages. Topical steroids may be used sparingly in resistant cases.

Seborrhoeic eczema is a red scaly rash affecting the scalp (dandruff), central face, naso-labial folds, eyebrows and central chest. This is due to *Pityrosporum ovale* infection. Extensive seborrhoeic dermatitis may be a manifestation of AIDS. Recommended allopathic treatment is to use antipityrosporal agents (ketoconazole shampoo) along with weak corticosteroids.

Discoid eczema is seen in elderly patients and in young men who use excessive amounts of alcohol. Lesions are discrete and coin-shaped and seen on the limbs.

Irritant eczema may be caused by detergents, alkalis (e.g. nappy rash due to irritant ammoniacal urine), solvents or abrasive dust. It is common in the elderly and in those with a family history of asthma, hay fever or eczema. Allopathy recommends avoidance of irritants, use of protective clothing and regular use of emollients.

Allergic contact eczema follows exposure to an allergen (e.g. nickel in jewellery, rubber chemicals, sticking plaster, hair dye, perfumes and cosmetics). A sensitizing agent produces an eczematous reaction on subsequent contact. The original site of the rash is important in the diagnosis. Allopathic treatments include avoidance of the allergen, use of emollients and protective clothing.

Asteatotic eczema is seen on the lower legs in elderly hospitalized patients due to dry skin caused either by over-humidity due to central heating, over-washing, or the use of diuretics. Allopathy recommends regular use of greasy emollients.

Gravitational oedema is swelling (oedema), reddish bluish discolouration, loss of hair, pigmentation and ulceration seen on the lower legs due to venous insufficiency. Allopathy recommends elevation of the legs, compression bandages and application of steroids confined to eczematous areas only.

ECZEMA:

Some herbs used in treatment

Aloe vera
Burdock
Calendula
Chamomile
Chickweed
Cleavers
Dandelion
Echinacea
Elder
Evening primrose oil
Figwort
Fumitory
Jojoba
Liquorice
Linseed
Nettle
Oregon grape
Plantain
Red clover
Sarsaparilla
Senega
Tea tree (topical)
Vervain
Witch hazel leaf extract
Yarrow

Several Chinese herbal medicines have been used in the treatment of eczematous conditions. It is necessary to seek the expertise of Chinese herbal practitioners as to the manner of use and dosages.

FUNGAL INFECTIONS OF THE SKIN – RINGWORM, ATHLETE'S FOOT

Ringworm is caused by a fungus that feeds off keratin, a substance found in the uppermost layer of the human skin. The infection appears as a small, circular itchy lesion and is highly contagious especially in warm damp conditions such as bathrooms and swimming pools. When ringworm appears on the feet it is referred to as athlete's foot and nails may become yellow and thick. Diagnosis can be confirmed by microscopic examination of skin scrapings or nail clippings. It should be treated with a fungicidal agent (an agent which kills fungi) applied directly to the affected areas (topically) or taken by mouth (systemically).

FUNGAL INFECTIONS OF THE SKIN – RINGWORM, ATHLETE'S FOOT:

Some herbs used in treatment

Aloe vera (juice)
Burdock (tea)
Chamomile (cream)
Cinnamon (tea)
Garlic
Ginger (tea)
Juniper – fungicidal against *Penicillium notatum*
Marigold (tea, cream)
Peppermint
Rose (tea)
Rosemary
Tea tree (topical)
Thyme (tea)

WARTS – VERRUCAS

Warts are skin-coloured papules seen on the hands, face, genitalia or areas of the arms or legs exposed to the sun. They are the result of an increase in the production of skin cells caused by a virus, which is infectious and can be transmitted to others by direct contact. When a wart occurs in the foot it is commonly referred to as a verruca. Verrucas have a rough surface and may cause pain and disability.

Spread of genital warts (warts in the region of the genitals) often follows sexual activity. Genital warts may predispose to cancer of the cervix.

Extensive and widespread (often painful) warts often occur in patients who have a low immunity (e.g. following organ transplantation or AIDS).

Most viral warts resolve spontaneously, but as this may be delayed for several years, patients are often compelled to seek treatment. Allopathic medicine recommends the use of salicylic acid or salicylic acid and lactic acid applications with regular paring for several months.

WARTS – VERRUCAS:

Some herbs used in treatment

Burdock
Celandine
Dandelion (topical)
Echinacea
Elder
Garlic
Jojoba
Liquorice
Marigold
Tea tree (topical)
Thuja (topical)

SCABIES

Many textbooks state that approximately 300 million people worldwide suffer from scabies, a skin lesion caused by mites. The mite lives in furrows in the skin and causes severe itching. Common sites are between the fingers, on the hands, wrists or elbows. Face and scalp are almost never involved except in infants. Scabies is highly contagious and it is absolutely necessary that all symptomatic family members should be treated at the same time. There are several agents in allopathic medicine (benzyl benzoate, permethrin, malathion) that can be applied to the affected areas. In some forms of scabies (hyperkeratotic or crusted or 'Norwegian') this topical treatment can be used along with ivermectin taken by mouth.

SCABIES:

Some herbs used in treatment

Anise
Balsam of Peru
Echinacea
Elecampane
Garlic
Lavender
Peppermint
Rosemary

LICE – NITS

It is estimated that 6–12 million cases of head lice infestations occur in the US annually at a cost of $363 million a year. Adult lice live on the scalp by attaching themselves to the base of hairs by strong crab-like claws. The lice are usually 3–4 mm long and dirty white or grey-black in colour. Adult lice are very difficult to dislodge, but once injured/damaged, they tend to die quickly. They readily resist washing by closing over their breathing apparatus. On an average, 5–10 lice infest a head and eggs are produced at a rate of 6–8 per day. During a lifetime of 30–40 days, up to 300 eggs are laid. These are placed within 1 cm of the scalp and are strongly cemented to the base of the hair, growing out at rate of 1 cm a month. Thus the duration of infection can be measured by the distance of the ovoid egg containers ('nit') from the scalp. It is highly contagious.

The lice suck blood through a stylet and their movement and the sucking of blood is most probably the cause of the intense irritation and itching that is the predominant symptom. Secondary infection following itching and irritation may cause lesions referred to as impetigo or furunculosis, which leads to enlargement of lymph glands in the neck.

Parents and teachers should be alerted to infestations if children are inattentive or are persistently scratching the scalp. Diagnosis is most commonly confirmed through the finding of the white empty nits firmly adherent to the hairs. Differential diagnosis includes dandruff, hair spray, soap flakes and cats' hairs, all of which are readily brushed off.

All affected or exposed children should be treated. In allopathic medicine, increasing resistance to DDT has made the organophosphorus insecticide malathion as a 0.5% alcohol lotion or shampoo the drug of choice. Malathion may be combined with dicophane. More recently, the less toxic and unrelated insecticide permethrin (0.5–1%) has been used as a shampoo. Head shaving is not necessary.

LICE:

Some herbs used in treatment

- Basil (topical)
- Cinnamon (topical)
- Lavender (topical)
- Neem shampoo (topical)
- Pawpaw shampoo with thymol and tea tree oil[1]
- Peppermint (topical)
- Rosemary (topical)
- Tea tree (topical)

PSORIASIS

Psoriasis is a non-infectious chronic skin disease characterized by dry silvery white scales on reddish well-demarcated areas of skin, usually on the scalp, back of the hands, and front of the legs. The nails may also be affected, showing 'thimble pitting' and separation of the nails from the nail bed, the space being filled by keratin.

It affects approximately 2% of European young adults and those between the ages of 50 and 60 years, but seldom affects those under the age of 5 years. Those who develop the disease during the teenage years and early adulthood usually have a family history of the disease: in general, if one parent suffers from psoriasis, the chance of a child being affected is 15–20%.

The initial presentation and clinical course tend to be severe in patients who develop the disease during the teenage years and early adulthood. Often this skin condition disappears for varying periods of time (remissions), which may last several years before recurring (relapse). Remissions followed by relapses are a feature of the clinical course of psoriasis.

The cause of psoriasis is unknown. It may develop in susceptible people following skin damage caused by scratching or surgery, or after exposure to ultraviolet light (sunlight). Other triggers include beta haemolytic streptococcal infections, emotional stress and drugs such as antimalarials, beta adrenergic blockers and lithium, which may also make the lesions more severe.

In the vast majority of cases, psoriasis is not life-threatening. However, the social consequences can be psychologically damaging. Individuals may be reluctant to pursue hobbies such as swimming, find sleeping with partners or spouses embarrassing and the presence of scales wherever they lie or sit could be a constant source of discomfort and unease. Thus counselling should be aimed at reassurance, and constant discussion may be necessary to persuade patients to follow treatment.

In allopathic medicine psoriasis is treated by preparations applied to the skin (topical agents) such as emollients, corticosteroids, vitamin D antagonists or weak tar compounds. In addition more intensive treatments can be given under medical supervision, which may use systemic medicines (taken by mouth) such as retinoids or immunosuppressives, and ultraviolet light therapy. Near total clearance of the disease has been achieved with some treatment schedules, with remission lasting a year or more before a relapse occurred, but in some instances the side-effects of treatment may be perceived as being worse than the disease.

PSORIASIS:

Some herbs used in treatment

Aloe vera	Linseed (flax)
Burdock	Oregon grape
Chickweed	Red clover
Evening primrose	Sarsaparilla
Goldenseal	Tea tree (topical)
Hydrocotyle (topical)	Yellow dock
Jojoba	

GENERAL DISORDERS OR SYMPTOMS

OBESITY

Adults being grossly fat or overweight have become a great concern particularly in developed or rich countries. This is also a concern in children.

Medical texts[2] state that 20% of adults in the UK and more than 30% in the US are obese and that the prevalence of obesity has increased three-fold in the last 20 years. In allopathic medicine, obesity is diagnosed following measurements of body weight and height to obtain a diagnostic parameter referred to as the 'body mass index' (BMI). Body mass index is the weight in kilograms divided by the square of the height in metres. Obesity is diagnosed when the body mass index is greater than 30 kg/m^2. An individual is considered to be extremely obese if the body mass index exceeds 40 kg/m^3.

The common and probably obvious causes of obesity are an inactive lifestyle and excessive intake of fatty food, frequent 'snacking', consumption of drinks high in sugar and fat content and excessive alcohol intake. Thus regular meal habits, increased intake of fruit and vegetables, particularly those with a high fibre content, frequent exercise regimens, and reduction in the intake of alcohol, which is a rich source of energy intake, would help most individuals to reduce their BMI.

However, it is known with some certainty that there are genetic factors that are responsible for individuals being obese. In addition, disease states such as overactivity of the adrenal glands in the body (Cushing's syndrome), decreased activity of the thyroid gland (hypothyroidism), tumours such as insulinomas or tumours in the hypothalamus in the brain also cause obesity. There are also some medications that cause increase in body weight.

Thus in the assessment of subjects with obesity, easily remediable factors should be sought (e.g. management of hormonal or endocrine disorders, elimination of medications that cause increase in body weight), and in others counselling and support to change lifestyle and diet should be encouraged.

Risks associated with obesity

The adverse health effects of weight gain include:

- Type 2 diabetes mellitus
- Hypertension – high blood pressure
- Stroke
- Hyperlipidaemia (increase in fat content in the blood which increases risk of heart attacks)
- Coronary heart disease – heart attacks
- Formation of stones in the gallbladder – gallstones
- Increased risk of certain cancers such as cancers of the bowel (colorectal)
- Shortness of breath, and chest diseases
- Menstrual abnormalities and hirsutism (abnormal growth of hair on a woman's face or body)
- Pregnancy complications
- Weight-related musculoskeletal disorders and osteoarthritis
- Stress incontinence
- Obstructive sleep apnoea
- Loss of self-esteem.

Benefits of moderate weight loss

The following are some estimated benefits of moderate weight loss:

- Fall in mortality
- Reduction in diabetes-related deaths and significant reductions in blood sugar levels
- Reduction in obesity-related cancer deaths (e.g. colorectal cancers in men, cancers of the breast and cervix in women)
- Fall in blood pressure – both systolic and diastolic
- Reduction in fat constituents in the blood which tend to increase the risk of heart attacks and strokes (e.g. blood cholesterol, low density lipoproteins, triglycerides)
- Increases in the fat components in the blood which are considered protective against heart attacks (e.g. high density lipoproteins).

Strategies for weight loss

Though it is now known with certainty that obesity increases the risk of ill-health and death, it is also important to know that the health risks associated with obesity are reversible.

Allopathic medicine employs the following strategies to manage obesity, aiming for a weight loss of 0.5 kg per week:

1. Give up smoking.
2. Promote weight loss in a group setting.
3. A diet of 600 kcal less than expenditure, assessed on sex, weight, daily activities and age. Starvation diets are potentially dangerous due to the risk of sudden death from heart disease exacerbated by profound loss of muscle mass and the development of heart arrhythmias attributed to increases in free fatty acids and harmful changes in electrolytes.
4. Behavioural modification therapy.
5. Promotion of an increase in physical activity.
6. Orlistat, which produces a 30% loss of absorption of dietary fat. Sibutramine which reduces food intake through beta adrenoceptor and 5-hydroxytryptamine receptor agonist activity (these are receptors for some of the chemical messengers or neurotransmitters in the nervous system). Side-effects of the latter include dry mouth, constipation, insomnia and increase in heart rate and blood pressure.
7. Surgical procedures, e.g. stapling of the upper part of the stomach (to decrease capacity of the stomach), bypassing the stomach (gastric bypass).
8. Obesity needs to be managed like any other chronic disease – with empathy and a non-judgemental professional attitude.[3] It is also important to inform obese individuals that a small (5–10%) reduction in weight over 3–6 months is an achievable goal that will bring about considerable benefits. Further it is necessary to emphasize the importance of maintaining a lower weight after such losses and to develop strategies with these individuals for achieving this.

OBESITY:

Some herbs used in treatment

Chickweed	Garlic
Cinnamon	Ginger
Cleavers	Linseed (flax)
Fennel	Pineapple
Fucus (kelp)	Plantain

ASTHMA – BRONCHIAL ASTHMA

Asthma is a disorder where there is difficulty in breathing, with wheezing, cough, chest tightness and shortness of breath, caused by obstruction to air flow due to narrowing of the small tubes in the lung (bronchi and bronchioles) through which oxygen enters the body and carbon dioxide leaves the body. The bronchioles become narrow when the muscle that surrounds the tubes contracts, or when they fill with secretions, or most commonly when they become inflamed.

Asthma may be caused by genetic factors, as shown by the higher prevalence of asthma in first-degree relatives of asthmatic patients. There are also several environmental factors which may act as triggers.

Environmental triggers of asthma

Indoor environmental pollutants	House dust mites, fungal spores and cockroach antigens, nitrogen dioxide (from cookers), sulphur dioxide (from open fires) and cigarette smoke.
Important outdoor pollutants	Nitrogen dioxide (from motor vehicles, fuel burning industries), sulphur dioxide (burning of fossil fuels and diesel engines), flower pollens.
Environmental pollutants encountered at work	Isocyanates, epoxy resins and wood dust.
Asthma-inducing drugs	Beta adrenergic antagonists (beta-blockers), which can induce asthma even when administered as eye drops; salicylates (aspirin) and non-steroidal anti-inflammatory drugs (e.g. Neurofen).
Viral infections and some bacterial infections	
Smoking during pregnancy	Believed to increase the risk of asthma in childhood.
Severe anxiety or stress	

Acute severe asthma can sometimes be life-threatening. Confusion, a slow heart rate and a 'silent chest' (where no breath sounds are heard on examination of the chest with a stethoscope) are life-threatening clinical features. If the pulse rate rises above 110 beats/min, the patient is unable to speak in sentences and the peak expiratory flow rate (the maximum amount of air expired) is less than 50% of the expected value, hospitalization is advised to prevent the patient developing cyanosis (becoming blue due to lack of oxygen), and becoming exhausted.

Asthma may reverse spontaneously or with treatment.

ASTHMA – BRONCHIAL ASTHMA:

Some herbs used in treatment

Aloe
Angelica – psychogenic asthma
Anise
Ashwagandha
Bee pollen
Betony
Bloodroot
Boswellia
Butterbur
Carline thistle
Celery
Chamomile
Chickweed
Drosera
Elder
Elecampane
Ephedra
Euphorbia
Evening primrose
Garlic
Ginger
Ginkgo
Hyssop
Iceland moss
Jamaica dogwood
Khella
Lavender
Lemon balm
Liquorice
Lobelia
Lungmoss
Magnolia
Maidenhair fern
Nettle
Oleander
Parsley
Passion flower
Pill-bearing spurge (Cat's hair)
Rosemary
Senega
Skunk cabbage
Yerba santa

HEADACHE

Headache is one of the most common conditions and most people suffer from a headache at least once a year. Most headaches last only a few hours and may be caused by excess intake of caffeine or relatively simple disturbances/disorders such as dehydration (lack of fluid in the body), or fall in sugar content in the blood. They are seldom associated with significant disease of the nervous system unless accompanied by other symptoms or neurological signs. Urgent neurological investigation may be indicated if the headache is described as:

- a 'dull ache' which is often mild and of sudden onset
- worse in the morning
- associated with 'morning vomiting'
- worse on bending forwards, coughing and straining.

Tension headache is the most common type of headache, experienced by the majority of the population. It is common in subjects who are depressed or are under continued stress. The pain is constant and generalized, often described as 'dull', 'tight' or 'like a pressure' but often radiates forward from the back of the head (occipital region). Unlike migranous headaches, tension headaches are not associated with vomiting or visual disturbances and may continue for weeks or months. Allopathic medicine recommends courses of muscle relaxation and stress management. The antidepressant drug amitriptyline may also prove to be useful.

Migraine headaches are often accompanied by nausea and vomiting and alterations in eyesight or vision, such as intolerance of light (photophobia) and seeing silvery zigzag lines moving across the field of vision. There is often a period preceding the headache where the individual feels irritable and off-colour (prodrome). Migranous headaches may be accompanied by sensations of numbness and tingling, which may spread from one part of the body to another over a period of about 15–20 minutes.

Migraine is most common in people aged less than 40 years old. There is often a family history and females are more affected than males. Women may have episodes of migraine during the menstrual cycle. Factors known to trigger migranous headaches are dietary constituents such as cheese, chocolate and red wine, and psychological stress. Allopathy recommends avoidance of precipitating/exacerbating factors and use of aspirin or paracetamol with an antiemetic (drug to stop vomiting). Long-term use of codeine is not recommended. Severe attacks are treated with drugs that constrict the blood vessels outside the brain. These include 5-hydroxytryptamine antagonists and triptans, e.g. sumitriptan. To prevent migranous headache, the drugs propranolol, pizotifen, amitriptyline and sodium valproate have been used.

Migranous headaches/cluster headaches. In contrast, migranous neuralgia or cluster headaches more often affect males (usually over 30 years old). They usually last for 30–90 minutes and are characterized by pain around the eye, which is often one-sided and accompanied by redness of the conjunctiva, tearing from the affected eye and congestion of the nose. Allopathy recommends the use of the drug sumitriptan or inhalation of 100% oxygen for migranous neuralgia attacks and the drugs verapamil, methysergide or corticosteroids for prophylaxis (prevention).

Other causes of headache

Headaches may also be caused by:

- Medical disorders such as trigeminal neuralgia, temporal arteritis and post-herpetic neuralgia, usually occurring in older people (>60 years). Medical investigation and treatment is needed if such a diagnosis is considered likely.
- Exposure to toxic substances such as lead, mercury, petrol fumes, benzene, sulphur dioxide, paints and solvents. The toxic effects of chronic exposure to low concentrations of

carbon monoxide can also cause headache and it is important to consider this possibility in cases of frequent headaches which tend to be associated with being in a particular place where exposure to carbon monoxide might occur (e.g. a home which has a faulty boiler).

- Monosodium glutamate, a flavouring agent used in many Chinese restaurants.

HEADACHE:

Some herbs used in treatment

Herbs with sedative properties or anxiolytic properties (e.g. chamomile, rose, lavender, lemon balm, lime flower and valerian) have been used for the management of tension headaches. Ginseng (*Panax ginseng*), Siberian ginseng (*Eleutherococcus senticosus*) and astralagus are reported to help in migraine by reducing underlying fatigue.

Angelica
Avens
Basil
Birch
Carline thistle
Celery seeds
Chamomile
Cramp bark, to relieve tension in muscles
Cumin
Damiana
Elder
Feverfew
Hawthorn
Hydrocotyle – Gotu kola
Jamaica dogwood
Kudzu
Lavender (topical)
Lemon balm
Lungmoss
Marjoram
Mate (*Ilex paraguariensis*), for psychogenic headaches
Meadowsweet
Milk thistle
Mint
Mistletoe, for headache due to hypertension
Night-blooming cereus
Pau d'arco
Peppermint
Rosemary
Sage
Siberian ginseng
Scull cap
Stone root
Thyme
Valerian
Vervain
Wood betony
Yucca

Some herbs known to cause headache

Blue flag (*Iris versicolor*)
Gentian
Ginger
Ginkgo – *Ginkgo biloba* may be used for the treatment of migraine.

PAIN

Pain is the most common symptom in medicine and always merits treatment. The International Association for the Study of Pain (IASP) defines pain 'as an unpleasant sensory and emotional experience associated with actual or potential tissue damage or described in terms of such damage'.

The commonest form of pain results from damage to tissues or occurs in situations where tissue damage is imminent. Such pain is referred to as nociceptive pain. Pain that is caused by damage to the sensory pathway of the nervous system by which pain impulses are transmitted to the brain is referred to as neuropathic pain. Different mechanisms are responsible for nociceptive and neuropathic pain, the latter being nearly always associated with irreversible damage.

Acute pain states include abdominal emergencies (e.g. acute appendicitis, perforated stomach ulcer, intestinal obstruction), trauma/accidents, heart attacks (myocardial infarction) and pain associated with labour. Pain from deep tissues such as abdominal viscera (e.g. intestines) is difficult to localize and diagnosis may be a problem.

Clinicians need to be aware of the possibility of referred pain, which is pain at a superficial site caused by a disorder at another site, often in deep tissues. If the diagnosis is missed, serious ill-health may continue.

Emotional stress can exacerbate physical pain. Therefore examination to detect physical and mental signs of anxiety and/or depression is essential. This should be followed by appropriate investigations to determine the underlying cause of the pain. Radiological imaging may also be necessary.

Neuropathic pain is chronic pain resulting from injury to the peripheral or central nervous system that may be caused by disease or surgery. It may present as a burning, stabbing or pulsating pain, spontaneous in origin and not associated with any ongoing tissue damage. The pain is usually in an area where there is loss of sensation and may be associated with a major neurological deficit. When there is severe pain in the area supplied by a nerve, the condition is known as neuralgia. For example, trigeminal neuralgia is a severe stabbing pain on the side of the face and the cheek, areas supplied by the trigeminal nerve (one of the nerves coming from the brain). Attacks of trigeminal neuralgia may be caused by chewing, certain facial movements or touching the face.

In post-herpetic neuralgia, which is caused by shingles, an infection due to the herpes virus, pain is localized in areas supplied by nerves that have been affected or damaged by the virus. Response to morphine-like (opioid) painkillers is poor, and local anaesthetic creams may prove to be helpful. Antiviral drugs such as aciclovir may reduce the duration and severity of post-herpetic neuralgia.

Specific therapy for neuropathic pain often requires the use of drugs usually used to control and prevent convulsions (anticonvulsant), such as gabapentin, or a drug usually used to treat depression, the tricyclic antidepressant amitriptyline. Surgery may be needed in some instances to bring relief from trigeminal neuralgia.

PAIN:

Some herbs used in treatment

Basil	Indigo
Birch	Mate
Capsicum	Myrrh
Comfrey (topical)	Red poppy
Daisy	Thyme
Devil's claw	Willow
Evening primrose	Wintergreen (topical)

GROWTHS – TUMOURS – CANCERS

Usually the growth and death of cells in the body occurs in what would be called a controlled manner. Growth and increase of cells occurs when a child is growing. Cell growth does not usually cause ill-health, but when cells begin to multiply in an uncontrolled manner, tumours result (swelling of a part of the body generally without inflammation/infection). A tumour may be benign or malignant. Malignant growths or tumours are commonly called cancers.

A benign tumour is one that remains localized to the site where cell growth occurred and does not spread to other tissues. Tumours are considered to be malignant when cells spread along blood vessels or lymph vessels to other parts of the body and cause damage to tissues and organs.

Benign growths may cause disfiguration and discomfort, depending on their location/site, and they may be associated with bleeding following injury and non-specific symptoms such as itching, excessive sweating or changes in pigmentation. Problems caused by benign tumours are usually due to pressure on neighbouring tissues as they grow in size. Pressure on vital structures such as the kidney, the ureters, spinal cord, brain, lymph and blood vessels can severely affect function. For example, the pressure of a benign tumour in the brain can decrease the functional capability of brain cells causing symptoms such as loss of memory, unstable gait and headache.

Benign tumours can become malignant, but this is rare. The change would be heralded by an increase in the rate of growth or by ulceration or pain. The growth of benign tumours should be constantly monitored with a view to surgical removal at the appropriate time, since it is very unlikely that either allopathic or traditional therapies would cause them to shrink or disappear.

Malignant tumours, by contrast, will spread and produce widespread dysfunction and serious ill-health unless removed surgically or treated with anticancer (antineoplastic) drugs (chemotherapeutic drugs) or radiotherapy. It is very unlikely that such tumours would respond to any traditional medicines. Reports of such occurrences are only anecdotal with no pathological evidence. However, it is common to hear of incidents when a diagnosis of a malignant tumour has ceased to cause ill-health or discomfort following several forms of alternative therapies and spiritual contact.

In most instances, it would be unwise and dangerous for patients to abandon antineoplastic drugs or radiotherapy in favour of traditional medicines which have neither been proved to decrease growth of the primary tumour nor to control its spread. However, traditional medicines, either alone or in combination with allopathic medicines, can sometimes reduce or control, to some degree, the numerous distressing side-effects suffered by patients receiving antineoplastic drug therapy or radiotherapy.

Malignancy can have both local and systemic features. The local signs and symptoms may be due to the pressure from the mass of malignant cells forming the tumour on surrounding tissues. The systemic effects may be the result of spread to other tissues (metastases) or effects of the malignancy on other organs, particularly those regulating hormonal activity, or may be due to the chemicals/hormones produced by the malignancy itself.

Local features of malignant tumours may include bleeding, which may sometimes be severe (haemorrhage) when the tumour is in the stomach, large bowel (colon) or lung. Slow blood loss from tumours of the large bowel may occur and go unrecognized/undetected for long periods of time until it results in anaemia. Patients with tumours of the stomach may vomit blood (haematemesis), while patients with tumours of the lung could cough up blood (haemoptysis). Tumours growing within tubes such as the tube draining urine from the kidney (the ureter) or the tube leading from the mouth to the stomach (the oesophagus) eventually cause an obstruction. Tumours in the oesophagus produce difficulty in swallowing (dysphagia) while obstruction to the ureter may result in an enlarged kidney.

Tumours within the bowel may partially obstruct the passage of the residues of digestion from the intestine, resulting in an alteration of bowel habits, or cause complete obstruction.

When tumours arise from bone or when tumour cells are deposited in bone from other sites (secondary deposits), there can be severe bone pain and increased risk of fractures.

Brain tumours can bring about changes in personality as a result of the destruction or malfunction of brain cells.

Often tumours within the abdominal cavity of organs such as the ovaries cause accumulation of fluid (ascites) and distension of the abdomen.

It is necessary to be aware of symptoms and signs which are not due to spread which would in many instances facilitate early diagnosis of malignant tumours. These include:

- loss of appetite (anorexia) leading to weight loss
- fever which is associated with malignancies of lymph gland (lymphomas)
- tiredness, loss of energy, fatigue and night sweats which occur with most malignant tumours
- changes in the pigmentation of the skin (e.g. acanthosis nigricans) in tumours of the gastrointestinal tract and the lung
- hormonal effects as seen in tumours of the lung
- alterations in muscle function such as weakness as seen with myopathies due to lung cancers.

Clinical assessment

It is essential to make a thorough clinical examination and investigate the:

1. nature and site of the primary tumour (site, type, pathology)
2. extent of the disease (stage)

3. patient's general condition and the presence of other diseases
4. available treatment options – surgery, drugs or radiotherapy.

Herbal drugs are increasingly used by cancer patients, often at the same time as allopathic medicines without any regard to the possibility of interactions, and often without consulting or informing their allopathic physicians beforehand.

GROWTHS – TUMOURS – CANCERS:

Some herbs used in treatment

Agrimony
Aloe
Anise
Arnica (topical only)
Bitter melon
Bloodroot
Burdock
Carline thistle
Cassia
Cat's claw
Celandine
Chamomile – Roman
Condurango
Dandelion (topical)
Echinacea
Fucus (kelp)
Garlic
Ginseng Panax
Goldenseal
Hydrocotyle (Gotu kola)
Holy thistle
Horsetail
Indigo
Marjoram
Mayapple (topical only)
Meadowsweet
Mint
Mistletoe
Motherwort
Myrrh
Nettle
Rosemary
Scull cap
St John's wort
Thuja
Wild cherry
Yucca

A herb that may cause tumours

Euphorbia

DIABETES – DIABETES MELLITUS

Diabetes is becoming increasingly common and is causing great concern to health professionals and policy makers. It is expected that approximately 300 million people will suffer from diabetes by the year 2010.

Diabetes mellitus is essentially a condition where the sugar levels in the blood are high (hyperglycaemia) due to an absolute or relative lack of the hormone which regulates blood sugar in the body (insulin), which is secreted by the pancreas.

The term diabetes is also used to describe another quite unrelated disorder – diabetes insipidus – where there is excessive passage of urine due to a variety of causes. This will not be discussed in this section.

There are, in allopathic medicine, many types of diabetes mellitus (1 to 4). Type 1 diabetes generally occurs in young individuals who have a normal or low body weight, usually without a family history of diabetes. The more common type 2 diabetes usually occurs in obese older individuals, who have a history of diabetes in the family.

Diabetes may be induced by allopathic drugs such as steroids and thiazide diuretics and may also be a feature of other diseases of the endocrine (hormonal) system like Cushing's syndrome (cortisol excess), or acromegaly (growth hormone excess).

The pronounced rise in incidence of diabetes mellitus seen among immigrants in industrialized countries (e.g. Asians and Afro-Caribbeans in the UK) has been attributed to changes in lifestyle, diet and eating habits and to stress.

Signs and symptoms

Signs and symptoms associated with diabetes are:

- Polyuria – frequent passing of urine
- Nocturia – increased passing of urine at night
- Thirst (polydipsia), dry mouth and dry tongue
- Tiredness, fatigue, irritability, apathy
- Recent change in weight
- Blurring of vision
- Nausea
- Headache
- Pruritus vulvae (itching of female genital organs), balanitis, genital candidiasis
- Skin infections
- Abdominal obesity.

Uncontrolled diabetes can lead to a wide range of serious and debilitating complications such as impaired vision, kidney failure, loss or impaired sensation in the limbs (peripheral neuropathy), muscle weakness, gastrointestinal problems and ulceration of the feet with wounds that tend to heal very poorly so that the feet may need to be amputated to relieve discomfort or stop the spread of infection.

There is also a high risk of heart disease. Type I diabetics can die suddenly without insulin treatment. In treated diabetics, heart disease (70%) is by far the most common cause of death. Other causes of death are kidney failure (10%), carcinoma (10%) and infections (6%).

While insulin is an absolute necessity for type 1 diabetics, type 2 diabetics can be managed initially with allopathic medicines that are taken by mouth (oral hypoglycaemic drugs), although sometimes insulin may be necessary as well.

Dietary measures are necessary in the treatment of all diabetics. Strict control of blood sugar is important to reduce the risk of diabetic complications and any form of treatment should include self-assessment of sugar control. Equipment for home-testing of urine and blood is affordable and widely available.

All diabetics need to be closely observed and monitored throughout their entire lives for the onset of complications, for example, by measuring kidney and heart function, and examining the eyes. To minimize life-endangering complications, target blood pressure and lipid levels (e.g. blood cholesterol) have been set at a lower limit than for non-diabetic patients. Particular care is also necessary when diabetics need surgery and it is often necessary to alter the treatment plan for the control of diabetes prior to, during and after surgery.

While traditional medicines have been used in the management of diabetes for centuries, the serious drawback of such treatment is the absence of continuous monitoring to determine whether the blood sugar remains within the acceptable ranges during treatment.

DIABETES – DIABETES MELLITUS:

Some herbs used in treatment

Alfalfa
Allspice
Aloe
Barley
Basil
Bilberry
Bitter melon
Ginger juice
Goat's rue
Indigo
Jambul
Java tea
Liquorice
Mate
Milk thistle
Myrrh
Nettle
Senega
Stevia
Vanadium (maximum dose 1.8 mg/day)
Yucca

Some herbs that may do harm in diabetics

Clivers
Cranberry
Ephedra
Willow

ACUTE SORE THROAT

Acute sore throat (pharyngitis) and tonsillitis are infections caused either by viruses or bacteria. They are very common in children and younger adults and are estimated to account for nearly 40 million visits to doctors every year.

Pharyngitis causes pain in the throat and difficulty in swallowing. These symptoms may be accompanied by a raised temperature and a feeling of general malaise. The symptoms of tonsillitis are similar but more severe. The throat is reddish on examination and the tonsils are usually swollen and may be coated with a membrane. Enlarged lymph glands may be felt under the jaw and in the neck. The patient may have sour breath.

In most cases the infection is caused by a virus, bacterial infections (mainly group A streptococci) being less common, and is spread from person to person by airborne droplets and contaminated hands. The incubation period is usually 2–4 days.

Sore throat may also be a symptom of other conditions such as glandular fever, but in such cases the sore throat is usually accompanied by other symptoms and lasts for more than 10 days.

Complications are unusual: they include secondary infections in the middle ear or sinuses. Streptococcal infections may cause a rash (scarlet fever) and, in rare cases, immunological diseases such as rheumatic fever and glomerulonephritis (a disease of the kidney).

The symptoms usually clear within a few days without treatment, but antipyretic (fever lowering) medications can be given to reduce temperature. Analgesics or topical anaesthetics can be given to relieve soreness (gargles often bring relief). Antibiotics are useful only for the small minority of patients with bacterial infection. It is advisable to take a swab from the infected area to identify the causative agent.

Herbs with demulcent properties may soothe and relieve sore throat by forming a mucilaginous coating on the irritated lining of the mouth and throat.

ACUTE SORE THROAT:

Some herbs used in treatment

Agrimony	Grapefruit seed extract
Avens	Liquorice
Bayberry	Marigold
Betony	Marshmallow
Bilberry	Myrrh
Boneset	Pau d'arco
Cleavers	Propolis
Echinacea	Rosemary
Elder	Sage
Eyebright	Savory
Garlic	Senega
Goldenrod	Thyme

RAISED BLOOD CHOLESTEROL

Atherosclerosis is a hardening and thickening of the arteries (the vessels that carry oxygen around the body) thought to be caused by fatty deposits (plaques) on the innermost lining of the artery walls. The deposits tend to increase in size over time, particularly if the levels of fats or lipids in the blood circulation are high, and they may become large enough to decrease or even completely obstruct blood flow.

Sometimes a clot (thrombus) forms on a fat deposit and further restricts blood flow. If clots break away they may partly or completely block other arteries, often distant from the site of the initial clot.

When the blood flow through the artery is restricted or blocked, cells are deprived of oxygen and other nutrients. Reduction in oxygen supply to the brain and heart is particularly serious, and causes strokes, heart attacks and other serious health problems that may lead to death.

Cholesterol is a type of fat known as a lipid and is carried in the blood by lipoproteins. The main types of lipoproteins in the blood are triglycerides, high density lipoproteins and low density lipoproteins.

Triglycerides and low density lipoproteins promote the formation of cholesterol-rich plaques within arteries, while high density lipoproteins take cholesterol away from the plaques. Low blood concentrations of cholesterol, triglyceride and low density lipoprotein, and high levels of high density lipoproteins, reduce the risk of atherosclerosis and the life-threatening events caused by atheromatous plaques.

Raised levels of cholesterol may be an inherited condition. High cholesterol levels are also associated with a sedentary lifestyle, a high intake of carbohydrates and fats in the diet, and medical conditions such as diabetes mellitus and hypothyroidism (decreased activity of the thyroid gland).

In allopathic medicine, among the most important measures to prevent formation of the potentially lethal fat-rich plaques are those which reduce the concentration of cholesterol in the blood. Of these, giving up of cigarette smoking is the best known preventive measure.

The concentration of lipids in the blood can be lowered by changes to diet and lifestyle and by allopathic drugs called statins. Patients with high cholesterol levels should be meticulously monitored and treated for the commonly associated spectrum of associated diseases: hypertension (high blood pressure), diabetes mellitus, obesity, and heart disease.

RAISED BLOOD CHOLESTEROL:

Some herbs used in treatment

Alfalfa	Myrrh
Artichoke	Plantain
Barley	Royal jelly
Evening primrose	Safflower
Garlic	Scull cap
Green tea	Soy
Gum Arabic	Vanadium (max 1.8 mg/day)

BLEEDING

Bleeding is usually caused by damage to a blood vessel wall following injury, but may also occur when a blood vessel wall is eroded, as can happen with a stomach ulcer or a rapidly growing tumour.

Three processes stop bleeding from injured blood vessels: narrowing of the blood vessels (vasoconstriction), formation of a plug by blood platelets and activation of blood clotting factors (mostly produced in the liver). Narrowing of a damaged blood vessel reduces the flow of blood, platelets stick to the injured area and form a plug, and at the same time clotting factors are activated to reinforce the platelet plug and form a clot.

There are many underlying causes of abnormal bleeding. If a clot does not form this could be due to a deficiency of the clotting factors. This is usually the cause of bleeding from muscle or joints and also occurs in the rare inherited disease known as von Willebrand's disease. Pinpoint haemorrhages (purpura) in the skin, prolonged bleeding from superficial cuts, nose bleeds and bleeding from the gastrointestinal tract are usually due to a deficiency or functional defect of platelets. Another common cause of bleeding is haemophilia (an inherited disorder of blood clotting) where spontaneous bleeding may occur into joints, causing severe pain. Recurrent bleeds into joints can result in disabling arthritis.

Recurrent bleeds at a single site suggest local factors such as a structural abnormality or a localized disorder. Other causes of bleeding include drug therapy with aspirin, warfarin or non-steroidal anti-inflammatory agents, e.g. ibuprofen (Neurofen), and systemic illnesses such as liver failure, renal failure and some connective tissue disorders.

The following investigations would be helpful in determining the cause of bleeding: platelet count, blood film and coagulation tests (prothrombin time, activated partial thromboplastin time and fibrinogen levels).

Acute blood loss from trauma is managed by compression of the vessel, allowing time for the natural clotting mechanisms to take effect. In severe cases lost blood is replaced by blood transfusions. Platelet disorders are treated by transfusion of platelets if the counts are dangerously low. Corticosteroids may be used in addition. Clotting factor deficiency is treated by replacing the deficient factor/s.

Bleeding from the gastrointestinal tract requires urgent investigations such as endoscopy and imaging techniques to locate the site of bleeding and to exclude malignancy, and the use of heat (cauterization) to promote clotting from the bleeding points in small blood vessels.

Bleeding from stomach ulcers caused by drug therapy is managed by withdrawing the offending drug and treating with a drug called a proton pump inhibitor that decreases acidity in the stomach and promotes healing of the ulcer.

Bleeding gums may be due to infection in the mouth or a deficiency of vitamin C.

BLEEDING:

Some herbs used in treatment

Avens	Lady's mantle
Beth root	Nettle
Betony	Notoginseng root
Bistort	Peach
Chinese rhubarb	Shepherd's purse
Goldenseal	Woundwort

Some herbs that may increase bleeding

Bilberry	Ginkgo biloba

FEVER

Measurement or assessment of body temperature is one of the oldest and earliest forms of investigation used in the treatment of disease in nearly all forms of medical practice throughout the world, because an increase in body temperature is one of the most overt and earliest signs of disease.

Body temperature is normally around 36.8°C with a variation between the day and night of 0.5°C. It is controlled by a section of the brain called the thermoregulatory centre which acts as a thermostat. Fever is a temperature above 37.5°C caused when the thermostat is reset to a higher temperature. Substances that cause fever are called pyrogens. They may be produced inside the body or outside the body, most commonly by bacteria and viruses. Death of tissue (necrosis) due to invasion of bacteria and viruses also causes fever.

When the thermostat is set at a higher point, normal body temperature feels subnormal. Patients with fever feel cold and tend to cover themselves, and the body attempts to generate heat by mechanisms such as shivering. Fever may be accompanied by rigors (episodes of shaking) which results in a rapid rise in body temperature. Fever may also be accompanied by delirium in young children and the elderly.

Sweating is a natural and effective process by which the human body loses heat, due to the evaporation of the sweat. Sweating is commonly associated with most fevers, but may also be due to non-infective causes such as alcohol misuse, anxiety, thyrotoxicosis (toxicity due to excess thyroid hormones) and diabetes mellitus. Fevers associated with night sweats are characteristic of tuberculosis and lymphomas.

Fever from any cause can provoke a headache. Fever with headache may be due to infection of the air-filled spaces in the skull around the nose (paranasal sinuses) when the fever is accompanied by pain in the sinuses, nasal discharge and sneezing. Severe headache accompanied by intolerance of light (photophobia) often suggests meningitis, infection of the layers (meninges) lining the brain. Infection with meningococci (meningococcal meningitis) is a serious and life-threatening illness. Presence of a purpuric or petechial rash associated with low blood pressure may point to its diagnosis.

Common causes of fever in children include ear infection, and tonsillitis or sore throat (pharyngitis), which is usually accompanied by enlargement of the lymph nodes in the front of the neck. Enlargement of the lymph nodes at the back of the head suggests glandular fever.

Fever accompanying vesicles on the skin indicates chicken pox or rarer viral infections (Coxsackie A virus infection).

Recurrent fever is commonly due to a focus of bacterial infection below the diaphragm, such as:

- infection of the gallbladder (cholecystitis)
- abscesses beneath the peritoneum or in a muscle such as the psoas muscle
- an infection of the urinary tract, indicated by frequent desire to pass urine and pain on passing urine, loin pain and discharge from the urethra, vagina or penis
- abdominal infections which are suggested by the occurrence of diarrhoea, weight loss and abdominal pain

Other causes of fever are infections such as malaria, an adverse reaction to allopathic medications such as penicillins, cephalosporins, sulphonamides, antituberculous agents, phenytoin, methyl dopa or quinidine, alcoholic hepatitis and liver cancer.

The causes of fever

1. ***Infections*** – intra-abdominal abscess (cholecystitis), cholangitis, urinary tract infection, prostatitis, dental and sinus infections, bone and joint infections, malaria, dengue, brucellosis, enteric fevers (typhoid), infective endocarditis, tuberculosis – particularly extra-pulmonary, viral infections (cytomegalovirus, infectious mononucleosis, HIV, toxoplasmosis), and fungal infections.
2. ***Malignancy*** – lymphoma, myeloma, leukaemia and tumours of the kidney, liver, colon, stomach and pancreas.
3. ***Connective tissue disorders*** – rheumatoid disease, polyarteritis nodosa, temporal arteritis, polymyalgia rheumatica, systemic lupus erythematosus, Still's disease and polymyositis.
4. ***Others*** – inflammatory bowel disease, cirrhosis, sarcoidosis, drug reactions, thyrotoxicosis, atrial myxoma, familial Mediterranean fever, lesions of the hypothalamus in the brain.

Allopathic treatment of fever

It is essential to treat the underlying cause of the fever. A detailed history is necessary, including drug therapy and information about travel to countries where infectious diseases such as malaria are common.

Drugs, e.g. paracetamol, can be used to reset the thermoregulatory centre and provide symptomatic relief. It is essential to bring the temperature down fairly quickly in children as they are prone to develop fits (seizures – febrile convulsions) and delirium. This can be achieved by tepid sponging, fanning, ice packs on groins and armpits and the administration of paracetamol. Aspirin also brings down fever but should not be used in children under the age of 12 years. It is essential to ensure that sufficient fluids are drunk during a fever.

FEVER:

Some herbs used in treatment

Barberry	Lemon balm
Basil	Lime flower
Boneset	Meadowsweet (hot infusion)
Borage	Mugwort
Bugleweed	Oregon grape
Carline thistle	Pau d'arco
Celery	Peppermint (infusion)
Chamomile (tea)	Prickly ash
Chickweed	Rose
Cleavers	Rosemary
Cinnamon	Safflower
Echinacea (tincture)	Southernwood
Elder (infusion)	Tansy
Ephedra	Vervain
Feverfew	Willow
Ginger	Wormwood
Goat's rue	Woundwort
Horse chestnut	Yarrow (infusion)
Horsetail	Yellow dock
Indigo	Yerba santa
Lavender (topical)	

MOUTH ULCERS

Mouth ulcers are usually small sores that tend to cause a great deal of discomfort and pain. They may be caused by:

- damage or irritation due to bad teeth or ill-fitting dentures
- stress
- hormonal changes such as those that occur in women before their periods
- vitamin deficiencies

- bacterial, fungal and viral illnesses. Such cases can be treated effectively by treating the disease state appropriately
- allopathic medicines (e.g. cytotoxic drugs)
- bowel diseases such as Crohn's and coeliac disease
- malignant diseases (carcinoma, leukaemia, Kaposi sarcoma)
- systemic lupus erythematosus
- skin diseases such as lichen planus, pemphigoid and pemphigus.

Pemphigus is characterized by blistering or lesions on other parts of the body and is associated with underlying malignant disease which occurs in people between the ages of 40 and 60 years.

Lichen planus is characterized by an intensely itchy rash (glistening discrete papules) that usually starts at the back of the wrists and tends to spread rapidly, and also by painful or uncomfortable mouth ulcers. It may be caused by hepatitis (chronic active hepatitis, hepatitis B and C) or by allopathic drugs such as sulphonamides, penicillamine, antimalarials, antituberculous drugs and diuretics. Allopathic or traditional medications containing gold or other heavy metals and chemicals used in industries such as the printing industry may also cause lichen planus. Although the disease is often self-limiting, oral lichen planus may persist for up to 10 years.

It is important to investigate the cause of mouth ulcers and to exclude the possibility of any other associated disease.

There are several mouthwashes and other preparations that can be used topically to relieve pain caused by mouth ulcers, and local applications of corticosteroids (triamcinalone) may reduce their duration. Ulcers due to bad teeth or ill-fitting dentures can be effectively treated by dental care.

Corticosteroids are used in the treatment of most of the underlying diseases causing mouth ulcers and these should clear if the underlying disease is treated appropriately.

MOUTH ULCERS:

Some herbs used in treatment

Aloe vera 'gel'	Marshmallow
Bilberry	Myrrh
Black catechu	Peppermint
Chamomile	Plantain
Ginger	Propolis
Goldenseal	Ragwort
Lavender	Thyme
Lemon balm	

VITILIGO

Vitiligo is characterized by sharply defined white patches on the skin due to absence of melanocytes, the cells that contain the melanin pigment that gives the skin its colour. The underlying cause is not properly understood, but may be associated with diabetes and diseases of the thyroid and adrenal glands. It can be precipitated by trauma and sunburn. It may run in families.

Vitiligo should be distinguished from albinism, a condition in which melanocytes are present in their usual numbers but fail to produce the pigment melanin. Albinism is an inherited condition while vitiligo is usually an acquired condition, although there may be a genetic cause in some instances.

The white lesions are symmetrical in generalized vitiligo but there is no loss of sensation in these areas. Hair may also be affected (on the scalp and beard area). The condition does not make people unwell and the affected areas are not sore or itchy.

Allopathic treatments cannot cure vitiligo and do not usually stop its spread. Phototherapy with PUVA or TLO1 phototherapy is sometimes able to restore skin colour. Camouflage cosmetics can improve appearance. People with the condition should protect the affected areas from exposure to sunlight to avoid sunburn.

VITILIGO:

A herb used in treatment

Khella

GOITRE

A goitre is a visible lump in the neck caused by enlargement of the thyroid gland. It is normal for this to occur temporarily at puberty or during pregnancy. Goitre may be due to lack of iodine in the diet, but this is rare except in communities living in regions where the iodine content in the water is low. Other causes are Hashimoto's thyroiditis and benign or malignant tumours of the thyroid gland.

The physiological enlargement that occurs during puberty or during a pregnancy may persist, and the goitre may become multinodular and grow large enough to press against the windpipe causing hoarseness and noisy breathing. The goitre may press against the oesophagus causing difficulty in swallowing (dysphagia).

In any patient with an enlarged thyroid gland it is necessary to exclude malignancy, which is commonly associated with small single nodules with or without enlargement of the lymph glands in the neck. Rapid enlargement of a thyroid growth may occur due to bleeding into the tumour. A needle aspiration biopsy and histological investigations are necessary in any instance of doubt.

Surgical removal of the goitre may be necessary if it is causing difficulty in breathing or swallowing or if malignancy is suspected.

GOITRE:

Some herbs used in treatment

Fucus (kelp) Nettle

HYPERTENSION (HIGH BLOOD PRESSURE)

Blood pressure is the force applied to the wall of the arteries as the heart pumps blood through the body. The measurement is dependent on the amount of blood pumped, which is in turn dependent on the volume of blood in the body, the force with which the heart pumps blood and the diameter and flexibility of the arteries.

There are two components to a measurement of blood pressure. The first is the maximum pressure exerted when the heart is pumping the blood (systolic pressure) and the second represents the pressure in the arteries when the heart is at rest (diastolic pressure). In normal people these measurements are recorded as 130/80 mm Hg. Hypertension is defined as a condition in which either the systolic blood pressure or the diastolic blood pressure or both are elevated when measured on at least two occasions.

High blood pressure (hypertensive heart disease) is one of the most common diseases of the modern world, mainly affecting middle-aged people, and can have serious consequences, including heart failure, kidney failure, strokes and heart attacks.

Factors affecting blood pressure

Several factors affect blood pressure, including:

- disease of the heart or blood vessels (cardiovascular disease)
- psychological factors such as stress, anger or fear
- kidney disease
- diseases of the nervous system
- pregnancy, when there is sometimes a marked and potentially dangerous increase in blood pressure (pre-eclampsia)
- several allopathic medications
- pain.

Also, in many people the visit to the doctor or the process of measuring blood pressure causes anxiety and an elevation of blood pressure, which is commonly referred to as 'white coat hypertension'. As many as 10–20% of individuals may experience white coat hypertension and be unnecessarily prescribed antihypertensive drugs for life.

It is necessary to make repeated measurements under conditions which have been specified as 'ideal' (relaxed, comfortably seated with the arm well supported, appropriate length and width of the blood pressure cuff applied etc), before a diagnosis of high blood pressure or hypertension is made.

Causes of hypertension

The most common form of hypertension, which accounts for about 95% of cases, is essential hypertension, i.e. there is no underlying correctable cause. The most common underlying cause of hypertension is kidney disease. Other causes include some endocrine (hormonal) diseases (acromegaly, Cushing's disease and Conn's syndrome), diseases such as renal artery stenosis and coarctation of the aorta, alcohol toxicity, cocaine abuse, diabetes mellitus and obesity.

Secondary causes of hypertension should be sought when:

1. the patient is young (<30 years)
2. raised blood pressure is detected for the first time in elderly patients
3. the blood pressure is very high (>180/110 mm Hg) and associated with organ damage
4. abnormal physical signs such as abdominal bruits are detected
5. the control of blood pressure becomes suddenly difficult
6. the blood pressure increases when ACE inhibitors (a class of antihypertensives) are added
7. blood test results are abnormal (e.g. raised creatinine and low potassium).

Such patients should be investigated extensively and referral to a specialist centre is warranted.

It is essential to investigate each patient to assess the extent of organ damage (heart, kidney and eyes) at the initial diagnosis and periodically thereafter. Clinical examination includes measurement of blood pressure in both arms and examination for target organ damage, i.e. heart enlargement, signs of heart failure and eye examination followed by examination for signs of secondary causes of hypertension. Investigations include: examination of urine for red cells and proteins, blood tests to assess kidney function and an ECG (electrocardiograph) to look for heart enlargement and ischaemic heart disease. Blood sugar and lipid profiles are measured routinely and relevant investigations to exclude secondary causes of hypertension may also be needed.

Measures for reducing blood pressure

Management of hypertension includes correction of the cause in the minority of patients where this is possible.

Lifestyle modifications that have been found to reduce blood pressure satisfactorily include:

1. A low calorie diet
2. Regular exercise
3. Relaxation therapy
4. Reducing alcohol consumption to <21 units/week in men and <14 units/week in women
5. Low salt (<6 g/day) diet.

These measures are indicated as initial therapy if the blood pressure is persistently elevated above 140/100 mm Hg.

Pharmacological agents (allopathic medicines) are indicated when:

1. Lifestyle changes fail to bring the pressure below 140/100 mm Hg.
2. The blood pressure is persistently elevated over 160/100 mm Hg from the beginning.
3. The initial blood pressure of 140/90 mm Hg is associated with clinical evidence of end organ damage or if the future heart attack and stroke risk is deemed to be high.

The aim is to bring the blood pressure below 140/90 mm Hg and to 130/80 mm Hg if an individual suffers from diabetes mellitus or kidney disease. The choice of drug for a given patient should be determined by the age, co-morbidity, race and side-effect profile.

Management to prevent future heart attacks and strokes is also important, including proper blood pressure control and managing levels of blood lipids and blood sugar. Small doses of aspirin may be indicated to reduce the risk of blood clots.

HYPERTENSION (HIGH BLOOD PRESSURE:

Some herbs used in treatment

- Aconite (only under medical supervision)
- Chamomile
- Cinnamon
- Evening primrose
- Fucus (kelp)
- Garlic
- Hawthorn (tea or tincture)
- Hydrocotyle (Gotu kola)
- Java tea
- Kelp
- Kudzu
- Lime flower (tea or tincture)
- Lysine
- Mistletoe
- Olive leaf
- Parsley
- Passion flower
- Rauwolfia
- Scull cap
- Stone root
- Rosemary
- Vervain
- Yarrow

Some herbs that may cause harm in patients with hypertension

- Agrimony
- Gentian
- Ginseng
  - *Eleutherococcus*
- Panax ginseng
- Nettle
- Liquorice – with pregnancy-related hypertension

ISCHAEMIC HEART DISEASE – ANGINA – HEART ATTACKS

Ischaemia means 'reduced blood supply'.

Every cell in the human body needs oxygen, supplied by the blood to function normally. All blood supplied to the heart muscle passes through the coronary arteries; there is no alternative source of supply. When the blood supply to the heart muscle is reduced (ischaemic heart disease) heart muscle cells are deprived of oxygen and serious ill-health or death may follow very quickly.

Ischaemic heart disease is the most common cause of death in most Western countries and it is considered responsible for one-third of all deaths in men and one-fifth of all deaths in women in the UK. In addition, many developed countries spend a considerable proportion of their health budgets on measures to prevent and manage the consequences of ischaemic heart disease as millions of working days are lost in these countries. Despite the development of new methods of treatment for heart disease, the incidence of heart attacks and resulting heart failure is still on the rise.

Most ischaemic heart disease is caused by atherosclerosis which was discussed in section on cholesterol.

Initially there is a sudden severe narrowing or closure of the arteries to the heart muscle, which may cause severe acute pain in the chest (usually behind the sternum) commonly referred to as angina. When the blood supply to the heart muscle is blocked by a blood clot (see section on atherosclerosis), the heart muscle is damaged. If the damage is temporary, there is severe pain and the state of ischaemia persists unless medical/surgical interventions are carried out very promptly. Damage to heart muscle may cause a loss of heart muscle activity leading to 'heart failure'. If the heart muscle dies as a result (acute myocardial infarction) this is very serious as the heart muscle does not have the ability to repair itself. If the damage to the heart muscle affects the initiation or conduction of electrical impulses that control the normal rhythmic contractions of the heart muscle, the heart beat may become irregular (arrhythmias). When the heart beats irregularly, its efficiency at pumping blood round the body is reduced, so that the oxygen supply to the cells including those in the brain is affected. Sudden death following coronary artery thrombosis is often due to arrhythmias.

Ischaemic heart disease (IHD) is a very serious medical condition and the emphasis in allopathic medicine is towards preventing it by identifying factors that increase the risk of it occurring.

These predisposing factors are also referred to as 'risk factors':

1. advancing age
2. gender: males are 3–4 times more at risk of developing IHD
3. positive family history
4. race
5. smoking
6. physical inactivity
7. stress
8. elevated lipids – high cholesterol diet – see section on cholesterol, p. 23
9. hypertension – see section on high blood pressure, p. 28
10. diabetes – see section on diabetes mellitus, p. 21
11. obesity – see section on obesity, p. 14
12. insulin resistance
13. hyper-homocysteinaemia.

Approximately 15% of all patients with acute myocardial infarctions die before they reach hospital and a further 15% die soon after. A significant proportion of those who survive the acute event are likely to die within a year. The elderly (>75 years) are especially at risk, 20% dying within one month and a further 30% dying within a year.

Following a heart attack the patient is acutely distressed, in severe pain, restless and sweating with a low blood pressure. Pulse rate may be irregular. There may be signs of heart failure. Urgent diagnosis should include an electrocardiogram and blood tests to detect markers of heart muscle damage; echocardiography can be helpful.

Patients are immediately treated with painkillers (morphine), aspirin, beta-blockers and nitrates, and assessed for the suitability of thrombolysis (dissolving of the clot or thrombus) or surgical treatment (primary angioplasty, insertion of stents or coronary artery bypass grafts) depending on availability. The patient should be managed in an intensive care unit in most cases. Some patients are given heparin as an anticoagulant and antianginal (drugs to relive the pain or angina) drugs.

Those patients who are thrombolysed and anticoagulated should soon be assessed with different types of cardiac stress tests and evaluated for coronary revascularization. Those who do not require surgical interventions are managed on several drugs including aspirin and monitored for life. All patients will be advised to stop smoking, and encouraged to lose weight and increase exercise. Optimal blood pressure and blood sugar control along with proper control of lipids is essential to prevent further heart attacks. There is good evidence that the addition of some drugs (ACE inhibitors) prevents or delays development of heart failure in the future.

ISCHAEMIC HEART DISEASE – ANGINA – HEART ATTACKS:

Some herbs used in treatment

Garlic Hawthorn

GOUT

Gout is a condition caused when there is more uric acid in the blood than can be removed from the blood by the kidney. The excess is deposited as crystals in the joints, to produce swelling, stiffness and inflammation (redness) and pain, particularly in the joint at the base of the big toe (first metatarso-phalangeal joint).

Gout is much more common in men between the ages 30 and 60 years and rarely affects women before the menopause. A considerable number of patients with gout have a family history of the disease.

The commonest cause of gout is a diet containing food such as red meat, cream sauces, beer and red wine, tomatoes, cheese and citrus fruits, which are broken down in the body to form excessive amounts of uric acid. Other causes include exposure to lead in the environment, allopathic medications such as levodopa which is used in the treatment of Parkinson's disease, ciclosporin and some diuretics.

In allopathic medicine, acute attacks of pain are treated with anti-inflammatory painkillers such as ibuprofen (Neurofen), and colchicine, a drug made from an alkaloid found in the autumn crocus, *Colchium autumnale*. However, prevention is the best course of action.

GOUT:

Some herbs used in treatment

Bilberry	Liquorice
Burdock	Meadow sweet (tea)
Celery	Milk thistle
Centaury	Nettle (tea)
Chickweed	Parsley
Cleavers	Rosemary
Dandelion	Sage
Echinacea	Sarsaparilla
Elder	Thyme
Fennel	Turmeric
Lime flower	Yarrow

CYSTITIS

Cystitis is inflammation of the lining of the urinary bladder usually caused by infection from bacteria normally present in the intestines. Accompanying symptoms include frequent and painful urination, abdominal pain and fever.

Cystitis is more common in women than men, particularly postmenopausal women in whom hormonal changes make the bladder more vulnerable to infection. It is also common in diabetics.

In allopathic medicine, the infection is treated with an increased intake of fluids, and antibiotics are often prescribed following bacteriological examination of the urine and after determining the sensitivity of the organisms to the antibiotic. Mild to moderate painkillers often bring relief. If recurrent infections occur, it may be necessary to investigate further by directly looking at the bladder and urethra using a cystoscope.

CYSTITIS:

Some herbs used in treatment

Agrimony	Hydrangea
Barley water	Lady's mantle
Bearberry	Lemon balm
Bilberry	Marshmallow root
Buchu	Matico leaves
Burdock	Meadow sweet
Chamomile	Nettle
Coriander	Parsley
Couch grass	Pellitory of the wall
Cranberry	Pipsisewa
Dandelion	Plantain
Fennel	Shepherd's purse
Garlic	Uva-ursi (Bearberry)
Goldenrod	Vervain
Goldenseal	Wild carrot
Hydrocotyle (Gotu kola)	Wild yam
Heather flowers	Yarrow

HIVES OR URTICARIA (NETTLE RASH)

Nettle rash, also known as uriticaria or hives, is a lumpy, itchy rash with red raised spots or pimples on the skin, sometimes called weals. They may cover the whole body or affect just one part. The Latin name urticaria is from the Latin word 'urtica' which means stinging nettle.

Hives or weals are different from blisters such as those caused by burns or by hand-held implements rubbing against the skin. A blister is a little sac filled with clear fluid which often breaks so that the liquid comes out and the sac becomes flat.

Urticaria usually lasts a few minutes or hours (acute urticaria). Sometimes it may persist for several weeks or even years (chronic urticaria) but this is uncommon.

In acute urticaria the inflammation is caused by chemical substances called histamines released from cells in the skin. The release of histamines is triggered by an allergic reaction to certain medicines (e.g. ibuprofen, aspirin and penicillin), foods (e.g. nuts, eggs, strawberries, shellfish and food additives) or local irritants including nettles and other plants, insect bites, latex and some chemicals.

Chronic urticaria is not caused by an allergy and the cause is not known. It may be associated with some systemic diseases such as systemic lupus erythematosus (SLE).

Acute urticaria is sometimes accompanied by swelling, known as angioedema, usually around the eyes, lips, or hands. There may also be some pain in the joints. Angioedema may last for 24–48 hours. Occasionally swelling of the inside of the mouth, tongue and throat makes it difficult to breathe or swallow and requires urgent treatment.

Urticaria is also a symptom of a life-threatening allergic reaction known as anaphylaxis which develops within minutes of exposure to an allergic substance. There is swelling over the whole body and a rapid fall in blood pressure. Swelling of the mouth, tongue, or throat may cause wheezing and difficulty in breathing. Anaphylaxis requires immediate treatment usually with injections of drugs such as adrenaline and corticosteroids. Such reactions may occur after bee and wasp stings.

Almost all urticaria gets worse in hot weather and some people develop urticarial reactions only in hot weather. Because of this, urticaria is often called a 'heat rash' but it is quite different from prickly heat which is an infection in the sweat glands often associated with poor skin hygiene. Other aggravating factors include pressure from tight clothing such as brassiere straps and belts (pressure urticaria), cold, and sunlight (solar urticaria).

If a cause is detected following consultation and specialized investigations, treatment become easier as it involves removing the cause.

In allopathic medicine, the first line of treatment is to give an antihistamine drug to counter the effects of histamine. Soothing lotions may be used to ease the irritation. Both doctor and patient should make an effort to identify aggravating factors accurately so that they can be avoided in future.

Anaphylaxis could be life-threatening and is treated with adrenaline by injection.

HIVES OR URTICARIA (NETTLE RASH):

Some herbs used in treatment

Aloe vera	Lemon balm
Burdock	Liquorice
Calendula	Marigold
Chamomile	Milk thistle
Chickweed	Nettle
Coriander	Rehmannia
Echinacea	Rose
Ephedra	Yarrow
German chamomile	Yellow dock

Some herbs to be avoided by patients with urticaria

Anise	Corn silk

LIVER AND GALLBLADDER DISEASE

JAUNDICE

Jaundice is a yellowish discoloration of the skin, whites of the eyes and mucous membranes. The name is derived from the French word *jaune* which means yellow. Jaundice is not a disease but is a clinical sign seen in many disease states, particularly of the liver. It is caused by increase in the blood of a pigment called bilirubin.

Bilirubin is produced in the liver, by the normal breakdown of red blood cells that carry oxygen round the body. Bilirubin is normally excreted in the bile.

Causes of jaundice

There are three conditions which could lead to excess amounts of bilirubin in the blood. Firstly, excessive destruction of red cells produces more bile pigment than the liver can process. This is haemolytic jaundice. Some of the excess bilirubin is excreted in the urine, which becomes darker (yellowish) than usual. The excessive destruction of red blood cells causes patients to become anaemic (haemolytic anaemia). This cause occurs in malaria, sickle cell disease where red cells are abnormal, and in people who lack an enzyme such as glucose-6-phosphatase dehydrogenase.

Secondly, bilirubin may be produced in normal amounts but accumulate in the blood because the liver cells that metabolize and excrete it are damaged. Liver cells may be damaged either by medications or infections (e.g. viral hepatitis) or following excessive consumption of alcohol. Alcohol is metabolized almost exclusively in the liver and the more alcohol a person drinks the more likely they are to develop liver damage. It is the most common cause of chronic liver disease in many societies. Women are more susceptible than men. Some genetic disorders can cause jaundice due to liver damage, e.g. haemochromatosis (a disorder caused by excess iron in the body) and Wilson's disease (a disorder caused when the body is unable to excrete copper).

Drugs that can cause hepatitis and liver failure include halothane (a volatile liquid to induce general anaesthesia but rarely used at present), rifampicin, isoniazid, chlorpromazine, ethambutol, oral contraceptives and anabolic steroids. Paracetamol can cause hepatitis and liver failure in overdose. The frequently prescribed cholesterol lowering statins and non-steroidal anti-inflammatory drugs (e.g. ibuprofen) can produce abnormal liver function tests. Methotrexate and vitamin A can cause cirrhosis; amiodarone and penicillamine may cause chronic hepatitis.

Damage to liver cells may be caused by the deposition of malignant cells from tumours outside the liver (secondary deposits). See section on growths and cancers, p. 19. Jaundice occurring in the newborn is due to the immature liver cells being unable to process the products of dead red cells efficiently.

Thirdly, bilirubin may accumulate in the blood if the bile duct is obstructed. Gallstones are a common cause of obstruction of the bile duct. A more serious cause is obstruction to the outlet of the bile duct by a cancer of the head of the pancreas. There are other less common causes which merit investigation if the common causes are not found.

JAUNDICE:

Some herbs used in treatment

Bistort	Chinese rhubarb
Barberry	Madder
Bayberry	Pareira
Betony	Pineapple
Black haw	Soapwort

VIRAL HEPATITIS

Several viruses infect the liver: hepatitis A virus, hepatitis B virus, hepatitis C virus, hepatitis D virus, hepatitis E virus, cytomegalovirus, Epstein–Barr virus, herpes simplex virus and yellow fever virus.

The overall mortality of viral hepatitis is about 0.5% in patients under the age of 40 years and may rise to 3% in patients over 60 years of age. WHO has estimated that approximately 3% of the world population have been infected with hepatitis C virus.

The most common forms of viral hepatitis are hepatitis A, hepatitis B and hepatitis C infections. Viral hepatitis A is mainly spread by ingesting food or water contaminated with faeces from infected people. Hepatitis B is spread by contact with infected blood or body fluids, or from contaminated needles. Hepatitis C is also spread by contact with contaminated needles and by infected blood. In the UK blood is screened for hepatitis C to prevent spread by blood transfusion. The hepatitis D virus is only found in people infected with hepatitis B virus, and hepatitis E is transmitted in a manner similar to hepatitis A by contaminated food and water.

Hepatitis A and E are short-term infections which are not usually serious. Hepatitis B and C are chronic (long-term) infections, and after many years may result in irreversible damage to the liver (cirrhosis) or liver failure resulting in death. There is also an increased risk of developing liver cancer. Some people with hepatitis B may remain well and not develop symptoms although they are still able to spread the virus.

People infected with hepatitis A virus excrete the virus for about 2–3 weeks even before they develop symptoms and thereafter for about two weeks. Thus spread of infection may occur unknowingly.

Acute hepatitis

The early symptoms of acute hepatitis may include malaise, nausea, vomiting, headache, diarrhoea, chills, anorexia and changes in perception of taste, e.g. distaste for cigarettes. Initially the physical signs are minimal and the liver may be slightly tender though not readily palpable on examination of the abdomen. There may be enlarged lymph nodes and the spleen is often enlarged in children. After 2–14 days these early symptoms disappear and jaundice develops, accompanied by pale stools and dark urine. Most patients recover in 3–6 weeks, although tiredness may persist for up to three months. In 5–15% of patients, symptoms may recur, but serious complications are rare. There is no specific treatment for acute viral hepatitis. Patients with severe vomiting may need intravenous fluids and nutrients. A nutritious diet aids recovery and alcohol and drugs such as sedatives should be avoided as these are metabolized in the liver.

Chronic hepatitis

Most people with chronic hepatitis remain well or develop symptoms similar to an acute infection lasting a few months. In some people symptoms such as tiredness, nausea, lack of appetite, aching muscles and joints, occasional pain above the ribs due to an enlarged liver, and jaundice persist. Eventually they may develop cirrhosis or liver failure.

There is no allopathic drug available to eradicate hepatitis B infections and no treatment is likely to be needed if there are few signs of liver inflammation.

When there are signs of liver inflammation hepatitis B infection may be treated with interferon and lamivudine. Hepatitis C is treated with interferon and ribavarin, with a success rate of 50–60%. However, these drugs are expensive and adverse effects are common.

Prevention

Hepatitis A infections are best prevented by improving sanitation and preventing overcrowding. Vaccines are available for active immunization against hepatitis A and B. Hepatitis B infection is prevented by avoiding exposure to infected blood. Accidental needle punctures, contamination with infected blood, contamination of mucous membranes or exposure to infected blood in the presence of grazes or cuts require immediate administration of hyperimmune serum globulin. Parenteral drug users (those who inject drugs of abuse such as heroin in to the veins), male homosexuals, newborn babies of infected mothers and regular sexual partners of infected individuals along with medical and nursing personnel (dentists, surgeons, obstetricians, anaesthetists, accident and emergency department staff, staff in intensive care units, liver units, oncology units and endoscopy units, laboratory staff) should receive hepatitis B vaccination.

VIRAL HEPATITIS:

Some herbs considered beneficial in liver disease

Angelica sinensis	Ginseng panax
Artichoke	Milk thistle
Boldo	Sarsaparilla
Dandelion	

Some herbs to be avoided or used with caution in patients with hepatitis

Black cohosh	Kava kava
Chaparral	Mistletoe
Chelidonium	

CIRRHOSIS

Cirrhosis of the liver (gradual destruction of the liver tissue preventing it from functioning normally) develops most commonly after 5–10 years of drinking excessive quantities of alcohol. The amount of alcohol that can cause liver injury varies considerably from person to person. The other important causes of cirrhosis are hepatitis B or C infection. Many patients with cirrhosis have no major symptoms during the early stages of the disease.

Symptoms which develop in advanced stages of the condition include jaundice, abdominal pain, fatigue and signs of malnutrition, accumulation of fluid within the abdomen (ascites) or in the legs (ankle oedema). Brain function may become affected causing apathy, confusion, inability to concentrate, disorientation and slurring of speech, progressing to changes in intellect, personality, emotions and consciousness. Increased blood pressure in the vein that takes blood from the gut to the liver may cause swellings in the blood vessels in the lower oesophagus or upper stomach. The swellings may bleed into the gut and the patient may vomit blood. This is very serious and may be fatal. Blood vessels in the rectum may also be affected and many patients with cirrhosis also have haemorrhoids.

Care should be taken when administering medications to patients with cirrhosis of the liver. Most medications are metabolized or inactivated by the liver, so liver cells which function abnormally take longer than normal to carry out these processes with the result that the medication is active for longer, and there is increased possibility of adverse effects.

GALLSTONES

Bile is made in the liver and stored in the gallbladder, entering the intestine through the bile duct when the gallbladder contracts. Bile contains mainly cholesterol, bilirubin and bile salts which aid digestion. Stones are formed from cholesterol (cholesterol stones) or bilirubin (pigmented stones), the former being more common. The stones can vary considerably in size and number.

People particularly at risk of developing gallstones are obese people, people with high blood cholesterol, women taking contraceptive pills, and people with chronic diseases which cause an increase in destruction of red blood cells (haemolytic diseases) such as thalassaemia and spherocytosis. Age and ethnicity may also have a role and explain why people over the age of 60 are more likely to develop gallstones, and why Native Americans and

Mexican Americans have higher rates of gallstones than other population groups living in the US.

The majority of gallstones do not produce symptoms but about 10% of patients with gallstones develop symptoms such as abdominal pain which is usually of sudden onset. Gallstones may also cause pain between the shoulder blades at the back or pain under the right shoulder. Other symptoms are rather vague, such as belching, gas and indigestion.

Colicky pain in the upper or upper right abdomen occurs when a gallstone is impacted in a duct (bile duct). The pain may be severe and similar to that observed after a heart attack which may cause some confusion in the diagnosis. When a duct is occluded by a stone, infection (cholecystitis) often follows and the patient may develop a high fever, chills, rigors and abdominal pain which may be referred to the tip of the shoulder. Accumulation of pus within the gallbladder may follow and very rarely abnormal channels (fistulae) may develop between the gallbladder and the adjacent parts of the intestine (e.g. duodenum, stomach or colon) if treatment is delayed. Cancer of the gallbladder is uncommon.

Rest in bed, relief of pain, antibiotics and maintenance of fluid balance are important aspects of allopathic management. Symptomatic gallstones are best treated surgically by removal of the gallbladder (cholecystectomy) though medical dissolution of gallstones is achievable. Fortunately, the gallbladder is an organ that is not essential for normal living. Losing it will not even necessitate a change in diet.

GALLSTONES:

Some herbs used in treatment

Boldo	Milk thistle
Chamomile	Rosemary
Dandelion	Vervain
Fennel	Wild yam
Lemon balm	Yarrow
Liquorice	

A herb that may cause harm in patients with gallstones

Devil's claw

DISORDERS OF BLOOD

ANAEMIA

Anaemia is a deficiency of red blood cells, which carry oxygen to the tissues.

Causes of anaemia

Causes of anaemia include:

- Deficiency of iron, vitamin B_{12} and folic acid which are needed to produce red blood cells.
- Disease in the bone marrow where red blood cells are made. The bone marrow can become diseased if invaded by cancer cells or other rapidly dividing blood cells which are not capable of carrying oxygen, e.g. white cells in leukaemias.
- Chronic blood loss as from haemorrhoids, heavy menstruation, polyps or growths in the bowel, erosions/ulcers of the stomach.
- Excessive breakdown of red cells by the spleen.

Signs and symptoms of anaemia

The symptoms and signs of anaemia are nonspecific and include tiredness, light-headedness, shortness of breath, ankle swelling, pallor of mucous membranes, increased rate of breathing, increased pulse rate and postural giddiness. Frequently murmurs are heard on auscultation of the heart.

A detailed history is essential to eliminate the common causes of anaemia (e.g. chronic blood loss, chronic diseases like rheumatoid arthritis, drugs that may cause blood loss). Clinical examination and investigations need to be meticulous to determine the cause and the severity of anaemia. It is important to consider cancer as a diagnosis in instances where the anaemia is unexplained.

ANAEMIA:

Some herbs used in treatment

Angelica sinensis	Pau d'arco
Elder	Vervain

LEUKAEMIA

Leukaemia is cancer of white blood cells. The bone marrow produces large numbers of abnormal white blood cells that accumulate and take the place of normal white and red blood cells and blood platelets. There are different types of leukaemia which affect different kinds of white blood cell in different ways.

Although the cause of leukaemia is unknown there are several factors that have been associated with its development: exposure to ionizing radiation produced by radiotherapy or atom bombs, cytotoxic drugs, occupational exposure to benzene, and retroviruses. There may also be genetic associations.

The incidence is approximately 10/10,000 per annum and about half of these are acute leukaemias. Men are affected more than women.

Acute leukaemia

In acute leukaemia the bone marrow produces large numbers of underdeveloped white blood cells which are unable to function properly. There are two types of acute leukaemia: lymphoblastic leukaemia affects the white blood cells known as lymphocytes; myeloblastic or myeloid leukaemia affects myeloid white cells from which neutrophils, eosinophils, monocytes, basophils and megakaryocytes are derived.

Acute myeloid leukaemia is more common in adults (median age at presentation is 60 years) while lymphoblastic leukaemia is more common in children, particularly between the ages of two and 10 years. It is possibly the most common malignant disease in children.

Acute leukaemia develops rapidly. The patient becomes weak, pale and tired due to anaemia, has abnormal episodes of bleeding, with fevers, chills or flu-like symptoms due to recurrent infections, weight loss, bone or joint pain and swollen lymph nodes that are tender to touch.

Leukaemias need to be distinguished from cancers of the lymphatic system (Hodgkin's and non-Hodgkin's lymphomas) which also cause swollen but painless lymph glands, night sweats, unexplained fevers, fatigue and weight loss.

Acute leukaemia can be treated with powerful drugs (e.g. vincristine, prednisolone, L-asparaginase, methotrexate, cytarabine, daunorubicin) to destroy the immature cells without affecting the cells from which normal blood cells multiply. If these are not appropriate, for example for elderly people or patients with other diseases, the patient will be given supportive care which may include blood transfusions to increase numbers of red blood cells and platelets, fresh frozen plasma for coagulation disorders, and intravenous antibiotics for infections when the white cell counts are low.

Without treatment, acute leukaemia progresses quickly and rapidly becomes worse over a few weeks. The chance of a good response to treatment depends on the exact type of leukaemia: for some types about 80% of adult patients under 60 years of age recover.

Chronic leukaemia

In chronic leukaemia there is an increase in production of abnormal white blood cells that cannot carry out all the functions of a normal white blood cell. They slowly replace normal white cells, red cells and blood platelets.

Chronic myeloid leukaemia

Symptoms include tiredness, lethargy, weight loss, shortness of breath, abdominal pain and discomfort, loss of appetite, sweating and bruising.

On examination, the spleen and liver are usually enlarged. Examination of the blood shows an anaemia and a massive increase in white cells.

Chronic lymphocytic leukaemia

This is the commonest form of leukaemia accounting for 30% of cases. Men are affected more than women and average age of onset is 45 years. The onset is insidious. Anaemia, painless enlargement of the lymph nodes (in contrast to myeloid leukaemia where lymph nodes are usually not enlarged) and recurrent infections are common presenting symptoms.

Treatment may not be needed, but drugs may be given if the patient is unwell, has enlarged lymph glands or is significantly anaemic. Radiotherapy is sometimes used. Bone marrow transplantation from suitable donors can be considered for some patients.

Patients treated conventionally have a 15% risk of death in the first 12 months and thereafter an annual risk of 20–25%. With drug treatment survival averages four or five years. No specific herbal remedies were found to treat lymphocytic leukaemia.

LEUKAEMIA:

Some herbs used in treatment of swollen lymph glands

Ashwagandha	Hydrocotyle (Gotu kola)
Burdock	Liquorice
Cleavers	Marigold
Dandelion	Red clover
Echinacea	

ABDOMINAL (GASTROINTESTINAL) DISORDERS

CONSTIPATION

Constipation is defined as infrequent passage of hard stools. Constipation is a symptom and not a disease.

The frequency of normal bowel movements differs from person to person, and may range from three times a day to three times a week. A working definition of constipation is when the bowel movements occur less frequently than three times a week accompanied by stools which are hard, dry, small in size and difficult to eliminate.

Constipation affects most individuals some time in their lives. However, it causes disproportionate distress to some and is considered to be responsible for nearly 2.5 million physician visits a year in the US.

Causes of constipation

Causes of constipation include:

1. Lack of fluid or fibre in the diet.
2. Drugs: opiates (e.g. morphine), anticholinergics, calcium antagonists, iron supplements, aluminium-containing antacids.
3. Irritable bowel syndrome.
4. Chronic intestinal pseudo-obstruction.
5. Neurological disorders – multiple sclerosis, spinal cord lesions, cerebrovascular accidents, parkinsonism.
6. Metabolic/endocrine disorders: diabetes mellitus, hypercalcaemia (elevated calcium levels in the blood), hypothyroidism (decreased activity of thyroid gland), pregnancy.
7. Any serious illness resulting in immobility especially in the elderly.
8. Depression.
9. Hirschprung's disease (a disorder due to abnormal nerve supply to the lower bowel) if neonatal in origin.

10. Cancer of the colon, developing in middle age; sometimes associated with intermittent diarrhoea.
11. Change in lifestyle, e.g. travel, ageing.

Signs and symptoms

Clinical examination should look for associated symptoms such as rectal bleeding, pain, weight loss, excessive straining, emotional distress and symptoms suggestive of irritable bowel syndrome. Rectal examination (examination of the anus and lower rectum by inserting a lubricated gloved finger in to the rectum) and perineal inspection should be carried out and a barium enema and colonoscopy should be considered. Investigations may include serum calcium, thyroid function tests and full blood count.

Treatment of constipation

In most cases, constipation can be successfully treated with judicious use of laxatives or extra dietary fibre. Insoluble fibre, found in fruits, vegetables and grain, cannot be digested so it adds bulk to the stools and helps the bowels to work well.

Constipation can be prevented by a diet that includes 20–35 g of fibre daily, and plenty of fluid (not caffeine or alcohol) and regular exercise to make stools soft and easy to pass.

CONSTIPATION:

Some herbs used in treatment

Artichoke
Basil
Black pepper
Boldo
Boneset
Burdock
Caraway
Carline thistle
Cascara sagrada
Chamomile
Damiana
Dandelion
Fenugreek
Fig
Frangula
Ginger
Glucomannan
Ispaghula
Lemon balm
Liquorice
Linseed (flax)
Marshmallow
Mugwort
Peach
Pineapple
Safflower
Senna
Sweet violet
Yellow dock

A herb that may cause constipation

Saw palmetto

DIARRHOEA

Diarrhoea is the frequent passage of increased amounts of watery stools. Gastroenterologists define diarrhoea in children over two years of age as passage of more than 200 g of stool daily. This means the passage of four or more stools a day.

Most people have episodes of diarrhoea from time to time, but it is not usually serious and they recover in a couple of days. However, in developing countries, acute diarrhoea due to lack of safe drinking water and due to poor disposal of sewage causes 5–8 million deaths per year particularly in infants. Some authorities say that seven children die of acute diarrhoea every minute.

Acute diarrhoea

Acute diarrhoea is almost always caused by bacterial, viral or protozoal infection and is short-lived.

Viruses and bacteria cause irritation to the lining of the small and/or large intestines which results in the stools becoming watery, and causes the bowel to contract more strongly than normal, which often results in colicky pain. Often the infection causes nausea and vomiting which results in additional loss of fluid from the body. There may also be a fever.

The bacteria that are most often the cause of diarrhoea are staphylococci, which are frequently found in wounds and sores on hands. People preparing food should cover cuts or wounds with dressings to avoid contaminating food with bacteria.

Food poisoning is usually due to infection by *Salmonella* bacteria. Amoebic dysentery is an important cause of diarrhoea in travellers and is due to infestation with *Entamoeba histolytica.* Cholera is not seen in the UK.

Diarrhoea may be a side-effect of medications such as cytotoxic drugs, drugs called proton pump inhibitors, anti-inflammatory analgesics and antibiotics. Antibiotics cause diarrhoea because they kill some of the normal bacteria in the bowel and the changes in the bacterial flora make the bowel function abnormally. This may occur even after the intake of antibiotics has ceased.

Other causes of acute diarrhoea include radiation sickness and rupture of an inflamed appendix.

Chronic or relapsing diarrhoea

Diarrhoea continuing for more than 10 days is considered to be chronic diarrhoea and is unlikely to be caused by an infection. Causes of chronic diarrhoea include:

- ***Irritable bowel syndrome***, which is the most common cause of chronic diarrhoea. Diarrhoea is most severe in the morning, before and after breakfast. There may be excessive wind passed and griping pain, and the bouts of diarrhoea may alternate with periods of constipation. Blood is never found in the stool.
- ***Inflammatory bowel disease***, which is characterized by inflammation of the colon; blood and mucus are found in the stools, and diarrhoea may be accompanied by cramping lower abdominal pain.
- ***Malabsorption***, which is the inability to absorb food from the gut, usually the small bowel (small intestine). This is caused by inflammatory disease of the pancreas (pancreatitis), cystic fibrosis, which affects secretion of pancreatic digestive enzymes, coeliac disease, tropical sprue, lymphoma, and lactose or fructose intolerance. Malabsorption results in steatorrhoea (an offensive, large volume stool that is difficult to flush down a toilet), undigested food in the stools, weight loss and nutritional disturbances.

When there is an alteration of bowel habit including diarrhoea, one should consider the possibility of malignant disease, such as cancer of the bowel. A hormone-secreting tumour is a rare cause of diarrhoea.

Prompt attention and investigation is required when blood or pus is present in the stools and when diarrhoea occurs in young children or in the elderly people. It is important that people with diarrhoea do not become dehydrated. Signs of dehydration include passing urine infrequently and in only very small amounts.

In allopathic medicine the main aim is to ensure adequate intake of liquids (3–4 litres a day) to prevent dehydration. Infestation of parasites (worms and amoebae) should always be treated using the appropriate medications.

The development and availability of oral rehydration fluid, a preparation containing sugar and salt to replace the excessive loss that occurs in diarrhoea, has been one of the most important life-saving products in medical history.

Investigations should include haematological tests (full blood count and clotting), and biochemical tests (urea, electrolytes, calcium, magnesium, etc.), sigmoidoscopy, colonoscopy, biopsy, ultrasound and CT examinations, barium follow through studies and measurement of gut hormone profile.

DIARRHOEA:

Some herbs used in treatment

Acidophilus
Agrimony
Allspice
American cranesbill
Barberry
Barley
Basil
Beth root
Betony
Bilberry
Bistort
Black catechu
Black haw
Black pepper
Boswellia
Burnet
Calumba
Carline thistle
Cassia
Chamomile – German, for nervous diarrhoeas
Chinese rhubarb
Cinnamon
Cola
Daisy
Elecampane
Fennel
Ginger
Goldenrod
Ground ivy
Guarana
Horse chestnut
Jambul
Lady's mantle
Lavender
Lemon balm
Lysine
Marshmallow
Meadowsweet – not recommended for use in children
Mint
Mugwort
Oregon grape
Peppermint
Pill-bearing spurge
Plantain
Pomegranate
Poplar
Quince
Rauwolfia
Red yeast
Rhatany
Sage
Savory
Scull cap
Shepherd's purse
Slippery elm
Sorrel
Stone root
Tangerine peel
Thyme
Tormentil
True unicorn root
Wild cherry
Wild yam
Woundwort
Yarrow

Herbs that may cause diarrhoea

Aloe
Bogbean
Broom
Elder
Goldenseal
Ispaghula
Lobelia
Saw palmetto

ABDOMINAL PAIN

Abdominal pain can be produced as a result of infection, distension, torsion and repeated contractions or stretching of any structure within the abdomen. Sharp and localized pain could be due to inflammation caused by infection or by cancer deposits in the thin covering of the abdominal cavity (peritonitis). Gallbladder pain may be referred to the shoulder tip. Non-specific abdominal pain without any organic cause could be due to depression or an associated psychological (somatization) disorder.

ABDOMINAL PAIN:

Some herbs used in treatment

Black pepper
Cinnamon
Caraway
Chamomile
Dill
Mint
Savory
Wild yam
Woundwort

A herb that may cause abdominal pain

Aloes

A herb contraindicated in patients with abdominal pain

Frangula

SEVERE ACUTE PAIN/DISCOMFORT IN THE ABDOMEN

Acute onset of pain in the abdomen accounts for approximately 50% of all urgent admissions to a hospital surgical unit.

Causes

The common causes are:

1. Inflammation – appendicitis, diverticulitis, cholecystitis, inflammation in the pelvis, pancreatitis, pyelonephritis, abscess within the abdomen.
2. Perforation/rupture – peptic ulcer, diverticular disease, ovarian cyst, aortic aneurysm, ectopic pregnancy.
3. Obstruction – intestinal obstruction, biliary colic, ureteric colic.
4. Rarely sickle cell disease crisis, acute intermittent porphyria, diabetic ketoacidosis, Addison's disease.

Investigation

Assessment consists of determining the duration and nature of the pain (colicky, constant, sharp, dull, intermittent or continuous, or occurring during the night), the site of pain and radiation, severity, precipitating and relieving factors, and associated features such as vomiting, dyspepsia and altered bowel habit.

Inflammation of the peritoneum (peritonitis) is indicated by a rigid abdomen which moves very sluggishly with breathing and very tender to touch, with involuntary guarding due to spasm of the abdominal muscles in an effort to minimize movement of the peritoneum.

Blood tests, X-rays of the abdomen and chest, ultrasound examinations and other imaging techniques such as CT scans should be used in cases where diagnosis is uncertain.

Treatment

Treatment includes antibiotics for inflammation, adequate rehydration and correction of metabolic abnormalities. Surgical removal of the inflamed structure may be necessary, and is mandatory if there is evidence of peritonitis. Perforations usually need to be closed surgically although some perforations can be treated conservatively with very close monitoring while obstructions should be relieved surgically.

CHRONIC OR RECURRENT ABDOMINAL PAIN

Chronic pain is usually associated with malignant disease and requires careful and thorough abdominal examination. Investigations could include endoscopy, colonoscopy, ultrasound examinations, contrast radiological studies (e.g. barium enema, mesenteric angiography, intravenous ureterography) and CT scans.

Psychological factors associated with chronic pain should be evaluated and treated with drugs, beginning with simple painkillers (analgesics) along with antidepressants, increasing strength and frequency when needed.

WEIGHT LOSS

Loss of weight in excess of 3 kg in six months in the absence of dieting, exercise and starvation, most often indicates disease.

Decreased intake of food may be caused by simple factors such as poor oral health or difficulty in chewing caused by problems with the teeth, especially in the elderly. Other causes include:

- psychiatric disturbances (anorexia nervosa, bulimia, depression)
- chronic illnesses (tuberculosis, brucellosis, recurrent chest and urinary tract infections, rheumatoid arthritis)
- parasitic and protozoan infestations
- general medical disorders, particularly those affecting hormones (endocrine disease) such as diabetes mellitus, Addison's disease or hyperactive thyroid
- growths in the upper intestinal tract (e.g. carcinoma of the oesophagus, stomach carcinoma) which can cause decreased intake of food due to difficulty in swallowing and associated loss of appetite (as with stomach cancer).

WEIGHT LOSS:

Herbs used in treatment

There are several herbal preparations available on the market for slimming which have been known to be contaminated with dangerous allopathic medicines and which have often resulted in liver failure. Some herbal preparations used for slimming or weight loss have also been known to contain, possibly mistakenly, dangerous plant alkaloids, e.g. aristolochic acid, which have caused kidney failure. It would be unwise for us to provide a list of herbs used for weight loss as there are many uncertainties.

MALABSORPTION

Before it can be digested, food needs to be broken down by enzymes to form smaller molecules that can be absorbed from the intestines. Some enzymes are produced by the stomach and intestines, others are produced by the liver and pancreas and sent to the stomach and intestines. The lining of the small intestine is covered with small finger-like projections (villi) which increase the surface area available for absorption.

Reduction in the surface area of the intestine or lack of certain enzymes reduces the ability of the body to absorb food (malabsorption). Malabsorption leads to loss of weight and nutritional deficiency.

Symptoms

Chronic diarrhoea of variable severity is a feature of malabsorption. Fat malabsorption produces bulky pale offensive stools which float in the toilet (steatorrhoea), a distended 'noisy' (borborygmi) abdomen and abdominal cramps. This may be accompanied by weight loss, lethargy and depression.

Poor wound healing, easy bruising or bleeding spots on the skin (purpura), night blindness, anaemia, bleeding gums and mouth and tongue lesions (which may cause a decrease in intake of food) may occur due to reduced absorption of vitamins and minerals necessary for the formation of blood cells (iron, folate, vitamin B_{12}) and constituents necessary for blood coagulation (vitamins C and K). In addition vision may be affected (due to lack of vitamin A) and tissue integrity and healing may be poor (due to lack of vitamin C, protein and zinc).

Osteomalacia and rickets may develop due to changes in bone metabolism caused by poor absorption of vitamin D and calcium leading to deformities or increased tendency to fractures of bones. Changes in the nervous system (loss of sensation leading to ulcers and loss of balance) may be caused by poor absorption of vitamin B_{12}, magnesium and calcium. Swollen ankles may develop due to lack of proteins.

Causes of malabsorption

Causes of malabsorption include:

1. Chronic pancreatitis characterized by acute abdominal pain progressing to chronic abdominal pain, weight loss and malnourishment

(common in middle aged alcoholics), causing deficiency of digestive enzymes mainly in the bile and from the pancreas.
2. Carcinoma of the pancreas (jaundice, cachexia, enlarged liver, vomiting, erythematous rash).
3. Cystic fibrosis (repeated lung infections, bronchiectasis).
4. Decrease in the absorptive area of the bowel following surgical resection.
5. Diseases such as coeliac disease (diarrhoea, malabsorption and failure to thrive in infants, growth failure in older children, tiredness, anaemia, weight loss in adults), tropical sprue, lymphoma of the intestine and lymphangiectasis.

MALABSORPTION:

Some herbs used in treatment

Burdock	Glucomannan
Chamomile	Guarana
Cinnamon	Lavender
Coriander	Lemon balm
Elderberry	Marshmallow
Elecampane	Rose
Fennel	Spirulina
Garcinia	Thyme
Ginger	

HAEMATEMESIS (VOMITING OF BLOOD)

Vomit containing fresh blood is bright red. When blood loss has been chronic, vomitus may be blackish (ground coffee). Haematemesis may be accompanied by the passage of black tarry stools (malaena).

Causes include:

1. Oesophagitis usually with a hiatus hernia.
2. Peptic ulcer.
3. Malformations of blood vessels.
4. Varices – dilatation of blood vessels in oesophagus and stomach.
5. Excessive retching.
6. Malignancy.
7. Erosions of the mucosa (lining) of oesophagus/stomach.

This common emergency requires close monitoring of blood pressure, pulse rate and urine output, and resuscitation with intravenous fluids/blood. A thorough clinical examination should include endoscopy to identify the site of bleeding and to arrest the bleeding. If the latter fails, surgery is necessary. Investigations should include full blood count, coagulation time and tests of liver and kidney function.

In the acute phase, there are possibly no indications for the use of traditional medicines.

HAEMATEMESIS (VOMITING OF BLOOD):

A herb used in treatment

Shepherd's purse

BLEEDING PER RECTUM

Blood in the stools may be visible or invisible (occult). Visible blood in the stools is often due to bleeding from the large intestine or anal canal and rarely from the small intestine. This bleeding may be acute and severe in diverticular disease or when the blood supply to the bowel is interrupted (ischaemia) as with occlusion (blocking) of the inferior mesenteric artery which is the main blood supply to the bowel. Such bleeding is accompanied by pain in the abdomen. Rarely bleeding may be due to developmental abnormalities of the gut and blood vessels in the gut (e.g. Meckel's diverticulum or angiodysplasia).

Chronic or sub-acute bleeding occurs with anal haemorrhoids or anal fissures, malignancies of the lower bowel, large polyps and some inflammatory diseases of the bowel and with angiodysplasia. Such bleeding also follows radiation-induced injury to the bowel (radiation enteritis). Radiotherapy is a form of treatment for bowel carcinoma.

Occult bleeding is commonly associated with colorectal malignancy and may be the earliest sign in the absence of other symptoms. Such bleeding often leads to iron deficiency anaemia. A negative occult blood test in the stools does not exclude malignant disease of the bowel and further investigations (e.g. colonoscopy) are necessary.

HAEMORRHOIDS (PILES)

Congestion and twisting of the veins around the anal canal gives rise to haemorrhoids (piles) which are usually associated with constipation and straining at stool. They may develop for the first time during pregnancy and resolve after the birth of the child. Bleeding occurs during or after defaecation. Some piles may prolapse and retract spontaneously while manual replacement may be required in some instances. Common accompaniments are pruritus (itching around anus) and a mucus discharge.

Prevention of constipation and straining is important. In allopathic medicine, piles are either thrombosed (sclerosed) or ligated (banding) or may require surgery for removal (haemorrhoidectomy), the latter being curative. All patients with rectal bleeding should undergo a colonoscopy to exclude malignancies in the lower gastrointestinal tract.

BLEEDING PER RECTUM:

Some herbs used in treatment

Aloe
American cranesbill
Balsam of Peru
Bilberry
Bistort
Burdock
Butcher's broom
Chamomile
Garlic
Hawthorn
Horse chestnut
Indigo
Ispaghula
Marigold
Oaks
Pilewort – locally as an ointment or suppository
Plantain
St John's wort
Stone root
Vervain
Witch hazel (topical)
Yerba santa

A herb to be avoided in patients with haemorrhoids

Willow

GASTRITIS AND PEPTIC ULCER DISEASE

Indigestion (dyspepsia), loss of appetite, nausea and vomiting with some discomfort or pain in the upper abdomen just beneath the rib cage are common symptoms during any individual's life time, often attributed to excessive alcohol consumption, or to eating spicy food. Such symptoms are most often due to inflammation of the stomach lining, and usually resolve with rest and medications to counter the acidity in the stomach (antacids) or to a decrease in the production of acid in the stomach (e.g. H_2-receptor antagonists), and avoiding the food or drink that caused the symptoms.

However, the inflammation may cause erosions in the lining of the stomach (mucosa) which may lead to bleeding. This may occur as a result of long-term use of medications such as non-steroidal anti-inflammatory drugs (e.g. aspirin or ibuprofen). Similar symptoms may occur during periods of severe stress and following burns and severe trauma. Certain viral infections (e.g. cytomegalovirus, herpes simplex virus in AIDS) may also cause similar symptoms and lesions. If relief is not obtained within a few days, it is necessary to investigate specifically to exclude ulcers or a malignancy.

The most common cause of non-specific chronic symptoms (chronic gastritis) is infection with *Helicobacter pylori* bacteria. Though most patients may remain without symptoms for long periods, many require treatment to eradicate this bacillus.

Peptic ulcers

Peptic ulcers occur in the lower oesophagus, stomach or duodenum, and may be acute or chronic. Around 90% of duodenal ulcer patients and 70% of gastric ulcer patients are infected with the bacteria *Helicobacter pylori*. The remaining 30% of gastric ulcers are due to non-steroidal anti-inflammatory drugs. Smoking increases the risk of gastric ulcers in particular and delays healing of the ulcer. Peptic ulcers are also considered to be associated with a certain type of personality, namely type A – ambitious, aggressive, active and result orientated.

The commonest symptom is recurrent episodes of pain in the upper abdomen, related to food intake. Other symptoms may include vomiting, loss of appetite, nausea and anaemia due to chronic blood loss from the ulcer.

All episodes of upper abdominal pain persisting for longer than a week merit investigation and endoscopy (passing a tube containing a light and a camera into the stomach to make it possible to see the lining of the stomach).

Eradication of *Helicobacter pylori* infection is the cornerstone of treatment for peptic ulcers. Two antibiotics are taken to kill the bacterium, at the same time as a drug to reduce acid secretion in the stomach, usually a proton pump inhibitor, or less commonly an H_2-receptor antagonist.

Antacids are often used for self-medication, but may cause either diarrhoea or constipation. Antacids also tend to cause retention of salt and worsen heart failure.

Surgery is indicated if an ulcer perforates or when there is haemorrhage from the ulcer. Occasionally surgery may be required if the ulcer causes obstruction to the passage of food.

To prevent recurrence, smoking and drugs that irritate the gastric mucosa (e.g. aspirin) should be avoided. Alcohol may be consumed in moderate amounts.

GASTRITIS AND PEPTIC ULCER DISEASE:

Some herbs used in treatment

Aloe	Irish moss
Burdock	Kudzu
Calumba	Liquorice
Carline thistle	Marigold
Cat's claw	Marshmallow
Chamomile	Meadowsweet
Coriander	Peppermint
Drosera	Plantain
Fennel	Rose
Fenugreek	Sage
Goldenseal	St John's wort
Hops	Turmeric
Iceland moss	Yarrow

Some herbs used to treat indigestion

Hops	Lemon verbena

A herb to be avoided in indigestion

Evening primrose

Some herbs contraindicated in patients with peptic ulcers

Devil's claw	Gentian

IRRITABLE BOWEL SYNDROME

Irritable bowel syndrome (IBS) is a disorder in which intermittent abdominal pain and chronic diarrhoea alternate with constipation. There may be excessive wind passed and griping abdominal pain. IBS is common in young people, between 20 and 30 years, and is twice as common in women.

Though the symptoms are distressing to the patient, IBS rarely leads to serious or life-threatening complications. Usually there is no blood in the stools and patients do not lose weight or have their sleep disturbed. The intestines appear normal on investigations and there is no certain cause for the disorder in allopathic medicine.

There is no single mode of therapy in allopathic medicine. A wide range of medications may be used to bring comfort to these patients. They include anti-diarrhoeal agents (e.g. loperamide), bulking agents (e.g. ispaghula husk), antimuscarinics (hyoscine) and antispasmodics (e.g. mebeverine) and some antidepressants.

IRRITABLE BOWEL SYNDROME:

Some herbs used in treatment

Usually combinations of herbs are used as teas

Continued

Carminative herbs (flatulence relieving herbs)

Angelica root	Fennel
Anise	Lemon balm
Asafoetida	Lovage
Caraway	Peppermint
Cardamom	Rosemary
Chamomile	Spearmint
Dill	

Herbs to aid bile output

Gentian	Wormwood
Hops	

Bitters

Artichoke	Milk thistle
Dandelion root	

Constipation remedies

Aloe vera	Linseed (flax)
Ispaghula	Psyllium seeds

Soothing herbs

Cinnamon	Marshmallow root
Fenugreek	Slippery elm
Ginger	

A herb to prevent loose stools

Arrowroot

MUSCULOSKELETAL SYSTEM DISEASES

JOINT PAINS

Bones are linked to each other by joints. Most people in the older age group (over 60 years of age) develop some stiffness and pain in one or more joints, and almost any joint in the body can be affected. In young men such symptoms are usually due to some injury or trauma, while in young women, although trauma is a cause to be considered, it is more often due to a connective tissue disorder.

Other causes of stiffness and pain in joints are the entry of foreign bodies such as thorns of plants. Foreign bodies entering a joint may also cause bleeding into the joint or around the joint (haemarthrosis).

However, there are certain disease states which need to be excluded if such symptoms cannot be related to trauma.

In middle-aged men, if pain occurs in the joint of the big toe, gout has to be considered in the differential diagnosis. The wrist and elbow may be involved in pseudogout which is more common in older women.

When a damaged joint becomes infected (septic arthritis), there is swelling of the surrounding soft tissues and the skin above may be reddened. Pain and stiffness may increase in a joint that is already abnormal. In this situation the diagnosis needs to be confirmed by an orthopaedic surgeon in allopathic medical practice and appropriate treatment started as soon as possible to prevent further damage.

Bleeding into joints often without any trauma or with minimal exertion is common in the bleeding disorder haemophilia where there is an inherited defect in one of the factors necessary for the clotting of the blood.

In allopathic medicine, aspiration of the joint may be required if there is suspicion of infection or of deposition of crystals.

JOINT PAINS:

Some herbs used to treat joint pains

Allspice	Celery
Arnica	Marjoram
Capsicum	Wild lettuce
Cat's claw	Woundwort

ARTHRITIS

Acute arthritis is sudden pain and swelling of one or more joints. Acute arthritis of a single joint (monoarthritis) is commonly caused by gout, trauma, bleeding into the joint or the entry of a foreign body. Bacterial infection of a joint, usually an injured joint, often causes an acute onset of pain in the affected joint.

In some people monoarthritis may be the first stage of diseases such as rheumatoid arthritis, psoariatic arthritis or erythema nodosum, but this is uncommon. Usually in psoriasis and rheumatoid arthritis more than one joint is affected and the term polyarthritis is used, particularly when more than five joints are involved.

Osteoarthritis is a common disorder which often occurs in old age and affects several joints. Certain infectious diseases such as mumps, chicken pox and hepatitis may also cause pain in several joints. In most of these infectious diseases, joint pains would be associated with the rash that is characteristic of the infection.

In allopathic medical management of infected joints it is recommended that the infecting organism is identified so that the most appropriate antibiotic can be used. This involves aspiration of the joint, a procedure which can be relatively painlessly carried out using a local anaesthetic.

Current management of arthritis, especially polyarthritis, involves specialists from many different disciplines, including rheumatologists, physiotherapists, occupational therapists, and social workers. Artificial joint replacements can be provided surgically for some joints such as the knee, hip and shoulder.

ARTHRITIS:

Some herbs used in treatment

Alfalfa
Aloe
Arnica
Ashwagandha
Bilberry
Burdock
Carline thistle
Cat's claw
Celery
Chaparral
Chickweed
Cinnamon
Cleavers
Comfrey (topical only)
Coriander
Cumin
Daisy
Dandelion
Devil's claw
Echinacea
Elderberry
Evening primrose
Fucus (kelp)
Galangal
Ginger
Hydrocotyle (Gotu kola)
Horsetail
Lavender
Liquorice
Lime flower
Mate
Meadowsweet
Mugwort
Mustard
Nettle
Night-blooming cereus
Nutmeg
Oregon grape
Pansy
Pareira
Peppermint
Ragwort
Rosemary
Sarsaparilla
Sassafras
Soapwort
True unicorn
Vervain
Wild yam
Willow
Yerba santa
Yucca

FIBROMYALGIA

Fibromyalgia is a diagnosis commonly made when there is pain in muscles, tendons and ligaments associated with fatigue and certain psychological disorders such as irritability, weepiness, poor concentration, loss of memory or forgetfulness. The condition affects mostly women between the ages of 30 and 60.

Pain is felt in several areas of the body, often specific regions such as the upper arms, thighs, neck and chest. People with fibromyalgia often wake up feeling tired despite having slept for a reasonable length of time. Many of them also have sleep problems. It is a distressing condition as these individuals find it difficult to cope with employment or carry out daily chores.

Detailed clinical examination usually fails to reveal any abnormal findings. The cause of fibromylagia is uncertain.

FIBROMYALGIA:

Some herbs used in treatment

The following have been used to treat the diverse symptoms of fibromyalgia:

Depression – St John's wort
Increase immunity – garlic, red clover, echinacea, astragalus
Sleep disorders – scull cap, valerian, passion flower, chamomile, evening primrose oil
Joint and muscle pain – capsaicin, cayenne – applied topically

OSTEOPOROSIS

Osteoporosis is a condition that affects the bones causing them to become thin, weak and more likely to break. It is more common in older people and is the usual reason why old people suffer fractures of bones easily with minimal trauma.

In women, this weakness in bones is thought to be due to the lack of the female hormone oestrogen. In older people, a diet low in calcium and inability to absorb calcium may be contributing factors. Long-term uses of steroids, low calcium intake throughout life, smoking and low body weight are risk factors.

In the early stages there may not be any symptoms, but as the condition develops patients may experience joint pain and difficulty in standing up straight.

Allopathic medicine recommends drugs to halt bone demineralization and calcium supplements, and measures to reduce the risk of elderly people falling.

OSTEOPOROSIS:

Some herbs used in treatment

Angelica	Nettle
Bilberry	Peppermint
Black cohosh	Plantain
Dandelion	Sage
Elecampane	Soy
Ginseng	Thyme
Hops	Wild oats
Liquorice	

BACKACHE

Back pain or backache is a very common symptom experienced by 60–80% of people at some time in their lives. In developed countries, low back pain ('lumbago') is the most common medical cause of inability to work. However, some people who have no other disease state but are unhappy with employment complain of chronic pain as an excuse to keep away from work.

Back pain may be due to spinal causes or non-spinal causes. In the great majority of patients it is due to abnormalities of joints and ligaments in the lower spine (lumbar spine).

Lesions of the spine that cause back pain may be due to mechanical or non-mechanical causes. In most instances, acute onset of back pain occurs in young active people often between the ages of 20 and 55 years, due to mechanical causes such as bending or lifting a heavy weight using an incorrect posture (positioning of limbs and spine). The pain is of sudden onset, predominantly on one side and is often in the lower region of the spinal cord (low back pain). Examination reveals tenderness in the region and some restriction of movement.

Mechanical back pain usually resolves in six weeks after rest, sleeping on a hard surface and other simple remedial measures such as use of painkillers and local application of non-steroidal anti-inflammatory drug ointments or gels. However, it is important to be aware that in a small number of people back pain indicates a definite or serious lesion in the spine, and that a complete history and examination is necessary to identify these patients.

Non-mechanical back pain is constant and does not vary with activity.

Serious spinal pain needs to be considered in people under the age of 20 or over the age of 50 with progressive pain. Particular care is needed if the pain is in the thoracic region of the spine (spine behind the chest).

Tuberculosis of the spine continues to be a concern and inquiries need to be made about symptoms such as night sweats, malaise and weight loss.

Loss of sensation in the lower limbs, muscle wasting and a spinal deformity are pointers to a serious condition affecting the spine.

Cauda equina syndrome is an emergency that needs immediate medical treatment. Between the vertebrae are discs which add stability and flexibility to the spine. These discs have a semi-solid or liquid inner area which is surrounded by a harder outer circumference. In this syndrome the softer inner part pushes itself through the outer harder layer – a process called herniation – and then presses on the nerves that leave the spinal cord at that site. The pressure of the herniated disc causes loss of sensation in the areas supplied by the nerves that are compressed and also muscle weakness in the muscles supplied by the compressed nerves. This often leads to difficulty in standing, and if the nerves to the bladder and/or anus are also compressed by the herniated disc, there may be difficulty in passing urine and faecal incontinence.

When pain spreads down the lower limb/s from the lower back it is often referred to as sciatica. The sciatic nerve is the largest nerve in the body and runs from the lower back through the buttocks and down the back of the thigh. When the nerve gets inflamed or is pressed by a disc in the spine, the pain may spread down to the heel. In allopathic medicine, surgery is often recommended to relieve the pressure on the nerve from the protruding disc in the spine. Plain X-rays of the spine are of little value in the diagnosis of lumbar disc disease. CT scans, especially using spiral scanning techniques, can provide helpful images of the disc protrusion and/or narrowing of the foramina through which the nerves exit the spinal cord. MRI is the investigation of choice if available, since soft tissues are well imaged.

All the above clinical features necessitate careful and detailed neurological and radiological investigations.

Non-spinal causes include gynaecological disorders, kidney disease, diseases of the pancreas, malignancy of the bowel (colon) or prostate gland and rarely an aneurysm of the aorta. To exclude the non-spinal causes, it is necessary to inquire and investigate for loss of appetite, abdominal discomfort (dyspepsia), change in bowel habit, signs of prostatism (symptoms accompanying an enlargement of the prostate gland), vaginal bleeding and any other symptom or sign that may indicate a malignant lesion which could cause non-spinal backache.

BACKACHE:

Some herbs used in treatment

Black cohosh
Chamomile
Devil's claw
Echinacea
Ginger
Hops
Lavender
Meadowsweet
Nettle
Passion flower
Pau d'arco
Rosemary
Scull cap
Vervain
Willow

SEXUALLY TRANSMITTED DISEASES

AIDS/HIV

Infection by the human immunodeficiency virus (HIV-1) is possibly the most common sexually transmitted disease today. Worldwide it is estimated that nearly 40 million individuals are infected with this virus. The disease state which causes death in such infected patients is acquired immunodeficiency syndrome, better known as AIDS. The number dying of AIDS annually is considered to be nearly 3 million.

Infection with this virus may also occur following the use of contaminated needles or syringes (used by subjects with the viral infection). Infection caused by blood transfusions is very uncommon today as blood is screened for HIV antibodies prior to transfusion in most countries. Pregnant women can transfer the infection to their baby while it is still in the womb.

To date, no other mode of transmission has been scientifically validated. It is fairly certain that mosquitoes do not transmit this virus. As the virus cannot survive well in the environment, environmental transmission is almost impossible. Further, there is no risk of infection being transmitted by HIV-infected individuals employed in food-service industries, other than by sexual contact. Of course such workers have to follow recommended standards for personal hygiene and food sanitation.

A closely related virus, HIV-2, causes a similar illness to HIV-1 but is less aggressive and restricted mainly to Western Africa.

Primary infection is symptomatic in 70–80% of cases and usually occurs 3–4 weeks after exposure. Early symptoms are similar to those of any viral infection – swelling of the lymph glands, fevers and night sweats, unexplained weight loss, diarrhoea and skin rashes.

Symptoms usually last 1–2 weeks, but occasionally up to 10 weeks. Following this, after many months to years, the patients can develop AIDS.

Patients with AIDS usually have recurrent fevers and rashes (reddish) and they tire easily. They have enlarged lymph nodes and develop muscle and joint pains and a range of other symptoms such as shortness of breath and difficulty in swallowing. More importantly, they are vulnerable to many organisms to which non-HIV infected patients are resistant. They frequently get infected with the fungus *Candida* and also develop pneumonias due to *Pneumocystis carinii* infection.

HIV infection can be confirmed by a blood test which identifies the presence of antibody and a test to detect the presence of HIV particles in the blood (the immunoblot assay). These tests can only be used once the anti-HIV antibodies have begun to appear in the blood (seroconversion), which takes about 3–12 weeks.

The HIV virus attaches itself to a type of white blood cells (lymphocyte) called CD4 T-cells, which are part of the immune system that protects the body against infection. The virus enters the cell and uses the genetic material in the cell to make copies of itself. It kills the lymphocyte and releases millions of viruses into the blood and these spread the infection, killing more lymphocytes. The body continues to make millions of new lymphocytes but eventually the immune system is weakened and becomes vulnerable to infections.

In allopathic medicine, drugs are used to interrupt the lifecycle of the HIV virus, by altering the HIV proteins so that the virus is unable to replicate itself. Drugs will also be needed to prevent what are referred to as opportunistic infections, e.g. hepatitis A and hepatitis B vaccination, pneumococcal vaccine and influenza vaccine.

It is important to watch for drug-related side-effects, which can be a problem, and to give the patient support that will maintain and improve their quality of life.

AIDS/HIV:

Some herbs used in treatment

There are three categories of herbs used in people with HIV infection. The first are herbs that are believed to directly kill HIV (antiviral herbs). The second are herbs that strengthen the immune system to better withstand HIV's onslaught (immuno-modulating herbs). The third are herbs that combat opportunistic infections (antimicrobial herbs). The following table summarizes each category and herbs that belong in each. Note that some herbs fall into more than one category.

Even though there is insufficient evidence to confirm antiretroviral activity of some herbs, those considered to show some degree of such activity are recorded below.

Category of herb	Supporting evidence from human trials	Supporting evidence from test tube studies
Some antiviral activity	Andrographis, boxwood, liquorice	Garlic
Immuno-modulators	Andrographis (possible antiretroviral), panax ginseng, bupleurum, echinacea, liquorice, mistletoe, sangre de drago, turmeric	Herbs: ashwagandha, eleutherococcus, schisandra Mushrooms: coriolus, maitake, reishi, shiitake
Antimicrobial	Garlic, tea tree oil	

Source: Health notes[4].

GONORRHOEA

Infection is passed from person to person during vaginal, oral or anal sex. Untreated mothers may infect their babies' eyes during delivery. In men, discharge from the penis (from the urethra) and pain on passing urine (dysuria) are the common symptoms. Rectal infection may not cause symptoms or may produce anal discomfort, anal discharge or rectal bleeding. Examination of the rectum by inserting an instrument to dilate the anus (proctoscopy) may not reveal any inflammatory change.

About 50% of women who have gonorrhoea have no symptoms. The lower genital organs are usually affected in females but lower abdominal pain, pain during sexual intercourse (dyspareunia) and bleeding between normal periods (inter-menstrual bleeding) indicate involvement of organs in the pelvis.

Pharyngeal gonorrhoea usually does not cause symptoms but may present with sore throat.

Gonorrhoeal infections of the eyes (gonococcal conjunctivitis, gonococcal ophthalmia) require urgent treatment to prevent blindness and other complications. Purulent discharge, swollen eyelids, pain in the eyes and intolerance of light (photophobia) are the common signs and symptoms.

Examination under the microscope of smears from affected sites confirms diagnosis. Usually the disease can be treated with a single dose of a suitable antimicrobial (e.g. ciprofloxacin, or ampicillin with probenecid).

GONORRHOEA:

Some herbs used in treatment

Cat's claw
Horsetail
Pareira
Pau d'arco
Pill-bearing spurge
Quince

SYPHILIS

Syphilis is caused by a bacterium (the spirochaete *Treponema pallidum*). The infection causes an ulcer and the disease is passed from person to person by direct contact with an ulcer (unprotected sexual contact), or passed through the placenta during pregnancy.

The characteristic ulcer, known as a chancre, develops at the site of infection after an incubation period of 14–28 days (may be longer) as a dull red pimple (macule) which becomes larger (papule) and erodes to form an ulcer with thickened edges (indurated ulcer). The lymph glands draining the region enlarge, become rubbery and are discrete. Both these lesions are painless. These lesions usually occur on the penis, vagina, and cervix but may occur on the lips, tongue, tonsil, nipple, fingers, anus or rectum. Without treatment the chancre will resolve in 2–6 weeks leaving a small scar.

The infecting organism remains in the body and spreads causing damage to several organs in the body. In this stage of the disease the patient may experience a mild fever, malaise, headache and a non-irritable rash which may be initially on the limbs and trunk but later becomes more generalized and involves the palms and soles. Untreated, the rash may persist for up to 12 weeks. The skin lesions (papules) may join up to form condylomata lata at warm moist sites such as the vulva or around the anus (perianal area).

A generalized enlargement of lymph nodes accompanies the rash. Lesions may appear on mucous membranes in the mouth, genitalia and pharynx and a characteristic lesion is the snail track ulcer in the mouth.

More severe disorders such as meningitis, paralysis of the cranial nerves, involvement of the eyes (uveitis), hepatitis, gastritis and glomerulonephritis may occur.

Most clinical lesions may resolve without treatment but may enter the phase of latency.

During the primary and secondary stages syphilis is contagious and can be transmitted by sexual contact, by transmission from a pregnant woman to the baby in her womb and rarely by transfusion of blood from infected people.

Syphilis in a latent form may persist for many years or for life, and without treatment over 60% of patients may be expected to suffer little or no ill-health. Between three and 10 years after infection, a tertiary form may develop involving the skin, mucous membranes (mouth, nasal septum, pharynx, larynx), tongue (which may subsequently lead to malignancy after formation of leukoplakia), bone, muscle or abdominal viscera. Single (gumma) or multiple lesions which heal poorly (tissue paper scars) may occur. Treating the active disease is possible even at this stage though some tissue damage may be permanent.

Cardiovascular syphilis may present several years after infection, affecting the aortic valve, aorta or openings of the coronary vessels. Aortic valve incompetence or aneurysms in the ascending aorta or aortic arch develop; they cannot be corrected by antibiotics and surgical intervention is necessary. The infection may also cause serious neurological damage (tabes dorsalis or general paralysis of the insane).

SYPHILIS:

Some herbs used in treatment

Boswellia	Sassafras
Condurango	Soapwort
Oregon grape	Yellow dock
Pau d'arco	

GYNAECOLOGICAL DISORDERS

AMENORRHOEA

Amenorrhoea refers to absence of menstrual periods. Primary amenorrhoea is failure to start menstruating; secondary amenorrhoea is the absence of normal menstrual periods for more than six months in a woman who previously had regular periods.

Primary amenorrhoea may be due to abnormalities in the development of the reproductive organs, including vagina, hymen, womb or ovaries. Rarely, it may be due to childhood infections (e.g. meningitis) or hormonal causes.

Secondary amenorrhoea is commonly due to pregnancy, breastfeeding, sudden and dramatic changes in the body weight, e.g. being severely underweight, cysts in the ovary, stress or hormonal disorders. Assessment should rule out life-threatening causes such as tumours in the brain, ovary or adrenal glands. Treatment depends on the underlying cause.

AMENORRHOEA (ABSENCE OF PERIODS):

Some herbs used in treatment

Agnus castus	Marjoram
Aloe	Mugwort
Black cohosh	Ragwort
Life root	Rue
Lovage	Squaw vine
Madder	True unicorn root

A herb that may cause amenorrhoea

Liquorice

INFERTILITY

Infertility (or subfertility) refers to the inability to conceive after 12 months of regular and unprotected sexual intercourse. It may be due to a variety of male and female factors. Common female causes include failure to produce an egg (ovulation) or problems in the genital tract that are detrimental to the sperm and egg meeting together to form a baby. Inability to produce sperms or to effectively deposit them in the vagina may result in male infertility. In up to 20% of couples, male and female causes may co-exist. However, in about 15% of couples, no specific cause may be identified.

Treatment is directed at the specific cause and generally involves drugs to bring about egg release (ovulation induction) or surgery to correct abnormalities of reproductive organs. In patients with blocked fallopian tubes, male infertility and unexplained infertility, 'test tube baby' treatment (*in vitro* fertilization or IVF) is recommended.

INFERTILITY:

Some herbs used in treatment

Ginseng
Noni juice (*Morinda citrifolia*)

Some herbs used to increase sperm count

Ashwagandha	Ginseng
Garlic	Liquorice
Ginger	Wild oats

DYSMENORRHOEA (PAINFUL MENSTRUATION OR PAIN WITH PERIODS)

Many women experience pain or discomfort at the time of their periods, but for most, the pain and unease is mild and does not interfere with daily life or require any special attention. However, for some women their monthly period is problematic and almost disabling because of the pain and inconvenience caused. They may have to take time off from school or work and stay at home for one or two days.

The natural pains are caused by contractions of the musculature of the uterus, stimulated by the release of the hormones (prostaglandins) which are produced by the lining of the uterus.

There are several causes of painful periods. These include emotional problems, muscular tension, stress and tiredness. Hormonal imbalances are also a cause. Painful periods are sometimes a sign of an underlying disease, but this is uncommon.

This condition often causes considerable distress and also fear and requires sympathetic evaluation and management. Often, relief is brought about by simple measures such as regular exercise and proper posture. Simple painkillers, in particular paracetamol or ibuprofen, naproxen or mefenamic acid, are often helpful. However, a varying range of therapeutic procedures (e.g. Mirena intra-uterine contraceptive device, vitamin B_1, transcutaneous electrical nerve stimulation) are available and need to be considered for each individual.

If the pains are not relieved by simple painkillers, a pelvic examination is necessary and this may have to be followed if indicated by an ultrasound scan or laparoscopy (where a small telescope is passed through a small cut in the wall of the abdomen allowing the pelvic organs to be viewed).

It is important to consider pelvic inflammatory disease, endometriosis or fibroids as a cause of dysmenorrhoea.

DYSMENORRHOEA (PAINFUL MENSTRUATION OR PAIN WITH PERIODS):

Some herbs used in treatment

Allspice
Angelica sinensis (Dong quai, Dong gui)
Black cohosh
Blessed thistle
Caraway
False unicorn root
Khella
Lady's mantle
Maidenhair fern
Marjoram
Mugwort
Oleander
Peach
Sage
Squaw vine
True unicorn root
Wild yam

ENDOMETRIOSIS

This is a condition where cells that normally line the womb (the endometrial cells) occur on other organs close to the uterus such as the ovaries and fallopian tubes and even the intestines. This results in bleeding into the abdominal cavity each month causing painful periods, scarring and infertility. Although the exact cause of endometriosis is unknown, it is thought that blood flowing backwards from the womb, down the fallopian tubes into the pelvis (retrograde menstrual flow), and changes in the immune system could play an important role. Endometriosis is a common cause of subfertility. There is also a risk of endometrial tissue becoming attached to adjacent structures or organs and causing obstruction within those organs.

No treatment is needed if the patient is asymptomatic. Medical treatment with birth control pills or hormonal injections can be given to encourage the tissue to stop growing. Patients with severe disease or those with fertility problems may require surgical treatment. This involves laparoscopy or open surgery to remove/destroy the tissue (laparotomy).

ENDOMETRIOSIS:

Some herbs used in treatment

Black cohosh
Chamomile
Cramp bark
Echinacea
Evening primrose oil
Ginger
Horsetail
Lavender
Liquorice
Marigold
Rose
Vervain
Wild yam
Yarrow

MENORRHAGIA (HEAVY PERIODS)

Menorrhagia or heavy periods are usually caused by hormonal imbalances or stress. However, some pathological changes in the uterus such as fibroids and endometriosis also cause menorrhagia. In some instances the insertion of a contraceptive device – the intrauterine coil – also causes menorrhagia. Other causes of menorrhagia include polycystic ovarian syndrome, uterine polyps, endometrial cancer and bleeding disorders including Von Willebrand's disease.

A detailed history and examination are necessary to find a cause, as prolonged blood loss can lead to anaemia, weakness and tiredness.

MENORRHAGIA (HEAVY PERIODS):

Some herbs used in treatment

Agnus castus	Lime flower
American cranesbill	Marigold
Beth root	Milk thistle
Bilberry	Nettle
Black cohosh	Plantain
Cinnamon	Rose
Dandelion	Wild yam
Hawthorn	Yarrow

MENOPAUSE

Menopause is the cessation of periods that occurs when the ovaries stop producing eggs and female hormones (oestrogens). It usually occurs between 49 and 51 years, although it sometimes occurs later. About 1% of women experience premature menopause before the age of 40. Genetic and environmental (drugs, chemicals, irradiation, chemotherapy, toxins and infections) are implicated in premature menopause. Removal of the womb (hysterectomy) or both ovaries (bilateral oophorectomy) causes 'surgical menopause'.

Symptoms of menopause include hot flushes, night sweats, mood changes and vaginal dryness that may lead to sexual dysfunction or painful sex. Long-term effects of menopause include 'weak bones' that are liable to fracture with minimal trauma (osteoporosis), loss of memory and possible heart disease. Treatment includes the use of hormones (hormone replacement therapy or HRT) and medications like clonidine that may be useful in hot flushes.

MENOPAUSE:

Some herbs used in treatment

Alfalfa	Ragwort
Black cohosh	Red clover
Clary	Royal jelly
False unicorn root	Sage
Hops	Soy
Liquorice	Wild yam

PREMENSTRUAL SYNDROME (PMS)

Premenstrual syndrome (also referred to as premenstrual tension or PMT) refers to a group of physical, psychological and behavioural symptoms that occur in the latter half of the menstrual cycle. It is believed to affect about 90% of female population, but severity varies and only about 5% of women suffer from severe PMS.

Physical symptoms include bloatedness, abdominal pain, constipation, discomfort and breast tenderness. Depression, anxiety, irritability and aggressiveness are the common psychological/behavioural symptoms. There is some evidence to suggest that there may be an increased tendency towards violence and crime during the premenstrual phase.

The exact cause is still unknown and there are a variety of treatment options, none of which is universally effective. Hormones may be used to alter the menstrual cycle or to prevent ovulation (release of eggs). Antidepressants (e.g. fluoxetine, Prozac) have been used in women with psychological symptoms. Yoga, reflexology and behavioural therapy have been recommended if there are behavioural symptoms. Very rarely, if all the medical treatments fail and the PMS is severe and debilitating, removal of both ovaries may need to be carried out as the last resort.

PREMENSTRUAL SYNDROME (PMS):

Some herbs used in treatment

Agnus castus	Fennel
Angelica sinensis (Dong quai or Dang gui)	Lemon balm
	Meadowsweet
Black cohosh	Milk thistle
Burdock	Peppermint
Chamomile	Rosemary
Chaste tree	Scull cap
Cleavers	St John's wort
Dandelion	Vervain
Evening primrose oil	Wild yam

NERVOUS SYSTEM AND MENTAL FUNCTION

DEPRESSION

Many life situations (e.g. death of a dear friend or close relative, divorce) bring about a sense of hopelessness, helplessness and/or a feeling of guilt. These senses by and large cause sadness and on occasions anxiety and withdrawal from society along with a loss of interest in hobbies or pleasures that were present at an earlier stage of life. When such symptoms persist and affect day to day living or employment the term depression is used medically.

Depressive illness is a common disorder and considered by many to be a leading cause of disability, particularly in developed countries. It is also a major cause of suicide. Some statistics from the US have indicated that nearly 20 million people suffer from depression in the US at any given time and that women are more affected than men.

It is important to be aware that depression can affect young people in adolescence when low self-esteem, a self-critical attitude and having little control over life events can cause distress, particularly when there are no understanding adults or parents to whom they can go to seek help or advice.

The use of certain 'substances of abuse' can also lead to depression.

Depressive illness is a disorder that may cause physical and psychological effects, including loss of appetite and weight loss in some people, or overeating and obesity in others. Sufferers may also complain of diverse but relatively common symptoms such as headaches, chronic pain and digestive disorders. These patients require a patient and detailed consultation including history taking and complete medical examination. It is also necessary to exclude certain diseases such as decreased activity of the thyroid gland which can also cause these symptoms.

Depression which is caused by a medical condition is suggested by lack of family history of psychiatric illness, no previous history of psychiatric illness and the absence of a precipitating cause for depression.

The current view in allopathic medicine is that depression runs in families and is caused by a combination of genetic vulnerability and environmental factors. The physiological basis is uncertain but is possibly related to a disturbance in the chemical messengers (neurotransmitters) in the nervous system.

In allopathic medicine, depression in the absence of another medical disorder can be managed using psychological processes such as cognitive behavioural therapy or antidepressant drugs or a combination of these. It is mandatory to ensure the co-operation of the patient and of the family. It is essential to ensure that patients have unrestricted access to counselling and medical opinion, particularly at times of severe distress. Suicide threats or attempts should never be ignored.

DEPRESSION:

Some herbs used in treatment

Aloe	Liquorice
Ashwagandha	Mate
Basil	Mistletoe
Chamomile	Mugwort
Clary	Parsley
Ginseng	Rose
Hydrocotyle (Gotu kola)	Rosemary
	Scull cap
Hops	St John's wort
Lavender	Vervain
Lemon balm	Wild oats

ANXIETY

In stressful circumstances or when there is uncertainty, it is natural for people to experience anxiety. Anxiety is also a common response in the presence of danger. However, when anxiety is severe or persists for no obvious or hidden reason and interferes with the day to day life of an individual, preventing them from doing their jobs properly or enjoying normal social activities, it should be recognized as a mental disorder which needs medical attention.

Physiologically, stress or danger brings on what is commonly referred to as a 'fight or flight' response. This response is due to the brain sending down impulses or messages to a part of the nervous system called the sympathetic nervous system which pours out substances such as adrenaline to prepare the individual for what is considered an appropriate response. Sometimes this 'adrenaline rush' improves performance. However, when it is a continuous and disproportionate state it can cause harm and bring about symptoms such as a dry mouth, rapid heart rate (tachycardia), palpitations (awareness of a rapidly beating heart), hand tremor, shortness of breath, dizziness, stomach discomfort, insomnia and a need to pass urine frequently.

It is stated that in contrast to depressed patients who wake up early in the morning, anxious patients find it difficult to fall asleep.

Phobias, which are abnormal or excessive fears of particular objects or situations which leads to avoidance of them, produce similar symptoms. It is common in medical practice to encounter individuals who have a phobia for needles and injections, the sight of blood or even for the masks used to administer oxygen.

Panic attacks are episodic attacks of severe anxiety which are not restricted to any particular situation or circumstance, and thus different from phobias, and are usually unpredictable. Somatic symptoms are common such as pain in the chest, palpitations, breathlessness, dizziness and numbness or tingling sensations. The symptoms are in part due to involuntary over-breathing (hyperventilation) and patients often fear that they are suffering from a serious acute illness. Fortunately, panic attacks do not last for long periods and subjects often develop their own methods of dealing with such attacks or even shortening their duration.

Explanation and reassurance are the cornerstones in the management of anxiety states. It is necessary to allay fears associated with medical illness after careful and detailed medical examination and investigation.

Techniques used in allopathic medicine include desensitization (gradually increasing exposure over a period of time to bring about a degree of acceptance or tolerance-graded exposures) to feared situations, relaxation exercises and cognitive therapy for panic attacks. Benzodiazepines have been used successfully to manage anxiety states of short duration (e.g. less than four weeks). Beta adrenergic blockers such as propranolol are useful to minimize or prevent physical symptoms and it is not uncommon, even among professionals, to use beta-blockers before examinations or delivering a lecture. In some patients, antidepressants may also prove to be useful.

A necessary consideration is that prolonged anxiety and tension may predispose to disease states such as high blood pressure (hypertension), stomach ulcers, bowel disorders and skin diseases.

ANXIETY:

Some herbs used in treatment

Ashwagandha
Chamomile
Clary
Cola
Cowslip
Ginger with ginkgo biloba
Ginseng
Hops
Hydrocotyle (Gotu kola)
Hyssop
Kava kava
Lady's slipper
Lavender
Lemon balm
Lime flower
Mugwort
Passion flower
Scull cap
St John's wort
Thyme
Vervain
Wild oats
Wild yam

Some herbs to be avoided by patients with anxiety

Ephedra
Mate

FITS – EPILEPSY

Fits or seizures should be distinguished from fainting. Fainting is often preceded by a feeling of light-headedness, diminishing of vision and some ringing in the ears due to a transient loss of adequate blood supply to the brain. Causes include events that produce an excessive degree of emotional discomfort (e.g. intravenous injections), pooling of the blood in the legs due to prolonged standing in the heat, or some defect in the pumping of the heart (e.g. heart block) or outflow from the heart during exertion (e.g. heart valve disease).

Fits or seizures are usually associated with some unusual sensations prior to loss of consciousness (aura) and during the period of loss of consciousness the subject may become blue (cyanosed) and may have jerky movements (fits). Patients usually pass urine and bite their tongue, and their eyes roll upwards during the period of unconsciousness. Following the period of unconsciousness, there is some degree of confusion, loss of memory of the event (post-ictal amnesia) and the patient may suffer from a headache.

There are several factors that precipitate seizures or fits. Causes include alcohol withdrawal, sleep deprivation, misuse of recreational drugs, physical and mental exhaustion, infection or disturbances in fluid and electrolyte balance in the body. In children, high fever is a common cause of seizures (febrile convulsions). However, the commonest pathological cause of seizures is epilepsy (tendency to have recurrent seizures), which is a symptom of brain disease rather than a disease itself.

The life-time risk of having a single seizure is about 5%, while the prevalence of epilepsy in European countries is about 0.5%. However, the prevalence in developing countries is five times higher.

Types of epilepsy

1. Idiopathic epilepsies, which make up about 10% of all epilepsies. Onset is always in childhood or adolescence. There is no structural abnormality and there is often a substantial genetic predisposition. In around 80% of people who develop epilepsy in childhood or adolescence, seizures go into remission in adulthood.
2. Other causes of epilepsy include:
   - inborn errors of metabolism
   - diseases where there are abnormalities in storage of body constituents
   - brain injury during childbirth
   - certain infections of the brain (meningitis, post-infectious encephalopathy)
   - hydrocephaly
   - alcohol and amphetamine withdrawal
   - changes in the content of electrolytes (hypocalcaemia, hyponatraemia, hypomagnesaemia) and glucose (hypoglycaemia)
   - kidney and liver failure
   - drugs, e.g. penicillins, isoniazid, metronidazole, chloroquine, mefloquine, ciclosporin, lidocaine, disopyramide, phenothiazines,

tricyclic antidepressants and lithium, can trigger fits in people who are epileptic.

After a single seizure, allopathic medicine recommends investigation using a CT or MRI. Electroencephalography is carried out if more than one seizure has taken place, to identify the type of epilepsy and to guide treatment.

In allopathic medicine, drug treatment is initiated if more than one seizure has occurred. After complete control of seizures for 2–4 years, withdrawal of medication may be considered.

The nature and cause of seizures should be explained to patients and their relatives, and relatives or carers should be taught first aid management. Until good control of seizures has been established, work or recreation above ground level and handling of dangerous machinery should be avoided. Patients should only take baths when a relative is in the house; they should not lock the bathroom door and the bath should be shallow. Open fires should be avoided. Cycling should be discouraged until a subject has been free for six months of seizures. Recreations requiring prolonged proximity to water (e.g. swimming, fishing and boating) should always be in the company of someone else who is trained in first aid management of seizures. In some countries (e.g. the UK) driving restrictions operate and they should be adhered to.

FITS – EPILEPSY:

Some herbs used in treatment

Blue cohosh	Oleander
Carline thistle	

Some herbs to be avoided by patients with convulsive disorders

Apricot	Rosemary
Damiana	Sage

IMPAIRMENT OF MEMORY AND DEMENTIA

Gradual onset of memory impairment is a normal consequence of ageing. A decline in mental function during old age generally begins with loss of memory for recent events (short-term memory loss). Dementia is a serious impairment of memory accompanied by personality changes and a decline in intellectual ability, caused by degeneration of the brain tissue. Dementia may follow a decrease in blood supply to the brain or frequent interruptions to blood flow from recurrent small strokes (multi-infarct dementia). Alcohol abuse, decreased activity of the thyroid gland and other disease states (Pick's disease, Levy body disease) also cause dementia.

An estimated 20 million people or more, worldwide, are known to suffer from dementia.

In Alzheimer's disease, possibly the best known form of dementia, cells in some areas of the brain are destroyed and other cells become less responsive to the chemical messengers (neurotransmitters) in the brain.

The distressing feature for carers and relatives is that the patients are often unaware of their disability.

IMPAIRMENT OF MEMORY AND DEMENTIA:

Some herbs used in treatment

Ashwagandha	Rosemary
Bilberry	Sage
Ginkgo biloba	Thyme
Hydrocotyle (Gotu kola)	*Uncaria sinensis*
Lemon balm	Wild oats

MALE AND FEMALE SEXUAL DYSFUNCTION

ERECTILE DYSFUNCTION AND IMPOTENCE

Erectile dysfunction (ED) is a common condition with a significant deleterious effect on the quality of life. The prevalence rate of ED is about 20–45% and its incidence in Western countries has been estimated to be from 25 to 30 cases per 1000 person per year. Two-thirds of men with ED report some embarrassment when discussing this problem with a physician and less than 25% seek medical advice.

Risk factors for ED are ageing, diabetes, cardiovascular disorders, urogenital disorders (carcinoma of the prostate or post-prostatectomy), psychiatric disorders (anxiety) and any chronic diseases (e.g. multiple sclerosis). Smoking, alcohol excess, hormonal factors and some drugs (beta adrenergic blockers, thiazide diuretics) may be associated with ED. Modifications of risk factors must be initiated before the age of 50 to prevent ED occurrence.

As a symptom of endothelial dysfunction, ED may be considered a premonitory sign of coronary or peripheral vascular disease and diabetes.

Management consists of avoidance of excess amounts of alcohol, cessation of smoking, psychotherapy for psychological disorders, use of drugs (e.g. sildenafil), self-administration of intracavernosal injections, use of urethral gel and use of vacuum devices.

ERECTILE DYSFUNCTION AND IMPOTENCE:

Some herbs used in treatment

Angelica sinesis (Dong quai or Dong gui)	Muira puama
Ashwagandha	Oats
Cantuba (Brazil)	Scull cap
Cinnamon	Suma (ginseng panax)
Damiana	Tongkat Ali (Asian Viagra – Malaysia, Thailand, Indonesia)
Ginkgo biloba	*Tribulus terrestris*
Ginseng	Yohimbine
Horny goat weed	
Maca (Incas – Peru)	

FEMALE SEXUAL DYSFUNCTION

In women lack of sexual activity usually develops during the onset of menopause and may be earlier due to surgical removal of ovaries (surgical menopause).

Female sexual dysfunction is a complex problem with multiple overlapping aetiologies. Androgens play an important role in healthy female sexual function, especially in stimulating sexual interest and in maintaining desire. Symptoms of androgen insufficiency include absent or greatly diminished sexual motivation and/or desire (libido), persistent unexplainable fatigue or lack of energy, and a lack of sense of wellbeing.

There are a multitude of reasons why women can have low androgen levels with the most common reasons being age, removal of ovaries (oophorectomy) and the use of oral oestrogens.

Although there is no androgen preparation that has been specifically approved by the FDA for the treatment of women's sexual interest/desire disorder or for the treatment of androgen insufficiency in women, androgen therapy has been used as unapproved therapy for low libido and sexual dysfunction in women over 40 years old. Most clinical trials in postmenopausal women with loss of libido have demonstrated that the addition of testosterone to oestrogen significantly improved multiple facets of sexual functioning including libido and sexual desire, arousal, frequency and satisfaction. In controlled clinical trials, women receiving testosterone therapy for up to 2 years tolerated it well and did not have any serious side-effects. The results of these trials suggest that low-dose testosterone therapy is effective for the treatment of this condition in postmenopausal women who are adequately oestrogenized. Based on the evidence of current studies, it is reasonable to consider testosterone therapy for a symptomatic androgen-deficient woman with women's sexual interest and desire disorder.

Decreased sexual desire may be due to marital problems, guilt, depression, anxiety or lack of confidence and it is important to consider this when assessing patients and take appropriate measures to manage such disorders before embarking on any specific drug therapy.

FEMALE SEXUAL DYSFUNCTION:

Some herbs used in treatment

Agnus castus	Rose
Ashwagandha	Wild oats
Ginkgo biloba	Wild yam
Ginseng panax	

Few drops (2) oil of basil or ginger or cinnamon or rosemary in a teaspoon of sesame oil for massage.

EYE DISORDERS

CONJUNCTIVITIS

Conjunctivitis or 'pink eye' or 'red eye' is a common eye disease that is characterized by the inflammation of the conjunctival membrane that covers the white of the eye and the inner aspects of the eye lids. Patients experience pain, blurring of vision, burning sensation and a discharge, which is often 'sticky'. There may be increased sensitivity or intolerance to light (photophobia). The most common type of conjunctivitis is caused by viral infections which are very contagious.

CONJUNCTIVITIS:

Some herbs used in treatment

Topical – eye washes	Fennel
Aloe vera	Goldenseal
Calendula	Liquorice
Chamomile flowers	Lime flower
Chinese rhubarb	Marjoram
Coriander	Marigold
Elder	Nettle
Eyebright	Oregon grape root

GLAUCOMA

Glaucoma is a condition in which the volume of fluid (aqueous humour) inside the eye increases, resulting in increased pressure within the eye (intraocular pressure). This may damage the optic nerve, which transmits the signals from the eye to the brain, and result in reduced vision, and blindness in severe cases.

The increase in volume of aqueous humour is most commonly caused either by excessive production, or by blockage of the channels that allow fluid to drain out of the eye.

Medications that are commonly used (eye drops and tablets) act either by decreasing the production of aqueous humour or by opening drainage channels.

GLAUCOMA:

Some herbs used in treatment

Aloe	Puerarin
Ginkgo biloba	Areca seed
Plantago	

Some herbs to be avoided by patients with glaucoma

Bloodroot	Ephedra

DIABETIC RETINOPATHY

This is a complication of diabetes mellitus, a condition characterized by excessive blood sugar due to absolute or relative deficiency of a hormone called insulin. Blood vessels in the retina (the light-sensitive cells at the back of the eye) become damaged leading to leakage of fluid and bleeding in and around the retina. As the disease progresses, scarring secondary to bleeding may pull the retina forward resulting in detachment of the retina. This can cause partial or total loss of vision.

Good control of blood sugar by regular exercise, diet and drugs that improve the sensitivity of the body to the hormone insulin are the mainstay of treatment. In severe cases, insulin injection and laser treatment to the areas of diseased retina may be required.

DIABETIC RETINOPATHY:

Some herbs used in treatment

Ginkgo biloba   Bilberry

EAR, NOSE AND THROAT DISORDERS

EARACHE AND EAR INFECTIONS

The ear, nose and throat are closely connected in the human body and earache may follow throat infections, infections of the nose or infections within the ear itself.

This is one of the commonest causes of ill-health in children and must be taken seriously and treated quickly and effectively because hearing may be impaired if the infection is not treated adequately. Hearing loss affects children's capacity to learn and may also affect their speaking. Ear infections may spread to adjacent areas in the head and have the potential to cause serious and long-standing ill-health.

The ear functionally has three parts: the outer ear, middle ear and inner ear. The outer ear or ear lobe collects sound and is separated from the middle ear by a membrane. In the middle ear, on the inside of the membrane are the tiny bones which transmit the sound to the inner ear, where mechanical vibrations are converted to electrical impulses which are sent to the brain. The chamber of the middle ear is connected to the nose by a small tube (the eustachian tube) through which fluid may pass into or out of the middle ear.

The middle ear is the part of the ear that most often gets infected. One or both of the Eustachian tubes may be blocked as a result of a cold or sore throat and as a result infected fluid builds up in the middle ear. The fluid thickens and presses against the membrane which separates the middle ear from the outer ear, causing extreme pain. The membrane may bulge and some times this membrane or the ear drum ruptures and pus drains out of the ear.

Infection of this middle chamber is referred to as otitis media. Otitis media may also occur and recur due to chronically infected adenoids and tonsils.

Small children often cannot specifically state that their ears are aching, but ear infection should be suspected when a small child repeatedly starts pulling or scratching the ear, develops fever, vomiting, cries excessively and is irritable. There may also be some evidence of hearing loss and a discharge from the ear. Older children may show some disturbance of balance or even complain of being dizzy.

In allopathic medicine it is essential to examine the ear and inspect the nose and throat, and to treat the infection promptly and aggressively because delays in diagnosis or treatment could interfere with the development of the child. Nasal decongestants may help to open up the blocked Eustachian tube. Sometimes it is necessary to make an opening in the ear drum and insert a small tube to facilitate drainage of infected fluid or pus.

Outer ear infections are often due to fungi and require appropriate antifungal treatment.

EARACHE AND EAR INFECTIONS:

Some herbs used in treatment

Chamomile	Lemon balm
Cleavers	Liquorice
Echinacea	Passion flower
Elder	Plantain
Garlic	Rose
Goldenseal	Scull cap
Lavender	Thyme

Herbs for pain relief

Oil from lavender/German chamomile applied locally

CATARRH AND SINUSITIS

Sinuses are air-filled cavities in the skull situated around the nose in the cheeks and in the forehead, above the eyes (frontal sinuses). They are lined by cells which secrete mucus (the mucous membrane) and are connected to the cavity of the nose by narrow tubes. Catarrh is a condition in which the mucous membranes of the nose and sinuses secrete excess mucus due to an infection or allergy. The condition is most often viral in origin. Secretions caused by an allergy decrease when exposure to the allergic agent stops.

If the membrane lining the sinuses becomes inflamed and swollen the condition is known as sinusitis. The swelling blocks the narrow tubes leading from the sinuses to the nose causing a build up of mucus. The symptoms are discomfort, headache, nasal stuffiness and pain around the sinuses.

Both catarrh and sinusitis may occur in a chronic form.

Allopathic medicine recommends the use of substances to relieve nasal congestion (nasal decongestants) and drugs to counteract the effects of histamine released following exposure to allergic agents (antihistamines). Infection of the mucous membrane likely to be due to bacteria should be treated with antibiotics.

When sinusitis tends to be recurrent and causes severe discomfort, it may be necessary to surgically drain the sinuses. Such procedures are carried out after proper investigations such as X-rays of the sinuses.

CATARRH AND SINUSITIS:

Some herbs used in treatment

Barberry	Goldenrod
Cayenne pepper	Goldenseal
Chamomile teas	Lime flower teas
Cinnamon	Liquorice
Coriander	Marigold
Echinacea	Marshmallow
Elder flower	Peppermint
Ephedra	Plantain
Euphorbia	Rose
Eyebright	Thyme
Garlic	Yarrow
Ginger	

TINNITUS

People with tinnitus hear noises/sounds such as ringing, buzzing, whistling or hissing, which are not produced by an external source. These sounds may be heard continuously or intermittently, in one ear or both ears. They are often distressing or disturbing, and sometimes the noises make it difficult to concentrate or to sleep, and may disrupt normal life. Stress, depression or anxiety often makes tinnitus more distressing.

Tinnitus is a symptom and not a disease.

It is estimated that tinnitus may be experienced by one in five individuals at some time of their life. It is commonly associated with the loss of hearing that occurs during the ageing process (presbyacusis). In most instances the causes are benign, but often the cause is unknown. In younger people it is often associated with persistent exposure to loud noises as from machinery (e.g. operators of pneumatic drills) and stereophonic sound systems (as with disc jockeys).

Very common causes of tinnitus include wax in the ear, infection of the middle ear and Meniere's disease, when it is associated with vertigo, dizziness, loss of hearing and nausea. Less common causes include hypertensive heart disease (high blood pressure); anaemia; systemic lupus erythematosus; allopathic medications such as aspirin, quinine and antibiotics such as streptomycin and other aminoglycosides; poisoning by some metals; disorders of the thyroid gland; and alcohol abuse. Benign tumours of the nerve that conducts hearing impulses to the brain (acoustic neuroma) would cause tinnitus in the ear on the side affected. Problems affecting the joint between the jaw and the skull, (the tempero-mandibular joint) could also cause tinnitus.

Management should include hearing tests. Unobtrusive devices called tinnitus maskers can be fitted into the ear. Therapy from a psychologist (cognitive behavioural therapy) may also help.

TINNITUS:

Some herbs used in treatment

Ashwaghanda	Hops
Black cohosh	Hydrocotyle (Gotu kola)
Chamomile	Lavender
Garlic	Passion flower
Ginkgo biloba	Scull cap
Hawthorn	Vervain

A herb to be avoided by patients with tinnitus

Uva ursi (bearberry)

TIREDNESS ALL THE TIME (TATT)

It is not unusual for nearly every individual to feel tired at some point of time of the day, week or month when the duties or chores to be performed bring about a sense of fatigue along with frustration, annoyance or despair. Feeling tired all the time is a common complaint that has its own acronym, TATT.

However, when tiredness is of such a degree and extent that it interferes with day to day life, there is a need to seek help from a medical practitioner to rule out some of the common medical causes of excessive tiredness such as:

- Anaemia
- Glandular fever
- Diabetes mellitus
- Thyroid disease
- Malignant disease – cancers.

Tiredness is common during menopause and also may occur for variable periods after viral infections such as flu.

In most instances tiredness may be due to individuals being very busy and stressed. Other factors are depression, boredom, poor sleep habits or poor eating habits.

In allopathic medicine, this wide ranging condition may require treatment to suit the individual when a medical cause has been conclusively eliminated.

Chinese medical practitioners consider tiredness to be due to a defect in the digestive system ('depleted of energy').

Allopathic medicine offers specific treatments for the detected medical disorder or as in most instances – i.e. nearly 95% of cases of TATT – dietary advice, relaxation techniques, exercise regimens and even psychotherapy.

TIREDNESS ALL THE TIME (TATT):

Some herbs used in treatment

Angelica	Oats
Black cohosh	Sage
Ginseng panax (Korean ginseng)	Siberian ginseng
	Wild yam

REFERENCES

1. McCrae CM, Ward SM, Paling CA, Fisher DA, Flynn PJ, McLaughlin JL. Development of a pawpaw herbal shampoo for the removal of head lice. *Phytomedicine* 2002;9:743–748.
2. Boon NA, Chilvers E, Colledge N et al. (Eds). *Davidson's Principles and Practice of Medicine*, 20th edn. Edinburgh: Elsevier Churchill-Livingstone, 2006.
3. Avenell A, Sattar N, Lean M. ABC of obesity. Management: Part I. Behaviour change, diet, and activity. *British Medical Journal* 2006: 333: 740–743.
4. Health notes. www.healthnotes.com. Healthnotes Inc, 2004.

BIBLIOGRAPHY

General

Eagles S. *Medicinal herbs and their uses*. www.richters.com/newdisplay.cgi-QandAMedicinal/Medicinal.html

Kong FY, Ng DK, Chan CH, Yu WL, Chan D, Kwok KL, Chow PY. Parental use of the term 'Hot Qi' to describe symptoms in their children in Hong Kong: a cross sectional survey 'Hot Qi' in children. *Journal of Ethnobiology and Ethnomedicine* 2006;2:2.

McIntyre A. *The top 100 Herbal Remedies*. London: Duncan Baird Publishers, 2006.

Zaffani S, Cuzzolin L, Benoni G. Herbal products: behaviours and beliefs among Italian women. *Pharmacoepidemiology and Drug Safety* 2006;15:354–359.

Cancer

Girgis A, Adams J, Sibbritt D. The use of complementary and alternative therapies by patients with cancer. *Oncological Research* 2005;15:281–289.

Hemalswarya S, Doble M. Potential synergism of natural products in the treatment of cancer. *Phytotherapy Research* 2006:20:239–249.

Meijerman I, Beijnen JH, Schellens JH. Herb–drug interactions in oncology: focus on mechanisms of induction. *Oncologist* 2006:11:742–752.

Mortel D, Bussieraes JF, Theoret Y, Lebel D, Kish S, Moghrabi A, Laurier C. Use of alternative and complementary therapies in children with cancer. *Paediatric Blood Cancer* 2005:44:660–668.

Dysmenorrhoea

BUPA's Health Information Team. Painful periods. June 2003. http://hcd2.bupa.co.uk/fact_sheets/html/Dysmenorrhoea.html

Owen P. Painful menstruation (dysmenorrhoea). http://www.netdoctor.co.uk/health_advice/facts/menstruationpainful.htm.

Malaria

Obeke TA, Okafor HU, Uzochukwu BS. Traditional healers in Nigeria: perception of cause, treatment and referral practices for severe malaria. *Journal of Biosocial Science* 2006;38:491–500.

Sickle cell disease

Sibinga EM, Shindell DL, Casella JF, Duggan AK, Wilson MH. Paediatric patients with sickle cell disease: use of complementary and alternative therapies. *Journal of Alternative and Complementary Medicine* 2006;12:291–298.

2

Commonly Used Herbs

Uses and Effects

This chapter brings together information about the uses, probable modes of action, adverse effects and known precautions for many commonly used herbs. The literature available to us on herbal medicines uses terminology which is quite distinct from that used in Western (allopathic) medicine. For consistency we have described disease states and other aspects using the terminology employed in traditional medicine texts although these may not be very familiar to allopathic clinicians. In most of the texts we have referred to, indications for use appear contradictory from the point of view of allopathic medical practice; for example, some herbs are described as both increasing and decreasing function or activity of organs or biological systems.

As regards constituents, evidence of pharmacological activity has been obtained mainly from in vitro ('test tube') laboratory experiments, using a series of in vitro models and there is no evidence that these would have the same activity and effect in humans. Some information on the effects of herbal medicines can be derived from studies of allopathic medicines containing the same, or chemically similar, active constituents. For example, the effectiveness of herbal medicines containing salicylic acid for specific disease states or symptoms could be deduced from the effect of salicylates in allopathic products. However, in the majority of cases the information available to us at present does not enable us to attribute the activities of herbal medicines to the specific herbal constituents. Further, the manner in which the herbal constituents are metabolized or handled by the human body may be different from their very similar allopathic counterparts.

We have followed the European tradition of referring to medicinal plants by the common name. However, this is not the most accurate system of identification as a common name can refer to several different plants so errors can occur.

The Latin binomial is more precise, and it is used here to aid identification; however, these are the accepted names from the current herbal medicinal literature, and have not been scientifically verified.

This chapter provides an overview and you are advised to refer to detailed texts on herbs and herbal products for further and possibly more specific information.

Commission E monographs were produced in Germany. They are reviews of safety and efficacy and were intended for use as package inserts in herbal medicines sold in Germany.

herbs

CONTENTS

ABSCESS ROOT

Polemonium reptans

The name polemonium is from a Greek word for war. Rarely used in herbal medicine at present.

Medicinal part: Dried root.

Uses: Fevers and inflammatory disorders.

Probable mode of action: Among the constituents are triterpene saponins. The herb is stated to contract cells (skin and other) following inflammation (astringent), induce perspiration (diaphoretic) and promote removal of secretions from the lung and upper airways (expectorant).

Adverse effects: No health hazards or side-effects are associated with the proper administration of recommended therapeutic dosages.

Precautions: None documented.

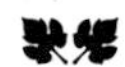

ACACIA – GUM ARABIC TREE OF INDIA

Acacia arabica

True gum Arabic is the product of *Acacia senegal*. The bark of *Acacia arabica* under the name of babul or babool is used in Scinda for tanning. In Ayurveda, babul is considered as a remedy for premature ejaculation.

The *Acacia* species is a spiritual icon and a symbol in freemasonry representing the eternal soul and the purity of the soul.

Medicinal parts: Bark, gum and fruit.

Uses: As a decoction for gum disease and inflammation of the mucous membranes of the mouth and throat.

Other uses: In Indian medicine, acacia is used as a decoction for treating diarrhoea, as an enema for haemorrhoids and also for vaginal secretions.

Probable mode of action: The constituents have been shown to contract cells (skin and other) following inflammation (astringent effect) and have antibacterial (antimicrobial) properties.

Adverse effects: Large doses taken internally may cause indigestion and constipation.

Precautions: None documented.

ADAM'S NEEDLE

Yucca filamentosa

The Catawba, Cherokee, Nanticoke and other native American tribes used *Yucca filamentosa* for food, medicine and even as a soap. The roots were used to treat gonorrhoea and rheumatism. The plant was used as a sedative to induce sleep. The leaves contain the strongest fibres native to North America and were used to make ropes, cloth, baskets and mats. It has also been used as a ceremonial medicine.

Medicinal parts: Leaves and roots of non-flowering plants.

Uses: Liver and gallbladder disorders.

Other uses: A poultice made from the roots was used in the treatment of sores, skin disorders and sprains.

Probable mode of action: Among the constituents are steroid saponins from the roots. The specific effects of the constituents are not known with certainty.

Adverse effects: No adverse effects have been reported following the use of recommended doses. But, rarely, injudicious intake can lead to stomach complaints because of the saponin content.

Precautions: None documented.

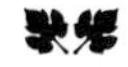

ADONIS – YELLOW PHEASANT'S EYE

Adonis vernalis

According to Greek legend, Adonis the beautiful youth was killed by a wild boar and the yellow flowers are supposed to have sprung up from his blood.

Approved by Commission E for:

- arrhythmia
- nervous heart complaints.

Medicinal parts: Roots and whole plants.

Uses: Mild impairment of heart function, especially when accompanied by nervous symptoms.

Other uses: In Russian folk medicine, the herb is used for dehydration, cramps, fever and menstrual disorders. For calming and diuretic effects.

Probable mode of action: The constituents include glycosides that act on the heart (cardiac glycosides) and coumarins and flavonoids. Acts in a manner similar to but not as effective as digitalis, but said to act faster. Animal tests have demonstrated that the constituents produce an increase in tone of the veins. Toxicity is attributed to the adonitoxin component.

Adverse effects: Despite the strong efficacy of the herb's glycosides that act on the heart, serious poisoning is unlikely following oral administration as the absorption of the constituent from the intestine is poor.

Precautions: Co-administration of digitalis and adonis is contraindicated. Adonis has to be used cautiously when there is depletion of body potassium, e.g. as in patients with chronic diarrhoea or in patients taking diuretics that cause loss of potassium.

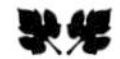

ADRUE – PIRI-PIRI

Cyperus articulatus

Piri-piri, as it is called by the Amazonian people, has a long history of use in herbal medicine systems in South America. It was a common remedy to treat nausea, vomiting, stomachaches and intestinal gas throughout the continent. In Peru, it is considered as an abortifacient, anticonvulsant, antivenin, carminative, contraceptive and haemostat. In Africa, piri-piri is used for malarial infections, toothache, headaches, diarrhoea, indigestion and coughs.

The indigenous Indian tribes of the Amazon ascribe magical properties to piri-piri. Women will cultivate the plant and bathe their children using it to prevent sickness and injury, and give it to their husbands to bring good luck in hunting and fishing.

Medicinal part: Root.

Uses: The root is used for digestive disorders (carminative), nausea, flatulence and as a sedative.

Other uses: In Chinese medicine, adrue is used for pre- and postnatal headaches, epigastric pain, vomiting with bleeding (haematemesis), blood in the urine (haematuria), white discharge from the vagina (leucorrhoea), menstrual irregularities, pain and tension in the breasts and amenorrhoea. Shipibo-Conibo Indians of the Peruvian Amazon ground up the fresh rhizome to extract the juice and use it as a nerve tonic for stress, mental disorders and epilepsy.

Used in the **West Indies** as an antiemetic.

Probable mode of action: The constituents include a volatile oil and alcohols which are reported to prevent vomiting (antiemetic) and to act as a carminative and as a sedative. Two constituents have been shown to possess activity in the laboratory against malarial parasites and also to inhibit, like aspirin and ibuprofen, prostaglandin synthetase.

Adverse effects: No health risks or side-effects have been recorded following the proper administration of recommended doses.

Precautions: None documented. Safety during pregnancy needs to be considered seriously as the herb has effects on menstruation.

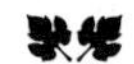

AFRICAN POTATO – *HYPOXIS HEMEROCALLIDEA* – MAGIC MUTHU

Hypoxis rooperi
Hypoxis colchicifolia
Hypoxis argentia

Has a long history of medicinal use on the African continent. The Sotho people use *Hypoxis* as a charm against lightening and storms. In times of famine, the roots of *Hypoxis argentia* are boiled or roasted by Sotho and Xhosa people as a source of food. Roots are used by Zulus for urinary tract infections, heart weakness, internal tumours and nervous disorders. *Hypoxis colchicifolia* is popularly used as herbal tea and tincture.

One of the two principal African herbal compounds used for HIV/AIDS treatment in sub-Saharan Africa, which has been recommended by the South African Ministry of Health for HIV management. The 14 member states of the South African Development Community (SADC), namely Angola,

Botswana, Democratic Republic of Congo, Lesotho, Malawi, Mauritius, Mozambique, Namibia, Seychelles, South Africa, Swaziland, Tanzania, Zambia and Zimbabwe, also support its use.

Medicinal part: Rhizome tuber.

Uses: For HIV infections and urinary tract infections. Also for weakness of the heart, internal tumours and nervous disorders.

Other uses: For prostatic hypertrophy, cancer and elevated blood sugar (hyperglycaemia). Used internally for urinary problems ranging from benign prostatic hyperplasia (benign enlargement of the prostate gland).

Used for bladder infections (cystitis) in **South Africa** and lung disease in **Botswana**.

Probable mode of action: Phytosterols are possibly the main ingredients; stated to have antioxidative effects in animal experiments. Hypoxoside is readily converted in the human gut to rooperol, the biologically active compound. The constituents appear to alert the immune system to produce more CD_4- or T-cells, lymphocytes which can destroy invading viruses like HIV. Also considered to slow viral replication rates in infected cells.

The beneficial effect of the herb on benign prostatic hyperplasia (reduction of the residual urine volume, improved flow of urine) is due to the ability of this constituent to inhibit an enzyme which is responsible for the hypertrophy of the prostate gland.

Sterols and sterolins found in the root have been found to have the potential to enhance immunity.

Adverse effects: There is evidence from one laboratory experiment (*in vitro* model) that the herb can interact with HIV drug-metabolizing enzymes. This could lead to drug resistance, drug toxicity and/or treatment failure. Other reported adverse effects are nausea, anxiety, vomiting, diarrhoea and suppression of the bone marrow. The rooperol constituent is believed to cause stimulation of the heart muscle due to its similarity to the chemical structure of substances like adrenaline (catecholamines).

Precautions: None documented. However, because of the potential to alter activity of drug metabolizing enzymes such as CYP3A4 in the liver and intestine, several drugs are likely to be affected to a degree to recommend avoidance of co-administration.

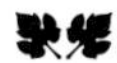

AGNUS CASTUS – CHASTE TREE

Vitex agnus-castus

Agnus castus is derived from the Greek word agnos (chaste) because the plant has been associated with chastity. Called agnos by the Greeks 2000 years ago, who considered the plant to calm sexual passion. Throughout Europe, the herb was used to relieve symptoms associated with female hormonal imbalances such as depression, cramps, mood swings, water retention and weight gain associated with the menstrual cycle.

Approved by Commission E for:

- premenstrual syndrome
- menopausal complaints.

Medicinal parts: Ripe dried fruit and the dried leaves.

Uses: For menstrual irregularity, premenstrual syndrome (e.g. breast swelling and tenderness, mood swings), menopausal symptoms. There are also claims of usefulness for inadequate lactation and acne.

Other uses: To control libido, reduce flatulence, suppress appetite and induce sleep. Other uses, mostly unproven, are to treat impotence, prostatitis, swelling of the testes, sterility, swelling of the ovaries. Chaste tree has also been used to induce menstruation. Pliny considered it effective for snake bites.

Probable mode of action: Constituents include flavonoids, glycosides and some that act like the male and female sex hormones. The sites of action of the constituents are considered to be the parts of the brain (pituitary and hypothalamus) responsible for releasing hormones or triggering hormonal responses in the reproductive system. It is likely that the constituents influence the balance between the two female sex hormones, oestrogen and progesterone, and have an effect on the hormonal levels in the production of ova by the ovaries (ovulation) and in supporting events in the luteal phase (after ovulation has taken place). Some believe that the herb increases the odds of pregnancy. Chaste tree constituents are considered by some workers to act like the chemical messenger dopamine (dopamine agonist).

Adverse effects: Headache, abdominal cramps and diarrhoea, increased menstrual flow, rashes and pruritus.

Precautions: Not recommended during pregnancy. Avoid if taking progesterone-containing drugs. Some workers have found the constituents to inhibit the secretion of the hormone which promotes milk production (prolactin), despite use for promoting milk production by some practitioners. Thus this issue is not resolved and it would be prudent to avoid this herb during lactation.

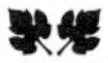

AGRIMONY

Agrimonia eupatoria

Agrimony is derived from agrimone, a word used by the Greeks for plants which were healing to the eyes. The Greeks used agrimony to treat eye problems. Agrimony is considered by some as a popular pre-event gargle for speakers and singers to soothe their throats. Anglo-Saxons referred to the herb as garclive and used the herb to treat wounds, snake bites and warts.

Approved by Commission E for:

- diarrhoea
- inflammation of the skin
- inflammation of the mouth and pharynx.

Medicinal part: The flowering plant, which is cut a few fingers' width above the ground and dried.

Uses: For mild non-specific diarrhoea, 'stasis' in the gallbladder and bile ducts (cholestasis), inflammation of the mouth and pharyngeal mucosa, inflammation of the kidney and bladder. Has a reputation for curing jaundice and liver complaints.

Other uses: Childhood bed wetting, diabetes. Topical application for poorly healing wounds, 'chronic pharyngitis', psoriasis and eczema. Hip baths for lower abdominal conditions. Used as a gargle and also as a tea, the former to relax the throat and the latter for looseness of bowels and for passive blood loss.

Probable mode of action: Agrimony is reported to contract cells (skin and other) following inflammation (astringent). The specific effects of the other constituents are not known precisely. The tannin content probably influences its use as a gargle and as an astringent application to indolent ulcers and wounds.

Adverse effects: Because of the constituent tannins, the intake of large quantities could lead to digestive complaints and constipation. Patients should be cautioned to avoid strong sunlight due to the possibility of photosensitivity (risk of photodermatitis).

Precautions: Contraindicated in patients with a history of hypersensitivity to plants of the rose family. Contraindicated in pregnancy and during lactation.

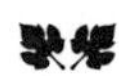

ALETRIS

Aletris farinosa

The Catawba people used a cold water infusion of aletris for stomachaches and as a remedy for snake bite. A bitter tonic and digestive aid and a uterine 'tonic'. Until the 19th century, the roots were collected and used medicinally to treat colic.

The commercial drug under this name found in markets may be the rhizome of *Chamaelirium* which is used primarily for abnormal conditions of the female reproductive organs.

Medicinal parts: Dried rhizome with roots. Leaves.

Uses: To induce vomiting (as an emetic) and as a cathartic. Mainly to treat disorders of the stomach, to increase motility and for loss of appetite, dyspepsia, flatulence and nervous digestive complaints. Also used as a tonic.

Other uses: In the US, the plant is used for gynaecological disorders or 'female complaints' particularly dysmenorrhoea, amenorrhoea and complaints associated with a prolapsed vagina.

Considered to be useful to treat habitual abortions. A tea from the leaves has been used to treat colic, stomach disorders and dysentery.

In **Argentina** it is used to treat chronic bronchitis.

Probable mode of action: Constituents include saponins, volatile oil, resins and starch, which are known to increase motility of the stomach. Some work suggests the presence of the female hormone (oestrogen) activity but this has not been confirmed. The root contains diosgenin which is considered to possess anti-inflammatory activity. In addition, though contentious, the root may have oestrogen-like activity.

Adverse effects: Small doses of the fresh root can cause abdominal discomfort (hypogastric). In overdose, colic, diarrhoea and vomiting could occur.

Precautions: As the herb is used to treat amenorrhoea, its use during pregnancy is not recommended. The fresh root is mildly poisonous.

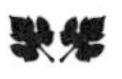

ALFALFA – BUFFALO HERB

Medicago sativa

Alfalfa was probably first used by the Arabs who called it the 'king of kings' of plants and the 'father of all food'. They fed alfalfa to their horses claiming it made the animals swift and strong. Widely used food crop for animals and humans in Southeast Asia.

Medicinal parts: Whole flowering plant or the germinating seeds.

Uses: For asthma, diabetes, gastrointestinal disorders (anti-ulcer), arthritis, to promote urination (diuretic).

Other uses: For allergies, to lower cholesterol levels. Also used to stimulate lactation, and for menstrual disorders. **In folk medicine**, the herb is used in the treatment of diabetes and for diseases of the thyroid gland.

Probable mode of action: There are several constituents, among which are saponins which are considered to act on the cardiovascular system, nervous system and digestive system. The cholesterol lowering effects are also attributed to the saponins. Alfalfa plant saponins and fibre bind significant quantities of cholesterol in *in vitro* experiments.

Alkaloids found in the seed produce effects on menstruation (emmenagogue) and on lactation.

Another constituent, L-canavaine, has been shown in laboratory experiments (*in vitro*) to induce abnormalities in the blood characteristic of SLE (systemic lupus erythematosus) in monkeys.

Adverse effects: Decreased blood cell counts (pancytopenia) have been caused following the ingestion of large amounts of ground alfalfa seeds. Alfalfa may cause increased faecal volume and promotes defaecation, which can cause frequent loose stools, diarrhoea, abdominal discomfort and increased production of gas in the intestine. Alfalfa seeds and sprouts can be contaminated with such pathogens as *Salmonella enterica* and *Escherichia coli*. The latter can lead to haemolytic uraemic syndrome with kidney failure particularly in children or in the elderly. High doses have caused pancytopaenia and lupus-like conditions.

Precautions: The FDA has issued an advisory indicating that children, the elderly and people with compromised immune systems should avoid eating alfalfa sprouts because of frequent bacterial contamination. Avoid during pregnancy and lactation. Patients with latent systemic lupus erythematosus have had relapses after the ingestion of alfalfa tablets. Avoid in patients with hormone sensitive cancer. Because of the content of purines, avoid in patients with gout. May cause uterine stimulation, so should be avoided during pregnancy. May antagonize the anticoagulant effect of warfarin due to the vitamin K content and may also interfere with the immunosuppressant effect of corticosteroids.

ALFAVACA – AMAZONIAN BASIL

Ocimum micranthum

Ocimum species were introduced to Brazil through Portuguese colonizers and other European immigrants. The plant has a long tradition of use in Brazil (to reduce fevers, as a diuretic, to treat intestinal disturbances), in Puerto Rico (as a carminative) and in Central and South America and the West Indies (to treat colds, bronchitis, eye infections, fevers). Has also been used to treat epilepsy, nervous symptoms and earache.

Medicinal part: Leaves.

Uses: An infusion of basil leaves is recommended for the urinary system for the treatment of kidney and bladder diseases, for the female reproductive system to relieve period pains and for the nervous system to help dizziness and the acute pains of neuritis.

Other uses: Basil leaves have been recommended in the treatment of cardiovascular diseases (hypertension, chest tightness and palpitations), chest diseases (shortness of breath), nutritional disorders (asthenia, anaemia, vitamin deficiencies), neurological and neuropsychiatric conditions (migraine, irritability, nervousness, hysteria, anxiety, depression and insomnia), skin diseases (hair loss, cracked feet, hands and nipples) and many other non-specific conditions such as cystitis, joint pains, cramps and sprains.

Traditionally used in **Bolivia** for the treatment of headaches.

Probable mode of action: Constituents include terpenes and essential oils which contain eugenol. Reviews have suggested pain relieving activity (analgesic properties), anticonvulsant activity, antispasmodic and antifungal activity. The precise effects of each of the constituents are not known with any certainty. The aromatic alcohols are considered to be effective against organisms such as *Escherichia coli* and *Pseudomonas aeruginosa.*

Adverse effects: Avoid in patients who may be hypersensitive to the constituents.

Precautions: Ethnopharmacological data document the use of the plant as an emmenagogue in Brazil, Piaui and Mevanhao. Best avoided during pregnancy. May enhance the action of diuretics.

ALISMA – ZE-XIE

Alisma plantago-aquatica

Alisma is the Latin name for water plantain and the ancient Greek name adopted by Linnaeus from Dioscorides.

Medicinal part: Fresh rhizome.

Uses: Diseases of the bladder (e.g. cystitis – inflammation of the bladder) and of the urinary tract. Used to treat kidney stones.

Other uses: In Chinese medicine, the herb is used in herbal formulae to lower blood sugar, blood pressure and blood cholesterol levels and as a diuretic. Has been used in the treatment of leprosy. Also has been applied topically to bruises and swellings.

Probable mode of action: Fresh leaf is a rubefacient. The root is rich in starch. The leaves are also considered to be antibacterial, anticholesterolaemic (lower blood cholesterol levels), diaphoretic, diuretic, hypoglycaemic (lower blood sugar) and hypotensive (lower blood pressure).

Adverse effects: No health hazards or side-effects are known to be associated with the proper administration of recommended therapeutic dosages.

Precautions: The fresh leaves and roots are toxic but the toxic principle is destroyed by heat or by drying. The seed is said to promote sterility. By contrast, there are suggestions that the whole plant may promote conception.

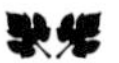

ALKANET

Alkanna tinctoria

Has been used as a dye. First reported use is by Theophrastus (300 BC), and around 77 AD Dioscorides described its properties in greater detail.

Used by the ancient Greeks to heal wounds.

Medicinal parts: Root (dried roots and rhizome).

Uses: Used externally to treat cuts, bruises and phlebitis (inflammation of the veins). Used internally to treat cough and bronchial catarrh, and in the treatment of skin wounds and diarrhoea.

Probable mode of action: All parts of the plant are demulcent and expectorant. Constituents have been attributed with effects against bacteria and other organisms (antimicrobial activity).

Adverse effects: Hepatotoxicity (liver toxicity) and carcinogenicity (ability to cause cancers) are expected, due to the pyrrolizidine alkaloids and other hepatotoxic constituents. The plant may have irritant properties from its rough hairs.

Precautions: Alkanet should not be taken internally for this reason and is recommended for external use only.

ALMOND

Prunus amygdalus dulcis
Prunus dulcis var amara

Before the cultivation and domestication of almonds occurred, wild almonds were harvested as food and were processed by leaching or roasting to rid them of toxicity. Domesticated almonds appear in the Early Bronze Age (3000–2000 BC). The fruits found in the tomb of Tutankhaman in Egypt (1325 BC) were probably imported from Levant.

There are two forms of the plant. One, often with white flowers, produces sweet almonds and the other, often with pink flowers, produces bitter almonds.

The almond is referred to in the Bible as *Shaqued* meaning hasten. It was a symbol of watchfulness and promise among the Hebrew Christians.

Medicinal part: Ripe fruit.

Uses: Bitter almonds were used in the past as a remedy for coughs, vomiting and nausea, taken as a bitter almond water. Bitter almonds are rarely used at present. Sweet almonds have an effect to relieve inflammation and irritation (demulcent effect) and have been used for skin care and as liniments. The fatty oil is used as an ointment base.

Probable mode of action: Constituents include mucilages (in bitter and sweet almonds) and fatty oils.

Adverse effects: There is no reliable information available.

Precautions: There is no reliable information available.

ALOE VERA

Aloe vera
Aloe barbadensis

Drawings of aloe have been found in the wall carvings of Egyptian temples erected in the fourth millennium BC. Called the 'plant of immortality' it was a traditional funerary gift for the Pharaohs. The Egyptian Book of Remedies (ca. 1500 BC) notes the use of aloe in curing infections, treating the skin and preparing drugs to be used as laxatives. The Bible (John 19:39–40) says that Nicodemus brought a mixture of myrrh and aloes for the preparation of Christ's body. Alexander is said to have conquered the island of Socotra to obtain control of aloe. The Greek physician Dioscorides in 74 AD recorded the use of aloe to heal wounds, stop hair loss, treat genital ulcers and eliminate haemorrhoids.

Approved by Commission E for:

- constipation.

Medicinal part: Dried juice of the leaves.

Uses: To build resistance against infections and to promote healing of minor burns and wounds; as a laxative, and for treatment of inflammatory bowel disease (ulcerative colitis).

Other uses: Promotes healing of skin affected by diseases such as psoriasis, seborrheic dermatitis and genital herpes in men. Also used for arthritis, chronic fatigue syndrome, diabetes, hair loss and as an abortifacient. The drug is used to facilitate painless or comfortable defaecation in the presence of anal fissures and after operations on the rectum and anus.

In European folk medicine, the herb is used for its ability to influence digestion.

In Chinese medicine, the most common use is for fungal diseases.

In Indian medicine, the herb is used for stomach tumours, constipation, colic, skin diseases, amenorrhoea, worm infestations and infections.

Probable mode of action: One of the constituents, the anthraquinones, exerts a laxative effect due to osmosis (promoting active movement of electrolytes and water into the lumen of the bowel). Absorption of electrolytes and water from the colon is also inhibited resulting in an increase in volume of the intestinal contents. This leads to an increase in pressure within the lumen of the bowel which stimulates intestinal peristalsis. There is some evidence to suggest that nitric oxide has a role in the diarrhoeal effect which usually takes place about 9 hours after ingestion.

Aloe vera depresses nerve activity at the neuromuscular junction (i.e. generation of electrical activity to cause contraction of muscle fibres). Also known to have pain relieving (analgesic) and anti-inflammatory effects. Aloe vera gel has been shown to contain substances that prevent ultraviolet light-induced skin changes. One of the major areas of studies associated with aloe is the effects on the skin.

Aloe vera also promotes healing of wounds. However, some workers have found that the use of Aloe vera has been associated with a delay in wound healing compared to standard treatment.

Animal and laboratory studies have shown that aloe taken by mouth may lower blood sugar and blood potassium levels.

Adverse effects: At recommended doses, aloe taken by mouth may cause cramping pain in the gastrointestinal tract and diarrhoea. If cramps occur after a single dose, the dose should be reduced. The laxative or purgative action may cause spasm of the gastrointestinal tract. Skin rashes have been reported with long-term use of aloe gel, particularly after long-term use or oral and topical preparations of aloe. Other adverse effects reported are blood in the stools and hepatitis. Rarer adverse effects are on heart rhythm, kidney damage and oedema. Prolonged use of aloe may lead to pigmentation in the intestinal mucosa (pseudomelanosis coli), a harmless side-effect, which usually reverses upon discontinuation of the herb. Long-term use can cause loss of electrolytes, in particular potassium. The loss of potassium may enhance the effect of drugs that act on the heart (e.g. digoxin).

Precautions: Except for the dried latex, aloe is not approved as an internal medication. People with allergies to aloe or plants in the Lilliaceae family (garlic, onions, tulip) should avoid use of aloe. Aloe should not be taken by patients with diarrhoea or if there is a possibility of intestinal obstruction. Subjects suffering from diabetes, kidney disease, heart disease or electrolyte abnormalities should only take aloe under supervision. Not recommended during pregnancy. Aloe leaves are best avoided during lactation. Bitter aloes should not be applied to the skin or be taken by mouth by patients suffering from kidney disease or haemorrhoids. Use of any laxative including aloe for more than seven consecutive days could make constipation worse or cause dependency. Should not be used by injection.

Aloe is contraindicated in children under the age of 12 years, in patients with inflammatory bowel disease and in elderly patients with suspected intestinal obstruction.

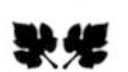

ALPINE RAGWORT – LIFE ROOT

Senecio nemorensis

Life root was used by the Catawba people in North America to treat gynaecological problems in general and to relieve labour pains in particular.

Dioscorides, along with Gerard and Culpeper, recommended ragwort to induce sweating and reduce fevers. It was also recommended for bile disorders (biliousness) and as a soothing agent for teething babies. Despite its historical background, the herb is not used frequently at present.

Medicinal part: Herb.

Uses: To treat urinary tract infections, gout, rheumatism and stone formation in the urinary tract. Also used to lower blood sugar.

Probable mode of action: The drug has effect against viruses (antiviral) and as a urinary disinfectant due to the tannin constituents. Reported to have hypoglycaemic (blood sugar lowering) properties. The flavonoid constituents have been reported to affect factors involved in inflammatory disease. Is being studied as a potential therapeutic agent to treat malignant disease.

Adverse effects: Avoid oral use as it contains pyrollizidine alkaloids, which may cause hepatotoxicity (liver poisoning) and carcinogenicity (cancers). Do not take excessive doses even for short periods of time.

Precautions: The herb is contraindicated in pregnancy and nursing and in children under the age of 12 years. Recommended only for external use and do not apply to broken skin.

AMARANTH

Amaranthus hypochondriacus

In ancient Greece, the amaranth was sacred and supposed to have special healing properties. As a symbol of immortality, the herb was used to decorate the images of gods and tombs.

Medicinal parts: The entire plant has been used.

Uses: Diarrhoea, ulcers and inflammation of mouth and throat.

Probable mode of action: The herb is considered to contract cells (skin and other) following inflammation (astringent effect), possibly due to constituents such as the saponins. There are no studies available on efficacy.

Adverse effects: No health hazards or side-effects are known to be associated with the proper administration of recommended therapeutic dosages.

Precautions: None documented.

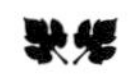

AMARGO

Quassia amara

Contains quassin, possibly the bitterest substance found in nature.

Medicinal parts: Wood of the trunk and branches.

Uses: Used in homeopathic medicine for gallbladder complaints, as a bitter tonic, purgative and antihelminthic (treatment of worm infestations).

Probable mode of action: Constituents have been shown to stimulate the secretion of gastric juice, increase appetite and aid digestion. May also increase production and flow of bile.

Adverse effects: Use of herbal extracts may cause dizziness, headaches and uterine pain. No health hazards or side-effects are known to be associated with use as a homeopathic remedy.

Precautions: Not to be used during pregnancy.

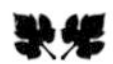

AMERICAN IVY

Parthenocissus quinquefolia

Native Americans used the plant to treat diarrhoea, difficulty in urination, swelling and lockjaw.

Medicinal parts: The bark, branch tips, fresh leaves, berries and resin.

Uses: For digestive disorders and as a tonic.

Probable mode of action: The plant induces perspiration (diaphoretic) and has an effect in contracting cells (skin and other) following inflammation (astringent).

Adverse effects: The berries contain oxalic acid and are considered poisonous. Older scientific literature describes the death of a child following intake of the berries. However no health hazards or side-effects are known to be associated with the proper administration of recommended therapeutic dosages.

Precautions: Do not use berries.

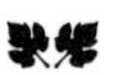

ANEMARRHENA – ZHI-MU

Anemarrhena asphodeloides

Used primarily in Traditional Chinese Medicine for fevers, inflammation, dehydration, diabetes and cough.

Medicinal part: Rhizome.

Uses: For agitation.

Other uses: In Chinese medicine, it is usually used as part of complex herbal formulae. Zhi-mu is used for febrile conditions and inflammation, diabetes, dry cough, 'bone fever' and general dehydration, and painful stools. Also used as a decoction for typhus, scarlet fever and tuberculosis.

Probable mode of action: Constituents include steroids, saponins, aglycones, water-soluble polysaccharides and many other chemical compounds. A variety of experiments have been able to demonstrate a fever lowering effect and an effect similar to the hormone from the adrenal cortex (cortisone) attributed to the steroid saponin content. In addition, it can interfere with clotting due to inhibition of platelet aggregation. Many other activities have been demonstrated in animal experiments.

Adverse effects: No health hazards are known to be associated with the proper administration of recommended therapeutic dosages.

Precautions: Not to be used in patients with diarrhoea. Safety during pregnancy is not known.

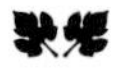

ANGELICA

Angelica archangelica

A Chinese herb with claims to be useful for many disorders. Considered to be 'cure-all' for gynaecological disorders. Its virtues are praised by old writers and folklore of all North European countries. From antiquity, it is considered to protect against contagion and as a blood purifying agent and possibly for every conceivable malady.

Angelica fruit is approved by Commission E for:

- fevers and colds

- infection of the urinary tract
- dyspeptic complaints
- loss of appetite.

Angelica root is approved by Commission E for:
- dyspeptic complaints
- loss of appetite.

Medicinal parts: Seed, whole herb and root.

Uses: Preparations of the seed are used internally for kidney and urinary tract disorders, intestinal and respiratory disorders, rheumatism and neuralgia. Preparations from the seed are also used to induce perspiration (diaphoretic) and have been used in the past for malaria. An ointment made from the seeds is used externally for body lice. The leaves have been used as diuretics.

Other uses: In folk medicine, the root was used to treat cough, bronchitis, menstrual complaints, loss of appetite, dyspepsia, liver and bile disorders.

Probable mode of action: Angelica leaves contain essential oils. Certain constituents are considered to stop cell division or growth (cytostatic) while others may increase photosensitivity (phototoxic). Other constituents are considered to reduce spasms (spasmolytic), stimulate the secretion of gastric juice and of bile.

Adverse effects: The essential oils and furanocoumarins from the leaves have a strong irritant effect on the skin and mucous membranes (angelica dermatitis). No health hazards or side-effects are known to be associated with the proper administration of recommended therapeutic dosages. Photodermatitis is possible following contact with the plant juice. The furocoumarins contained in angelica root sensitize the skin to light and can lead to inflammation of the skin in combination with ultraviolet (UV) rays. It is therefore advisable to avoid sunbathing and intensive UV radiation for the duration of treatment with angelica or its preparations.

Precautions: Preparations are not to be used during pregnancy.

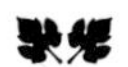

ANGELICA SINENSIS

Angelica sinensis

See Dang gui – Dong quai, page 135.

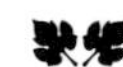

ANGOSTURA

Galipea officinalis

A Venezuelan shrubby tree acclaimed in folk medicine.

Medicinal part: Dried bark of the tree.

Uses: Used in **folk medicine** for diarrhoea; also used as a febrifuge.

Probable mode of action: Angostura stimulates gastric juices and acts as a tonic. In larger doses, angostura also has an emetic (causes vomiting) and strong laxative effect. Constituents have been studied for activity against malaria.

Adverse effects: The administration of large doses can lead to nausea and vomiting.

Precautions: None known.

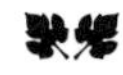

ANISE

Pimpinella anisum

Hindi (Indian) name: Saunf

Approved by Commission E for:
- common cold
- cough and bronchitis
- fevers and colds
- inflammation of the mouth and pharynx
- dyspepsia
- loss of appetite.

Medicinal parts: Essential oil from the ripe fruit and the dried fruit.

Uses: Used internally for stomach ailments (dyspepsia). Used both internally and externally for catarrh.

Other uses: In **folk medicine**, anise is used internally for whooping cough, flatulence, colic-like pains, as a digestive and for menstrual disorders, liver disease and tuberculosis.

Probable mode of action: Aniseed oil has been shown in animal experiments to have effects against bacteria, viruses (antibacterial, antiviral) and an insect repellent effect. Other animal experiments have shown the herb to promote removal of secretions from the lung and upper airways (expectorant), spasmolytic (relieve spasms) and female hormonal (oestrogenic) activities.

Adverse effects: Sensitization has been observed very rarely.

Precautions: Contraindicated in patients allergic to anise and anethol.

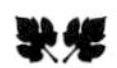

APRICOT

Prunus armeniaca

Apricot seeds were used to treat cancers in the 5th century. In the 17th century, apricot oil was used in England against tumours and ulcers.

Medicinal parts: Kernel.

Uses: During the late 1970s and early 1980s there was considerable interest in the possibility of a constituent being an effective treatment in cancer. However, continued research has not supported this probability.

Other uses: Traditionally the oil has been incorporated into cosmetics and perfumery products such as soaps and creams.

Probable mode of action: Amygdalin is a glycoside present in apricot. The exact effects of the constituents are not known with certainty.

Adverse effects: Laetrile and apricot kernel ingestion are the most common sources of cyanide poisoning. Cyanide is rapidly absorbed from the upper gastrointestinal tract and causes respiratory failure if untreated. Symptoms progress rapidly from dizziness, headache, nausea, vomiting and drowsiness to shortness of breath (dyspnoea), palpitations, marked fall in blood pressure (hypotension), convulsions, paralysis and death.

In chronic poisoning, blindness, disturbances in gait (ataxia) and mental retardation may occur along with disorders of thyroid gland function.

Precautions: Apricot kernels are toxic and should not be ingested. Laetrile-containing products are best avoided during pregnancy. Oral doses of 50 g of hydrogen cyanide (HCN) can be fatal. This is equivalent to approximately 30 g of kernels which represents about 50–60 kernels and approximately 2 mg HCN/g kernel.

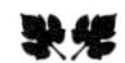

ARECA NUT – BETEL NUT

Areca catechu

First century Sanskrit medical writings claim 'betel possesses thirteen qualities to be found in the region of heaven. It is pungent, bitter, spicy, sweet, salty and contracts cells (skin and other) following inflammation (astringent). It expels wind, kills worms, removes phlegm, subdues bad odours, beautifies the mouth, induces purification and kindles passion'. There are only three drugs (caffeine, alcohol [ethanol] and nicotine) consumed more widely than betel. About 450 million people throughout the western Pacific basin, Southeast Asia, India and Indonesia chew betel nuts and leaves because of their intoxicating properties. Fresh slices of the nut are part of the 'betel titbit' in Eastern Asia.

Medicinal part: Nut.

Uses: Betel nut is no longer prescribed frequently in human medicine. It was used in the treatment of glaucoma and as a mild stimulant and digestive aid. There appears to be no appropriate medicinal use for betel nut.

In Chinese medicine, betel nut is used for chronic hepatitis, oedema, reduction in the passing of urine (oliguria), diarrhoea and digestive problems. **In Indian medicine**, the juice of young seeds is used as a laxative. A decoction of the root is used for cracked lips.

An oily extract of leaves containing phenolic active ingredients is claimed to be useful for respiratory symptoms and as a gargle for sore throats and cough.

Other uses: As a vermifuge (treatment of worm infestations) in horses and cattle.

Probable mode of action: The nuts contain at least nine structurally related alkaloids including some related to tobacco alkaloids such as nicotine. Betel nuts contain a tannin which inhibits a hormone secreted by the kidney in a manner similar to the allopathic medication captopril (angiotensin-converting enzyme [ACE]) which is associated with high blood pressure.

The constituent arecoline is a stimulant of the parasympathetic nervous system and stimulates the vagus nerve. It stimulates secretion in the salivary, bronchial and intestinal glands and causes tremors and bradycardia (slowing of the heart rate). Also found to produce euphoria. Arecaidine and arecoline are potentially carcinogenic. Arecoline is a veterinary antihelminthic (effective against worm infestations) and is also cathartic.

Adverse effects: Central nervous system stimulation, facial flushing, gingivitis, periodontitis, red staining of teeth and oral cavity, and resorption of gums. Long-term use of betel nut can result in malignant tumours of the oral cavity through the formation of nitrosamines. In a review of 17 cases reported to the Taiwan Poison Centre, tachycardia, tachypnoea/dyspnoea, sweating and a fall in blood pressure were the common adverse effects. Vomiting, dizziness, chest discomfort, abdominal colic and coma were also reported. There was one fatality; the patient developed an acute myocardial infarction ventricular fibrillation and died despite repeated cardiac defibrillation.

Precautions: Betel nut is contraindicated in patients with known hypersensitivity reactions to any of its components and is best avoided by subjects in whom there is a likelihood of overactivity of the parasympathetic nervous system/vagus nerve, i.e. subjects with slow pulse rates. Chronic betel chewing may increase a person's risk of certain oral cancers. Use during pregnancy is contraindicated.

ARENARIA RUBRA

Spergularia rubra

Medicinal part: Herb.

Uses: The herb is used for conditions of the urinary tract such as bladder infections (cystitis), painful urination (dysuria) or urinary calculi. Also has a diuretic effect.

Probable mode of action: Active ingredients – the resins probably act as a diuretic.

Adverse effects: No health hazards or side-effects are known to be associated with the proper administration of recommended therapeutic doses.

Precautions: None available.

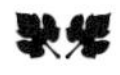

ARJUN TREE

Terminalia arjuna

Indian name: Kahu

Has been associated with Svati, a star of the zodiac. The early Sanskrit literature refers to the tree as Nadisarija and the use of the bark for heart disease has been attributed to Vagbhatta, an eminent physician of ancient India.

Arjuna is one of the heroes of the Hindu epic Mahabaratha. In 1869, J.L. Stewart writing about plants in the Punjab, India reported that the bark of the Arjun tree was used to cure sores.

Medicinal parts: Bark and fruit.

Uses: In Indian medicine, the Arjun tree is used for fractures, ulcers, discharge from the urethra, whitish discharge from the vagina (leucorrhoea), diabetes, anaemia, heart disease, hyperhydrosis (increased sweating), asthma, bronchitis, exhaustion, tumours, dysentery, haemorrhages (internal and external), cirrhosis of the liver and high blood pressure.

Related plants, *Terminalia belerica* and *Terminalia chebula* have been used orally for cardiovascular conditions such as angina, hypertension and hyperlipidaemia, and digestive disorders, including both diarrhoea and constipation and indigestion.

Terminalia chebula is also used orally for dysentery. Topically, *Terminalia belerica* and *Terminalia chebula* are used as a lotion for sore eyes. *Terminalia chebula* is also used topically as a mouthwash and gargle. Intravaginally, *Terminalia chebula* is used as a douche for treating vaginitis.

Probable mode of action: Constituents include tannins, steroids, flavonoids and many others. Clinical experiments with the bark powder have demonstrated efficacy against congestive cardiac insufficiency (heart failure which results in congestion in the heart and blood vessels). Various extracts caused lowered blood pressure, slowing of the heart rate (bradycardia) and a stimulating effect on heart muscle contraction (positively inotropic) in animal experiments. Spasmolytic (relief of spasms) activity has also been described. The substance is said to be sedative and to potentiate the activity of barbiturates (a type of sleeping tablet). Weak evidence for effectiveness against amoebic infections. *Terminalia chebula* is known to improve lipid profiles, but to a lesser degree than *Terminalia arjuna*. *Terminalia belerica* and *Terminalia chebula* are attributed with the ability to correct bowel movement irregularities and indigestion. An alcoholic extract of *Terminalia chebula* containing gallic acid and its ethyl ester may have activity against methicillin-resistant *Staphylococcus aureus*. *Terminalia chebula* may also act against cytomegalovirus, herpes simplex I, *Streptococcus mutans*, *Salmonella* sp., *Shigella spp.* and retroviral reverse transcriptase. Both *Terminalia belerica* and *Terminalia chebula* may have activity against HIV.

Adverse effects: No health hazards are known in conjunction with the proper administration of designated therapeutic dosages.

Precautions: Safety in young children, pregnant or nursing mothers or in people with severe liver and kidney disease has not been established.

ARNICA

Arnica montana

Arnica has a history of use in folk medicine in North America, Germany and Russia (where it was used externally to treat wounds, black eye, sprains and contusions). A mountain plant whose parts have been used as a means of assassination.

Has a history of use in the treatment of blood loss from the uterus (uterine haemorrhage), inflammations of the heart muscle (myocarditis), pain of ischaemic heart disease (angina – pain due to poor blood supply to the heart muscle) and heart failure (cardiac insufficiency).

Arnica was listed in the US Pharmacopeia from early 1800s until 1960.

Approved by Commission E for:

- fever and colds
- inflammation of the skin
- cough/bronchitis
- inflammation of the mouth and pharynx
- rheumatism
- common cold
- blunt injuries
- tendency to infection.

Medicinal parts: Oil extracted from the flowers, the dried flowers, the leaves collected before flowering and dried. The root and the dried rhizome.

Uses: In folk medicine, used externally to treat swelling, haematomas (collections of blood) and contusions that follow injury or trauma. Also used to treat rheumatic joint and muscle problems.

Other uses: Inflammation of mouth (oral) and throat, furunculosis, inflammation caused by insect bites, inflammation of the veins (phlebitis).

In Russian folk medicine, the herb is used to treat uterine bleeds (haemorrhages). Other uses include heart ailments such as myocarditis (inflammation of the heart muscle), arteriosclerosis (narrowing of the arteries), angina pectoris (pain in the chest due to decreased blood supply to the heart muscle), cardiac insufficiency and exhaustion, sprains, contusions, hair loss.

Probable mode of action: Contains several constituents including flavonoid glycosides, lactones, choline, tannins and volatile oils.

Arnica preparations have an anti-inflammatory, analgesic (pain relieving) and antiseptic effect when applied topically, mainly attributed to the lactone component, and are considered to be beneficial in inflammations. Some constituents had an effect against bacteria (antimicrobial) in laboratory experiments. Other attributed effects are: increase in uterine tone, increase in force of contraction of the heart muscle (inotropic) and countering respiratory depression (respiratory analeptic). The extract of arnica has been shown to stimulate the action of white blood cells in animal studies, increasing resistance to bacterial infections such as typhoid caused by *Salmonella*.

Adverse effects: Mouth ulcers, nausea, vomiting, hypertension, cardiac dysrhythmias, central nervous system depression, muscle weakness, hepatic failure, arnica-induced Sweet's syndrome.

The plant is considered toxic when taken orally. Gastroenteritis has occurred with high doses. The flowers and roots of the plant have caused vomiting, drowsiness and coma when eaten by children.

Poisoning caused by ingestion of excessive doses is characterized by severe mucous membrane irritation (vomiting, diarrhoea, bleeding from mucous membranes) and a brief stimulation of the activity of the heart followed by heart failure. Dyspnoea (difficulty in breathing) and cardiac arrest (stoppage of beating of the heart) may occur.

Allergy-related skin rashes with itching, blister formation, ulcers and superficial necroses can result from repeated contact with cosmetics containing arnica flowers or other composites (for example tansy, chrysanthemums, sunflowers). External application of very high concentrations can also result in primary blister formation and necrosis. The constituent helenalin is considered to be the allergic component that causes contact dermatitis.

Precautions: Arnica is deadly in large quantities. The herb or essential oil should not be ingested (taken by mouth). The essential oil has to be diluted before used externally and should not be applied to broken skin. Alcoholic extracts of arnica can cause toxic effects on the heart and raise blood pressure.

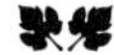

ARRACH – WORMSEED

Chenopodium vulvaria

Has a distinctive unpleasant smell. The name comes from the Nahuatl word for skunk.

Used as a food and remedy (for asthma and dysentery) by the Aztecs. For centuries, the Maya of Central America used wormseed to expel worms – hence its name. The Catawba people of North America used the plant for poultices to detoxify snake bites and other poisonings.

The long history of medicinal use has been across Europe, North Africa and the Caucasus to relieve menstrual cramps and promote menstruation. Considered the first line of defence against round worm and hookworm infestations in Mexico.

Medicinal parts: Aerial parts, flowering tops.

Uses: Has been used as an anti-inflammatory agent and as an antispasmodic. Used initially and to date to expel worms from the bowel. Also used for fungal infections and as a stimulant for the heart (cardiac stimulant). Form of treatment for acute gout.

Other uses: Internally and externally to relieve cramps and as an emmenagogue (promote menstruation). As a digestive aid (tonic). **In Chinese medicine**, wormseed oil is used for rheumatism, eczema and bites.

Probable mode of action: Constituents include volatile oil (which also contains some methyl salicylate) and triterpenoid saponins. Specific effects of the constituents are not known with certainty.

Adverse effects: No health hazards or side-effects are known to be associated with the administration of recommended therapeutic dosages. The offensive smell often precludes continued use.

Precautions: No information available.

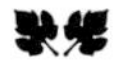

ARROWROOT – OBEDIENCE PLANT

Maranta arundinaceae

Studies show evidence of arrowroot cultivation 7000 years ago. Probably derived from the Caribbean word *aru-aru* which means 'meal of meals'.

Medicinal parts: Rhizome tubers and dried rhizome.

Uses: Dietary supplement for children during convalescence or for treatment of gastrointestinal disorders and diarrhoea.

Other uses: In **Indian folk medicine**, arrowroot is used in the treatment of dysentery, diarrhoea, stomach ailments (dyspepsia), bronchitis and coughs, and as a nourishing food for children, in the chronically ill and during convalescence.

Probable mode of action: The fresh bulbs contain approximately 25–27% starch, but other significant constituents are not known. May reduce cholesterol due to an action on bile acids. In humans, the drug relieves inflammation or irritation (demulcent) and is used as a soothing agent.

Adverse effects: No health hazards or side-effects are known to be associated with the administration of recommended therapeutic dosages.

Precautions: No information available.

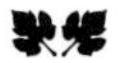

ARTEMISIA VULGARIS – MUGWORT ROOT

Roman soldiers put mugwort in their sandals to protect their feet against fatigue. Has been used in Asian Traditional Medicine to correct breech presentation (when the presenting part of the child at birth is the buttock and not the head). This method was termed moxibustion. The plant was also much used in witchcraft.

Medicinal parts: Root and aerial parts of the plant, particularly the dried branch tips.

Uses: Orally, for gastrointestinal problems such as colic, diarrhoea, stomach ulcers, constipation, cramps, weak digestion, worm infestations and persistent vomiting.

Other uses: To stimulate gastric juice and bile secretion, as a laxative in cases of obesity, as a liver tonic, and for hysteria, epilepsy, convulsions in children, menstrual problems (delayed or irregular menstruation), to promote circulation and as a sedative. Orally, *Artemisia vulgaris* is used as a tonic in individuals with diminished strength and energy. In combination with other ingredients, mugwort root is used for psychoneuroses, neurasthenia, depression, hypochondria, autonomic neuroses, general irritability, restlessness, insomnia, and anxiety – all of which are considered to be neuropsychiatric disturbances. It is an abortifacient and is also used to treat asthenic states as a tonic.

In **Chinese medicine**, mugwort is used to treat female complaints and ulcers and burns.

Probable mode of action: Several constituents including lactones, lipophilic flavonoids. A complex volatile oil has been isolated. Some evidence suggests mugwort can stimulate uterine activity, possibly due to the thujone content. Other evidence suggests the aqueous extract and the volatile oil have effects against bacteria and other organisms (antimicrobial).

Adverse effects: People allergic to members of the Asteraceae/Compositae families may have an allergic reaction to *Artemisia vulgaris*. These plants include ragweed, daisies and marigolds. People who are sensitive to birch, celery or wild carrot may also be sensitive to mugwort. People who are allergic to tobacco may have a reaction to mugwort pollen. It could theoretically cause a reaction in people allergic to honey.

Precautions: Probably unsafe for pregnant women as it might stimulate the uterus to contract and induce abortion/ preterm delivery.

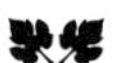

ARTICHOKE

Cynara scolymus

Artichoke was used as food and medicine by ancient Egyptians, Greeks and Romans. In the first century AD, Dioscorides (40–90 AD) recommended applying mashed artichoke roots on the body to sweeten offensive odours.

Ancient Greeks and Romans considered artichoke as an aphrodisiac. Artichoke was also attributed to being effective in securing the birth of boys.

Approved by Commission E for:

- liver and gallbladder complaints
- loss of appetite.

Medicinal parts: Dried whole or cut basal leaves and the dried or fresh herb.

Uses: Dyspepsia, prophylaxis against the return of gallstones (by increasing bile production).

Other uses: In folk medicine, artichoke is also used for digestive complaints and as a tonic during convalescence. Has been used to lower blood cholesterol and triglycerides to prevent atherosclerosis and heart disease.

Probable mode of action: Much of the pharmacological activity of the leaf has been attributed to the presence of constituents such as cyanaroside, which are believed to possess cholesterol lowering properties. Artichoke is a good source of essential polyunsaturated fatty acids containing stearic, palmitic, oleic and linoleic acids. Numerous enzymes, phytosterols, tannins and sugars have been isolated from artichoke. The flavonoid constituents have been reported to possess antioxidant activity. The flavonoids and some other derivatives are considered responsible for the gastrointestinal soothing effects. Caffeoylquinic acids are also considered important for the actions of artichoke.

Adverse effects: Can cause allergic reactions (dermatitis) in sensitive individuals due to the lactones. There is cross-reactivity with other members of the Compositae family (e.g. chrysanthemums, *Arnica*, *Pyrethrum*).

Precautions: Generally regarded as non-toxic. Use with caution in cases of biliary obstruction (if there are stones in the gallbladder or bile duct). May hinder breastfeeding (lactation). Contraindicated in patients allergic to plants belonging to the Asteraceae family.

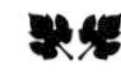

ASAFOETIDA – DEVIL'S DUNG

Ferula assafoetida

Indian name: Hing

Many unusual medical claims have been made for the resin from the belief that its foetid odour acts as a deterrent to germs. In the days of the Wild West, asafoetida mixed with other strong spices was used in cures for alcoholism. In ancient India, it was reputed to expel wind from the stomach. Used especially by the followers of the faith Jainism in India who are not permitted to eat onions.

Medicinal parts: Oily gum resin extracted from the plant.

Uses: As an aphrodisiac, carminative (in chronic gastritis and irritable colon), diuretic and sedative.

Other uses: Antidote for flatulence, dyspepsia, asthma and whooping cough. **In Chinese medicine**, the herb is used for infestations with intestinal parasites. **In Indian medicine**, it is used in the treatment of whooping cough, asthma, flatulence, constipation, diseases of the liver and spleen. It has also been used as an antidote to opium.

Probable mode of action: Has a mild intestinal disinfectant effect. Effectiveness as a sedative is unproven. Asafoetida is composed of volatile oil, resin and gum. The organic sulphur-containing active ingredients in the oil produce the unpleasant effects. A component of the resin may have an effect that protects against cancers. Shown to have antitumour effects.

Adverse effects: Topical use may cause skin irritation. There is report of methhaemoglobinaemia in a five-week-old child after ingestion of glycerated asafoetida solution. This folk remedy is now considered potentially life-threatening.

Precautions: Do not use solutions orally. Should be avoided in pregnancy because there is a theoretical risk of increased bleeding at delivery.

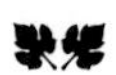

ASHWAGANDA – INDIAN GINSENG

Withania somnifera

Three varieties of the plant have been identified, one Indian and two Israeli. Clinical research data do not support the use of ashwaganda for any condition. However, it is a major herb in Ayurveda where every part of the plant is used, despite the plant being considered toxic if eaten. In Hindi (the official language of India), ashwaganda means 'horse smell'. Though 'Indian ginseng' is the common name, Ashwaganda does not belong to the true ginseng family.

Medicinal parts: The root, leaves, berry and seeds.

Uses: The root is used in Ayurveda as a sedative and diuretic. The seeds and leaves are used for relief of pain and to kill lice. Is considered to influence the immune response of the body. Use as a cytotoxic agent (ability to destroy cells, particularly cancer cells) has been studied in animals.

Other uses: Ashwaganda is considered in Ayurveda to be an adaptogen, a substance that enhances and regulates the ability of the body to withstand stress and enhance performance in a non-specific manner.

Probable mode of action: Active constituents are reported to have analgesic, antipyretic, sedative, hypotensive, anti-inflammatory and antioxidant effects. It may also cause smooth muscle relaxation and stimulate the formation of the thyroid hormone. Effects on the immune system are unclear.

Adverse effects: No available information.

Precautions: Can induce dependence. Likely to be unsafe during pregnancy because it has been reported to induce abortions. May decrease effectiveness of allopathic immunosuppressant drugs (drugs used after transplants to prevent rejection of the transplanted organ). Best avoided with sleeping tablets (barbiturates).

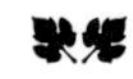

ASTRAGALUS – HUANG-QI

Astragalus membranaceus

An ancient Chinese remedy listed in the Chinese Pharmacopeia. An important component of

Chinese Fu Zheng herbal therapy in which the aim is to restore immune system function. Used primarily as a tonic and for the treatment of diabetes and nephritis.

Medicinal part: Roots.

Uses: Restoration of immune function after cancer chemotherapy and for HIV infections. In Western herbal medicine, astragalus is primarily considered a tonic for enhancing metabolism and digestion and is often consumed as a tea.

Other uses: Respiratory infections, heart failure, prevention of the common cold, diuretic, uterine relaxation, liver and kidney disease. **In Chinese medicine**, the herb has been used alone and in combination for liver fibrosis, acute viral myocarditis (inflammation of the heart muscle due to viral infection), heart failure, small cell lung cancer, amenorrhoea (absence of periods) and as an antiviral agent.

Probable mode of action: Saponins are capable of stimulating growth of isolated human lymphocytes (white blood cells), which are involved in immunity. The aqueous extract of the root stimulates phagocytosis (engulfing of foreign material like bacteria by white blood cells) and increases the production of other blood cells such as monocytes. May help to reduce infections in patients with AIDS. Saponins also produce a diuresis due to local irritation of the kidney lining (epithelial) cells.

Adverse effects: Little or no information. Due to the selenium content, toxic doses may result in neurological dysfunction leading to paralysis.

Precautions: Safety and efficacy during pregnancy and lactation is not established. Should be used cautiously in immunosuppressed patients (in whom the immune response is inhibited by drugs or disease), for example those who have received transplants or who have AIDS.

AVENA SATIVA – OATS

Avena sativa

Historically considered to be an inferior grain as bread cannot be made from it. However, it is held in high esteem in Scotland. Oats originated in England, France, Poland, Germany and Russia. It is now cultivated worldwide, even in Iceland. Used as a food for humans and as fodder for animals.

Oat straw is approved by Commission E for:

- inflammation of the skin
- warts.

Medicinal parts: The fresh or dried above-ground plant, the ripe dried fruits and the dried threshed leaf and stem.

Uses: Wild oat herb is used for anxiety (acute and chronic), bladder weakness (atonia of the bladder), when there are deficiencies in the healing of tissues (connective tissues), excitation, gout, old age symptoms and for withdrawal from opium and tobacco. Other uses include rheumatism, skin diseases, sleeplessness and stress.

Oat fruit is used for gastrointestinal complaints and for gallbladder and kidney diseases. Also used for diabetes, constipation, diarrhoea, tiredness and rheumatism.

Oat straw is used externally for skin disorders and itching. Also used for gastrointestinal disorders, bladder disorders, rheumatism, eye ailments, frostbite and gout.

Other uses: Oat straw is used as a foot bath for cold and tired feet. Also used as a tea for flu and coughs.

Probable mode of action: There is little information on the efficacy of oat straw. Dehusked oats have been shown to lower cholesterol levels. Oat straw contains sugars, flavonoids and saponins.

Adverse effects: None documented with recommended doses.

Precautions: None documented.

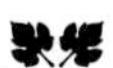

BAEL FRUIT – STONE APPLE – BENGAL QUINCE

Aegle marmelos

Indian name: Bel, Siriphal
The bael tree is held sacred by the Hindus. The history of this tree has been traced to the Vedic period (2000–800 BC) and has great mythological significance. It is commonly found planted close to Hindu temples. The leaves of the tree are used as a sacred offering to Lord Shiva, the God of Health. It is one of the most widely used medicinal parts in India.

Medicinal parts: Stem, bark, root, leaves, fruit.

Uses: Laxative; also used for chronic diarrhoeas and dysentery where there is no fever.

Other uses: Treatment of peptic ulcer (stomach and duodenal ulcers). The root was used for ear problems. Oil from the leaves was used for recurrent colds and respiratory infections.

Probable mode of action: Reported to contract cells (skin and other) following inflammation (astringent), and an effect on the digestive system.

Adverse effects: Excessive intake of the fruit causes heaviness of the stomach.

Precautions: The ripe fruit should not be taken regularly as it leads to atony of the intestine.

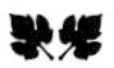

BAIKAL SKULL CAP – HUANG-QIN

Scutellaria baicalensis

Baikal skull cap and combinations are used in Asian medicine to improve brain function and to treat headaches and inflammatory conditions ranging from dermatitis to inflammatory bowel disease.

Medicinal part: The root.

Uses: For treatment of prostate cancer, respiratory and gastrointestinal infections.

Probable mode of action: Constituents include wogonin and baicalin which are considered to possess anti-inflammatory activity. Some studies have suggested that baikal skull cap helps to relieve nausea and gastric lesions that may follow treatment with irinotecan (anticancer drug) and ritonavir (antiviral drug used to treat HIV).

Adverse effects: Has been reported to cause liver toxicity (hepatotoxicity).

Precautions: Safety during pregnancy is unknown.

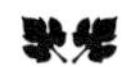

BAMBOO

Arundinaria japonica

Bamboo is the hardy woody stem of bamboo plants. Bamboo cups were used in cupping therapy or the 'horn method' in ancient China. Today the Chinese still use cupping therapy to stimulate circulation through the tissues, manage pain and enhance healing.

Cane and bamboo have been used for orthotic and prosthetic appliances (limb splints, wheel chairs, bamboo walkers, crutches).

An ancient all-purpose medicine, tabasheer was extracted from the lining inside the bamboo and has since been shown to be an antidote for food poisoning and to possess some sex hormonal activity.

Medicinal parts: Young shoots of the plant.

Uses: In Chinese medicine, bamboo is used orally for asthma, coughs and gallbladder disorders. In **India**, the leaves of the bamboo tree are used to treat spasmodic disorders of the stomach and to arrest bleeding. The tender shoots were used for treatment of respiratory disorders.

Other uses: The leaves have also been used as an aphrodisiac. A decoction of the leaves is considered to be an emmenagogue and has been used to regulate menstruation. The leaves have also been used to treat threadworm infestations.

Probable mode of action: Leaves contain chlorogenic acid, caffeic acid and other constituents which have been shown to possess both anti-oxidant and pro-oxidant activity. Some experiments in rats have shown that the constituents may possess activity against that of the thyroid hormone. Constituents include silicic acid. The precise effects of constituents are not known as yet.

Adverse effects: The shoots may contain toxic cyanogens (compounds that release the very toxic compound cyanide).

Precautions: Do not use during pregnancy. Bamboo shoots have been used to induce abortions. Bamboo shoots should be cooked before eating to rid them of the toxic cyanogens.

BANYAN

Ficus bengalensis – Indian banyan

Indian name: Bar
In Hindu mythology, the banyan tree is also called Kalpavriksha, meaning 'wish fulfilling tree'. It represents eternal life because of its seemingly ever expanding branches. It is the national tree of India. Its origin is from India, Pakistan and Sri Lanka.

Medicinal parts: Leaf buds, bark, latex, roots.

Uses: Leaf buds were used in the treatment of chronic diarrhoea and dysentery. The latex mixed with milk is used to treat bleeding piles (haemorrhoids).

Other uses: Tender roots have been used to treat female sterility. Aerial roots are used for cleaning teeth and preventing teeth and gum disorders. Infusions have been used to treat diabetes.

Probable mode of action: The leaves of the banyan tree yield ficusin and bergaptene. The precise effects of the constituents are not known with certainty.

Adverse effects: Have not been reported in the literature available.

Precautions: The latex of the tree is very toxic and should be used only under medical supervision.

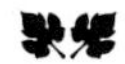

BARBERRY – EUROPEAN BARBERRY

Berberis vulgaris

Also referred to as holy thorn, as it is thought to have formed a part of the crown of thorns for Christ. The bark of the root is used as a dye in Poland.

Medicinal parts: Fruit and the root bark.

Uses: Constipation, appetite stimulant, heartburn, stomach cramps.

Other uses: Decreases susceptibility to infections; used for feverish colds, diseases of the urinary tract, liver disease (the bark), gallbladder disease, jaundice, gout, rheumatism, arthritis, leishmaniasis, malaria, opium and morphine withdrawal.

Probable mode of action: Considered to be a source of vitamin C. The acid constituents produce a diuretic effect. The root bark contains berberine and other alkaloids which have been shown to lower blood pressure, and there are reports that these extracts could increase the force of heart muscle contraction and increase the flow of bile.

Adverse effects: If the bark is taken in doses in excess of 4 mg, stupor, nosebleeds, vomiting, diarrhoea and kidney irritation may occur.

Precautions: Contraindicated during pregnancy because of risk of abortion. Use only in recommended doses.

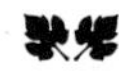

BARLEY

Hordeum vulgare

Has been cultivated by man for centuries. The ancient Greeks used the mucilage derived from the cereal to treat gastrointestinal inflammation. Gladiators ate barley for strength and stamina. The Roman physician Pliny used barley as a cure for boils.

Historically barley has been used for boils, inflammatory disorders of the gut and for increasing strength and stamina.

Medicinal part: The grain.

Uses: For bronchitis and diarrhoea, and as a source of folic acid and vitamin B_{12} and vitamin B_6.

Other uses: Prevention of colon cancer, to lower blood sugar and blood cholesterol, and for weight loss. Also as a carminative and digestive aid.

Probable mode of action: Active constituents include fibre, starch and also selenium, copper, manganese and phosphorus. May have an effect on the viscosity of the intestinal contents and delay the absorption of cholesterol. Meals high in soluble fibre have been shown to reduce the rise in postprandial blood sugar (blood sugar levels after a meal) and insulin concentrations.

A constituent is reported to influence the rate and degree of absorption of carbohydrates and fats and to decrease appetite by prolonging the feeling of fullness, possibly by delaying the emptying of the stomach. Reported to have a protective effect on the mucosal membrane of the gut.

The fibre in the grain is possibly responsible for decreasing blood cholesterol and blood sugar levels.

Adverse reactions: Exposure to barley flour can cause asthma. Several cases of hypersensitivity to barley have been reported, including life-threatening recurrent anaphylaxis. Constituents have been implicated as a trigger for coeliac disease. Beer contains hordein (a constituent) at a concentration of 1.12 g/serving, sufficient to exacerbate symptoms of coeliac disease in some individuals. Theoretically the fibre can reduce the absorption of certain medications.

Precautions: Avoid in coeliac disease as the gluten content of barley can aggravate the condition. Avoid concomitant use of sympathomimetics (substances similar to adrenaline) as barley contains a sympathomimetic component (hordenine).

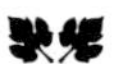

BASIL

Ocimum basilicum

Basil originated from India, where the Hindus believed that the Hindu Gods Krishna and Vishnu gave basil its protective and inspirational properties. Held sacred by the Brahmins.

Medicinal parts: Fresh or dried herb and the oil extracted from the aerial parts.

Uses: For flatulence, appetite stimulation and an aid to digestion, to relieve colic, constipation and to treat nausea; also used as a diuretic.

Other uses: In Chinese medicine, basil is used for kidney disease and for gum ulcers. **In Indian medicine**, basil is used for earache, rheumatoid arthritis, anorexia (loss of appetite), itching, menstrual disorders (amenorrhoea, dysmenorrhoea) and malaria. Hot basil tea has been used to reduce fever and clear phlegm from the chest and nose.

Probable mode of action: The main constituents are chavicol methyl ether (estragole), linalool and eugenol. The specific effects of the constituents are not known with certainty.

Adverse effects: No adverse effects have been documented with use of recommended doses.

Precautions: The herb contains an essential oil with estragole, which has potential carcinogenic and mutagenic properties (ability to cause cancers and mutations in genes). Basil should not be taken during pregnancy. Basil oil should not be given to infants or small children.

BAYBERRY – WILD CINNAMON

Myrica cerifera (L)

Native Americans took a decoction of the stems and leaves for fever. It was known to contract cells (skin and other) following inflammation (astringent).

The wax from the berries was used in candle making. The wax was introduced to medicinal use in the 18th century.

Medicinal parts: Root bark, berries, leaves and wax.

Uses: Orally for diarrhoea, mucous colitis (a disorder of the bowel due to excess mucus) and colds. Topically as a gargle for sore throats, and as a douche for whitish discharge from the vagina (leucorrhoea). The powdered bark may be used as a poultice for wounds and cuts, bruises and slow-healing ulcers.

Other uses: Dysentery, excessive menstrual bleeding or postpartum haemorrhage (bleeding after childbirth).

Probable mode of action: Constituents include tannins, flavonoid glycosides, resins, gum and volatile oil. The wax is said to contract cells (skin and other) following inflammation (astringent), to be a circulatory stimulant, to induce perspiration (diaphoretic) and to be a tonic. It stimulates flow of bile.

Adverse effects: Myrica causes vomiting in large doses. The constituent myricadiol is reported to cause salt retention and potassium excretion. The tannin constituents may cause gastrointestinal irritation and liver damage. The powder may induce coughing.

Precautions: Because of the effect on salt retention and potassium excretion, it should be avoided in patients with high blood pressure and with kidney disease.

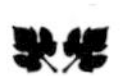

BEARBERRY – UVA-URSI

Arctostaphylos uva-ursi (Spreng.)

Marco Polo reported in the 13th century that the Chinese were using this herb as a diuretic. Uva-ursi was used in the 13th century by the Welsh Physicians of Myddfai. It was described by Clusius in 1601 and recommended for medicinal use in 1763 by Gerhard of Berlin. It appeared in the London Pharmacopoeia in 1788, though was probably in use long before. The tannin in the leaves was used in the past to tan leather in Sweden and Russia and an ash-coloured dye is said to be obtained from the plant in Scandinavia. Cattle avoid it but bears relish the fruit.

The leaves from *Arctostaphylos glauca* (manzanita) from **California**, *Arctostaphylos polifolia* from **Mexico**, and *Arctostaphylos tomentosa* (madrona) are also used medicinally. Continues to be a popular herb in Poland.

Medicinal parts: Leaves. The evergreen leaves may be collected throughout the year, but preferably in September or October.

Uses: Urinary tract infections of the bladder and urethra (cystitis, urethritis) and bronchitis.

Other uses: For fluid retention and bedwetting, profuse bleeding during menstruation, diarrhoea and toothache. Has also been used to treat arthritis. Claimed to strengthen the heart muscle and urinary tract and to return the womb to its normal size after childbirth.

Probable mode of action: Constituents probably have a diuretic effect. Also known to contract cells (skin and other) following inflammation (astringent), have an effect on lower digestive tract, be a urinary antiseptic and relieve inflammation or irritation (demulcent). Arbutin is the principal constituent attributable for the effects against bacteria.

Adverse effects: Large doses may lead to nausea and vomiting due to the high tannin content. Tinnitus (ringing in ears), nausea, vomiting, shortness of breath, convulsions and collapse are known to follow overdose. May cause passage of greenish urine and may give rise to a bluish grey skin which is harmless.

Precautions: *Arctostaphylos* is contraindicated during pregnancy due to its properties on the uterus.

Treatment should be of short duration (seven days) and an alkaline diet (high in vegetables, potatoes and milk) should be taken during treatment. Long-term use may produce toxic effects as large doses of hydroquinone are poisonous, though therapeutic doses of uva-ursi should not be a risk to health. The herb should perhaps be avoided if the kidney itself is affected. Not recommended for use in children under the age of 12 years.

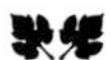

BENNET'S ROOT – OLD MAN'S WHISKERS

Geum urbanum

The word geum is from the Greek word *geno* which indicates that it yields an agreeable smell. Was believed to have the power to ward off evil spirits and venomous beasts.

Has been used to flavour ale.

Medicinal parts: Herb, root.

Uses: The herb is rarely used at present. Considered to be an astringent, antidiarrhoeal, antihaemorrhagic and a febrifuge. The powdered root had a great reputation as a substitute for quinine in the treatment of intermittent fevers. **In folk medicine**, the root has been used for digestive disorders and diarrhoea, and for fevers. Also used for nerve and muscle pain and as a bath for haemorrhoids. Used essentially for gastrointestinal disorders (for digestive complaints such as loss of appetite and diarrhoea).

The root has been used **in folk medicine** for digestive complaints such as loss of appetite and diarrhoea.

Other uses: The root has been used as a gargle for inflammation of the mouth and gums. Also used in a bath for frostbite, haemorrhoids and skin diseases.

Probable mode of action: The herb contracts cells (skin and other) following inflammation (astringent properties) and hence its use in baths for haemorrhoids. The plant contains tannins, volatile oil (mainly eugenol), a bitter principle, flavone and organic acids.

Adverse effects: None recorded with recommended doses.

Precautions: No information available.

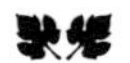

BETEL LEAF

Piper betle

Indian name: Pan

The plant originated in Malaysia. Plays an important role in Hindu, Sri Lankan and Vietnamese cultures. In Vietnam it is considered to 'begin conversation'.

The use of the betel leaf can be traced back 2000 years and is described in the most ancient historic book of Sri Lanka – the Mahavansa, written in Pali. In India, Sri Lanka and other parts of South East Asia, the leaves are chewed with mineral lime (calcium oxide) and the areca nut.

Medicinal parts: Leaf, stem.

Uses: As a diuretic, to relieve nervous exhaustion and debility.

Other uses: Applied locally, betel leaves have been considered to be beneficial in the treatment of arthritis and orchitis. The juice of the leaves has been applied to heal wounds. Has been prescribed by Ayurvedic physicians as an aphrodisiac (pan-supari).

Also used as a mild stimulant and as a digestive aid and as a breath freshener. Used in **Malaysia** to treat headaches, arthritis and joint pain. In **China** and **Thailand**, betel leaves are used to relieve toothache. In **Indonesia**, betel leaf is used as an antibiotic.

Probable mode of action: The oil obtained from the leaves has several constituents (e.g. chavicol, estragole, methyl eugenol, terpenes and sesquiterpenes). The precise effects of these constituents are not known as yet.

Adverse effects: There is no information in the literature on the local effects of betel leaves.

Frequent chewing with other ingredients may cause staining of the teeth.

Precautions: There are suggestions that a carcinogenic potential of betel is possibly affected by hormonal changes that occur during pregnancy.

BETH ROOT – INDIAN BALM

Trillium erectum

Beth root is also known as birth root as Native Americans used the herb to aid childbirth. The whole plant was also used as a poultice for the treatment of ulcers, tumours and skin inflammations.

Medicinal parts: The rhizome, dried root and leaves.

Uses: For long and heavy menstrual periods. Has been used to treat uterine prolapse and for bleeding from uterine fibroids (benign tumours in the uterine wall).

Other uses: Externally for varicose veins, haematomas and bleeding haemorrhoids.

Used as ain aid during childbirth **in folk medicine**.

Probable mode of action: The active constituents contract cells (skin and other) following inflammation (astringent) and promote removal of secretions from the lung and upper airways (expectorant).

Adverse effects: Can cause nausea in high doses and also promote labour and menstruation. Local application can cause irritation.

Precautions: Should not be used during pregnancy.

BETONY

Stachys betonica (L)

Stated to have been used in every continent for nearly all ailments. The physician to the Roman emperor Augustus claimed that betony could cure at least 47 different ailments. In the past it was believed to possess the power to dispel evil and to protect the wearer from 'visions and dreams'. Parkinson wrote, 'it is said also to hinder drunkenness being taken beforehand and quickly to expel it afterwards'.

Medicinal parts: Aerial parts, which should be collected during flowering in June and July.

Uses: Treatment of headache, vertigo, anxiety states, hysteria, neuralgia. Specifically used to treat certain forms of headaches.

Other uses: To contract cells (skin and other) following inflammation (astringent). The tannin constituents make it a suitable compress for wounds and bruises. The **French** recommend *Stachys* for liver and gallbladder complaints. Taken internally, it stimulates the circulation.

Probable mode of action: The constituents (alkaloids, choline, tannins, saponins) are considered to be sedative, bitter and aromatic, and to contract cells (skin and other) following inflammation (astringent). The alkaloid trigonelline is believed to have a hypoglycaemic action (lower blood sugar).

Adverse effects: Large doses can cause gastrointestinal irritation.

Precautions: Best avoided during pregnancy.

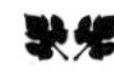

BILBERRY

Vaccinium myrtillus

Native Americans used bilberry teas and a tincture to treat symptoms of diabetes. There are unconfirmed reports that, during, World War II, British pilots ingested bilberry preserves to enhance their night vision. Also called black hearts in Southern England during the 19th century.

Medicinal parts: Dried leaves, ripe, dried fruit and ripe fresh fruit.

Uses: Fruit has been used for acute diarrhoea and mild inflammation of the mucous membranes of the mouth and throat. The leaf was used to treat diabetes and gastrointestinal disorders, kidney and urinary tract disorders, arthritis, gout and dermatitis. Topically the leaf has been used for inflammation of the mucous membrane of the mouth, inflammation of the eye, burns and skin diseases.

In folk medicine, bilberry is used internally for vomiting, bleeding and haemorrhoids. Used externally for poorly healing skin ulcers and to promote wound healing.

Probable mode of action: The constituent tannins are reported to contract cells (skin and other) following inflammation (astringent) and to have an anti-diarrhoeal action. Constituents are also reported to promote healing of wounds. This is probably by stimulating the formation of healing tissue or connective tissue. However, such an effect on the eye is considered to promote damage in diabetics. Reported to influence inflammatory responses by preventing leakage of fluid from blood vessels (antiexudative) and by protecting blood vessels from damage.

Adverse effects: The high tannin content may cause digestive disorders, and prolonged use or high doses should be avoided. The signs of poisoning observed in animal experiments include cachexia (wasting of the body), anaemia and jaundice. Poisoning which occurred after prolonged use was attributed to the tannin content.

Precautions: Avoid in pregnancy. Should not be used by patients on anticoagulant therapy (e.g. warfarin).

BIRCH

Betula species

In the past, the birch was referred to as the 'mother tree' as it facilitated a habitat for all trees and plants because of its endurance. The birch is the national tree of Russia where it used to be worshipped as a goddess during the Green Week in early July. Commercial oil of wintergreen (methyl salicylate) was made from *Betula lenta*. Silver birch (*Betula pendula*) is the national tree of Finland.

Leaves are approved by Commission E for:

- infections of the urinary tract
- kidney and bladder stones
- rheumatism.

Medicinal parts: Bark, leaves and buds.

Uses: The leaves are used as a 'flush out' for bacterial and inflammatory diseases of the urinary tract and for 'gravel' in the kidney. They are also used as adjuncts in the therapy of rheumatic disorders. Externally the leaves are used for hair loss and dandruff.

Other uses: The birch tar has been used externally for parasitic infestations of the skin with subsequent hair loss and also for the treatment of rheumatism, gout (as an ointment), dry eczema, psoriasis and other chronic skin diseases. Birch tar is a constituent of 'Unguentum contra scabiem' that is used in the treatment of scabies. **In folk medicine**, the leaves are used as a blood purifier and for gout and rheumatism. The oil from the bark keeps away insects and gnats.

Probable mode of action: Birch leaves are antipyretic (reduce fever). In animal tests they have been shown to increase the amount of urine formed and passed. Birch bark contains betulin and betulinic acid, both of which have been investigated as potential allopathic medications. Birch tea contains vitamin C.

Adverse effects: The aromatic and aliphatic hydrocarbons in birch tar are irritating to the skin.

Precautions: Do not use in patients with oedema or in patients with poor kidney or heart function.

BISTORT

Polygonum bistorta (L)

The name Bistort is derived from Latin words *bis* and *tortilis* meaning twice-twisted, referring to the character of the rootstock. In the past, the roots and leaves had a reputation as a remedy for wounds, and the plant was cultivated both for its medicinal uses as well as a vegetable. The seeds were often used to fatten poultry. As the roots contain starch, it has been consumed in Russia (including Siberia), and in Iceland at times of food scarcity.

Medicinal parts: Dried rhizome and root; fresh leaves collected in the autumn.

Uses: Digestive disorders including diarrhoea, and for internal bleeding. Externally as a mouthwash (gargle) for mouth and throat infections. As an ointment for wounds and anal fissures. As a douche for whitish discharge from the vagina (leucorrhoea).

Other uses: The powder directly applied to a wound will stem bleeding. **In Chinese medicine**, preparations from the rhizome are used for epilepsy, fever, tetanus, carbuncles, snake and mosquito bites, scrofula and cramps in hands and feet. Bistort has been considered useful in diabetes. The root has been used externally as a poultice.

Probable mode of action: Active ingredients are found in higher concentrations in the root. Leaves are considered to contain vitamin C. Bistort causes an increase in the secretion of mucus and also contracts cells (skin and other) following inflammation (astringent).

Adverse effects: No health hazards or side-effects have been reported with the proper administration of recommended therapeutic doses.

Precautions: None documented.

BITTER MELON

Momordica charantia

Considered by Asians, Panamanians and Colombians to be helpful in the prevention of malaria. Used in the Philippines as a tea to control blood sugar. It is known in Ayurveda as 'plant insulin'.

Medicinal parts: The fruit, seeds and, less commonly, the leaves and roots.

Uses: As an abortifacient and in the treatment of diabetes, gastrointestinal disorders, cancer, HIV and psoriasis. As it is also a bitter, it is used to stimulate digestion.

Probable mode of action: Constituents include a substance similar to bovine insulin which is sometimes referred to as p-insulin or polypeptide P. Another constituent has an antiviral effect. Flavonoids may have a cholesterol lowering effect. There is some evidence that the preparations may increase haemoglobin and white cell counts in the blood. Some laboratory studies have suggested beneficial effects in malarial infections and HIV infections.

Adverse effects: Generally well tolerated. Some may experience headaches. People with glucose-6-phosphate deficiency may experience adverse effects because of the inability to break down a component of the bitter melon seed. Reported to have caused convulsions in children and reduced fertility in laboratory experiments on mice.

Precautions: Should be avoided in pregnancy because it can cause abortion. May lower blood sugar levels and increase the risk of hypoglycaemia in patients taking antidiabetic drugs.

BITTERSWEET NIGHTSHADE – TRUE BITTERSWEET

Solanum dulcamara

Bittersweet is a poisonous plant that has a long history of use in the treatment of skin diseases, warts and tumours. Dulcamara is a composite of the two Latin words meaning sweet and bitter respectively.

Used for medicinal purposes by herbalists in the 19th century in the US.

Approved by Commission E for:

- eczema
- furuncles (boils)
- acne
- warts.

Medicinal parts: The dried stem. The liquid obtained by steeping dried herb in boiling water is taken orally as a tea or used topically as a compress.

Uses: Main usage has been for disorders of the skin, mucous membranes and membranes lining the joints (synovial membranes). **In folk medicine**, bittersweet nightshade is used internally for nosebleeds, rheumatic conditions, asthma and bronchitis. It is also used to stimulate the immune system. Externally the herb is used for herpes, eczema, abscesses and contusions. Has been used for heart conditions.

Probable mode of action: The main constituents are steroid alkaloid glycosides which are considered to stimulate white blood cells to engulf foreign or toxic substances that enter the bloodstream (phagocytosis). These constituents also possess haemolytic (ability to destroy red blood cells), cytotoxic, antiviral and anticholinergic (antagonistic effects on the chemical messenger or neurotransmitter acetylcholine) and local anaesthetic properties. Also contains solasodin, which has a cortisone-like effect (cortisone is a hormone secreted by the adrenal gland). Contains saponin which probably contributes to its effects to promote removal of secretions from the lung and upper airways (expectorant). Fruit marinated in vinegar has been applied to cancerous sores.

Adverse effects: Nausea, vomiting, diarrhoea and dilated pupils. Toxicity from ingestion of the stem is unlikely because it contains only low concentrations of alkaloids, but children have been poisoned by eating unripe berries. Toxic effects may include tightness in the chest and difficulty in breathing, chest pain and skin rashes (hives). Overdose may cause paralysis of the central nervous system, slow the heart and breathing (respiration), lower temperature and cause vertigo, delirium, convulsions and death.

Precautions: Contraindicated during pregnancy and lactation. The fruit, which resembles small bright tomatoes, is poisonous as is the foliage. Prevent children from eating the berries. This herb should only be used under the supervision of a medical practitioner.

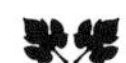

BLACK CATECHU – CATECHU

Acacia catechu

This tree is indigenous to Eastern India, Bangladesh and Myanmar.

In Bangladesh, it is a constituent of an antifertility pill.

Medicinal parts: Dried extract from the heartwood.

Uses: Treatment of catarrh, dysentery, bleeding. Externally, catechu is a constituent of tooth tinctures, mouthwashes and gargles, for gingivitis, stomatitis, laryngitis and pharyngitis, and as a dressing to control bleeding. Tinctures have been used for cracked nipples.

Other uses: In Indian medicine, catechu is used to treat mouth ulcers, throat infections and toothache. **In Chinese medicine**, catechu is used for poorly healing ulcers, weeping skin diseases, oral ulcers with bleeding and injuries following trauma. Has been used as a douche for vaginal discharges and topically to stop bleeding.

Probable mode of action: The constituents (mainly tannins) are known to contract cells (skin and other) following inflammation (astringent) and have antiseptic properties.

Adverse effects: May cause lowering of blood pressure. Another recorded side-effect is constipation. The lowering of blood pressure has been attributed to the release of a compound similar to bradykinin.

Precautions: Caution when using in patients on treatment for high blood pressure (hypertension). Do not administer together with iron tablets as absorption of both agents will be poor.

BLACK CATNIP – SHATTER STONE – STONE BREAKER

Phyllanthus amarus

Spanish name: Chanca piedra
Indian name: Bhunmalaki
The Spanish name of the plant, chanca piedra, means 'stone breaker' or 'shatter stone'.

Generations of indigenous Amazonian people used the herb to get rid of gallstones and kidney stones.

The herb has been used in Ayurveda for over 2000 years. Traditional uses in Ayurveda include the use of the whole plant for jaundice, gonorrhoea, frequent micturition and diabetes mellitus. Was used topically as a poultice for skin ulcers, sores, swellings and itchiness (scratching).

In Brazil, the plant is known as quebra-pedra or arraca pedra which is a translation of break-stone.

Medicinal parts: The whole dried herb, leaves, roots.

Uses: Main uses have been in the treatment of kidney and gallbladder stones. The herb is used for fever (**Cuba** and **Nigeria**), for malaria (**Cuba** and **Bahamas**), for diarrhoea, tachycardia and female sterility (**Congo**), for constipation with spasms and colic and as a diuretic (**Nigeria**) and for diabetes (**Dominican Republic**).

Other uses: In Indian medicine, black catnip is used for stomach conditions, ascites (fluid in the abdominal cavity), jaundice, diarrhoea, dysentery, intermittent fever, scabies, eye diseases and wounds. Considered to protect the liver and lower blood sugar. A related plant, *Phyllanthus niruri*, is reported to be effective against viral infections, mainly hepatitis B.

Probable mode of action: Constituents include tannins and lignans which have been shown to have effects against bacteria and viruses (antimicrobial and antiviral effects). The constituent with the antiviral activity is not known with certainty. *Phyllanthus* is considered to block DNA polymerase, the enzyme needed for hepatitis B virus to reproduce. Constituents also relieve spasms (antispasmodic).

Research has shown that the herb acts primarily on the liver.

Adverse effects: May increase the effects of drugs used in the treatment of diabetes mellitus, high blood pressure and for a diuretic effect.

Precautions: Not to be used during pregnancy.

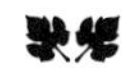

BLACK COHOSH

Cimicifuga racemosa

A traditional Native American remedy for menstrual pain and menopausal 'hot flushes' and to ease childbirth – hence the name 'squaw root'.

Approved by Commission E for:

- climacteric (menopause) complaints
- premenstrual syndrome.

Medicinal parts: Fresh and dried root.

Uses: Treatment of menopausal and premenstrual symptoms.

In folk medicine, the herb is used for rheumatism, sore throats and bronchitis. The tincture is also used as a sedative, for choreic states (involuntary rapid movements due to a brain disorder), fever, lumbago and snake bite.

Other uses: Treatment of high blood pressure, tinnitus (ringing in the ears), asthma, whooping cough and dyspepsia.

herbs

Probable mode of action: Active constituents include glycosides, isoflavones and salicylic acids. The compounds in the root are reported to bind to the oestrogen receptor. The effect is similar to that of the female hormone oestrogen which prevents symptoms such as hot flushes and psychological disturbances. Known to have an effect on the uterus. Also reported to have central dopaminergic activity (activity similar to a chemical messenger in the brain – dopamine).

There have been recent concerns about substitution of *Cimicufuga racemosa* with other American or Chinese species, which may have implications for mechanisms of action, efficacy and safety.

Adverse effects: Gastrointestinal disturbances, hypotension, nausea, headaches. Overdose can cause dizziness, vertigo and irritation of the central nervous system. Hepatitis has been reported. In 2006, the European Medicine Agency required labelling on black cohosh to carry warnings about liver damage.

Precautions: Not recommended during pregnancy or while breastfeeding. May interfere with therapy of breast carcinoma. Should not be taken concomitantly with iron. Some herbalists recommend that black cohosh should not be taken continuously for more than six months.

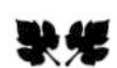

BLACK HAW

Viburnum prunifolium

Was used by Cherokee and Delaware American Indian tribes as an antispasmodic for complaints associated with the female reproductive system. Reported to have been used by slave owners to forestall abortions in female slaves trying to abort using cotton root bark.

Was included in the US Pharmacopeia from 1882 to 1926.

Medicinal parts: Bark of the trunk and the root.

Uses: Dysmenorrhoea (painful menstruation).

Other uses: Has been used to lower blood pressure and as an antispasmodic in asthma.

Probable mode of action: The herb is recorded to have spasmolytic effects and an undefined effect on the uterus.

Adverse effects: Symptoms of black haw overdose that have been reported include nausea, dizziness, fits (seizures), visual disturbances, increased perspiration and a reduced pulse rate. Rarely allergic reactions may occur.

Precautions: Should be avoided during pregnancy because of its effects on the uterus.

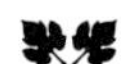

BLACK PEPPER AND WHITE PEPPER

Piper nigrum

The name pepper is derived from a Sanskrit word pippali. This gave rise to the Greek *peperi* and Latin *piper*.

Trading routes that followed the wars of Alexander the Great in Central Asia brought pepper to Europe and this became a very important item of commerce.

Became a status symbol of cookery during Roman times.

Black pepper is native to Malabar (Kerala state in India) and has been cultivated for millennia. The dried fruits are known as peppercorns. Depending on the harvest time and processing, peppercorns can be black, white, green or reddish.

Medicinal parts: Dried berry-like fruits. Black pepper is the dried unripe berry; white pepper is the dried ripe fruit from which the outer pericarp has been removed.

Uses: In folk medicine, pepper is used for stomach disorders and problems with digestion, neuralgia and scabies.

Other uses: In Chinese medicine, black pepper is used for vomiting, diarrhoea and gastric symptoms. **In Indian medicine**, uses include arthritis, asthma, fever, coughs, catarrh, dysentery, stomach ailments (dyspepsia, flatulence), haemorrhoids, hiccoughs, urethral discharge and skin damage. Also used as an insecticide.

Probable mode of action: Black pepper contains about 3% essential oil (including monoterpene hydrocarbons, sesquiterpenes). The essential oil content of white pepper is lower (1%). The constituents are considered to stimulate the temperature receptors and also increase the secretion of saliva and gastric mucous. Reported to have an effect against bacteria. Acts on the liver and is thought to have other metabolic effects.

Adverse effects: Not known.

Precautions: Not known.

BLESSED THISTLE

Cnicus benedictus

A popular folk remedy used by monks during the Middle Ages. In Renaissance Europe, blessed thistle gained a reputation as a 'cure-all' and was believed to have fought off the plague.

Medicinal parts: Dried leaves, upper stems and flowering parts.

Approved by Commission E for:
- dyspepsia (indigestion)
- loss of appetite.

Uses: Loss of appetite, fever and colds.

Other uses: Diuretic. Uses **in folk medicine** include management of loss of appetite (anorexia), fever and colds, and as a diuretic. Externally it has been applied to wounds and ulcers. Has been included in the unproven herbal remedy Essiac. The herb has been tested in the laboratory for treatment of cancers and inflammation.

Probable mode of action: The terpenoid constituents are considered to have an action against bacteria (antimicrobial) and against malignant cells (cytotoxic and antitumour effects), and to increase the flow of saliva and gastric juices. An antioedema (prevention of swelling) effect has been demonstrated in animals.

Adverse effects: May cause allergic reactions (contact dermatitis following direct contact) in individuals sensitive to the members of the Asteraceae/Compositae family. May also cause irritation to the eyes. If taken in excess of 5 g per cup of tea, stomach irritation and vomiting may occur. Cross-reactivity may occur with mugwort and echinacea. Cross-reactivity may also occur with bitter weed, blanket flower, chrysanthemum, colt's foot, dandelion and marigold.

Precautions: As the herb is considered to increase stomach acid secretion, it should be used with caution in patients with gastric ulcers and heartburn. As laboratory studies have also shown a tendency to increase bleeding, care should be taken in patients on anticoagulants or blood thinning agents. Avoid in patients awaiting surgery. No evidence of safety, so should not be used in pregnancy.

BLOOD ROOT

Sanguinaria canadensis

The root has been used by American Indians as a dye for their bodies and clothes. The US FDA has approved the inclusion of one of the active constituents, sanguinarine, in toothpaste as an antibacterial and antiplaque agent.

Has been traditionally used to stimulate menstruation and abortion.

Medicinal part: Roots.

Uses: Bronchitis, asthma, croup, laryngitis, pharyngitis.

Other uses: To promote menstruation and removal of secretions from the lung. Also to lower the pulse rate and to treat palpitations. The extract has been used to treat ringworm and as a local application to treat eczema. To improve circulation, for nasal polyps and in dental hygiene to decrease plaque formation and bleeding from gums.

Probable mode of action: The constituents are reported to have effects against bacteria (antimicrobial) and antiseptic effects. Also reported to prevent or relieve spasms (spasmolytic) and to promote removal of secretions in the chest by coughing (expectorant). Initially the constituents may produce a narcotic (inducing sleep) effect and cause severe cramping, followed by local paralysis of sensitive nerve endings.

Adverse effects: None documented for blood root. In animals, high doses of one of the constituents (sanguinarine), has caused diarrhoea and disturbances in gait (ataxia). Liver toxicity has been reported in animals after intra-peritoneal injections. Toxic doses cause burning of the stomach, intense thirst, vomiting, faintness and dimness of eye sight.

Precautions: Because of the pharmacologically active constituents, blood root is best avoided during pregnancy and lactation.

BLUE COHOSH – PAPOOSE ROOT

Caulophyllum thalictroides

Papoose root is a traditional herbal remedy of many North American Indian tribes and was used externally by them to facilitate childbirth.

The roasted seed is a substitute for coffee.

Medicinal part: The root.

Uses: Menstrual disorders such as amenorrhoea, dysmenorrhoea, threatened miscarriage. Also used to treat contraction-like spasms (spasmolytic), rheumatic symptoms and particularly for uterine atonia.

Other uses: In Indian medicine, the herb is used mainly for gynaecological disorders. In British and American medicine, the herb has been used since the beginning of the 20th century for worm infestations, dehydration, menstrual ailments and cramps, and during labour mainly to stimulate contractions and act as an antispasmodic. Recommended for rheumatism of hands and fingers.

Has also been used as a diuretic (increases passage of urine) and to aid in the removal of secretions from the chest (expectorant).

Probable mode of action: Constituents include alkaloids such as methylcystine (1/40th potency of nicotine) and glycosides. The glycoside constituent is thought to have an oxytocic effect (similar to oxytocin which stimulates uterine contractions). Other constituents have a weak oestrogenic effect (an effect similar to the female hormone oestrogen). N-Methylcysteine is considered to raise blood pressure and stimulate breathing (nicotinic effects – effects of one component of the parasympathetic nervous system).

Adverse effect: Excessive doses may cause high blood pressure and symptoms similar to nicotine poisoning. Overdose may cause nausea, vomiting, headache, thirst, dilated pupils, muscle weakness, incoordination and narrowing of blood vessels to the heart muscle. Powdered root can have an irritant effect on mucous membranes.

Precautions: Should not be used during the first three months of a pregnancy. The alkaloid constituents may cause teratogenic (abnormalities during the formation of organs) effects. As blue cohosh increases blood flow to the pelvis, avoid in subjects with heavy menstruation. Has inhibited ovulation in rat experiments. Contraindicated in patients with ischaemic heart disease (angina and heart attacks) and in patients with high blood pressure.

BLUE FLAG – HARLEQUIN BLUE FLAG

Iris versicolor

Was a symbol of majesty. Its shaping originated

the sceptre, invented by the early Egyptians. Provincial flower of Quebec, Canada.

Medicinal parts: Dried rhizome – decoctions and liquid extracts are made from it.

Uses: Skin diseases, bile duct (biliary) disease and constipation.

Other uses: Liver disorders. Has been used to treat syphilis and used externally to treat eczema.

Probable mode of action: Not known. Constituents include salicylic acid and many others, the precise effects of which are not known with certainty.

Adverse effects: Fresh root can cause nausea and vomiting. The volatile oil furfural is irritant to mucous membranes and causes lachrymation (tears) and inflammation of the eyes. Irritation of the throat and headache has also been reported. The sap can cause dermatitis.

Precautions: Should not be used internally except in small doses. There is a risk of nausea and vomiting with the dried root. Should not be used by people with allergies or sensitivities. Best avoided during pregnancy because safety in pregnancy has not been established. The species has been implicated in several poisonings in humans.

BOGBEAN – BUCKBEAN

Menyanthes trifoliata

Was considered very useful in the treatment of scurvy.

Medicinal part: Dried herb.

Uses: Stomach ailments (dyspepsia), loss of appetite (anorexia).

Other uses: Rheumatism, rheumatoid arthritis, muscular rheumatism with asthenia and treatment of dropsy (swelling usually of the ankles).

European folk medicine used bogbean for diseases of the digestive system and fevers.

Probable mode of action: Constituents include caffeic acid and salicylic acid. Bogbean is a bitter that stimulates gastric secretion and secretion of saliva. The salicylic acid and P-hydroxybenzoic acid constituents are thought to be responsible for the antiarthritic effect. Laboratory experiments have demonstrated an effect against bacteria (antimicrobial effect).

Adverse effects: Large doses may cause abdominal pains, nausea, diarrhoea and vomiting. There have been reports of red cell damage (haemolysis). Some of these effects may be due to the salicylic acid constituent.

Precautions: Safety in pregnancy has not been established, so is best avoided during pregnancy particularly as bogbean can cause diarrhoea.

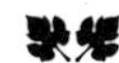

BOLDO

Peumus boldus

One of the most widely used medicinal plants in Chile. Fossilized boldo leaves more than 13,000 years old imprinted with human teeth have been found in Chile. Used as a herbal tea in Chile, Argentina, Brazil and many Spanish speaking countries.

Approved by Commission E for:

- dyspeptic complaints (indigestion).

Medicinal part: Leaves.

Uses: Dyspepsia (e.g. loss of appetite, flatulence, constipation, digestive difficulties), digestive disturbances (spastic gastrointestinal complaints), gallstones, pain in the liver or gallbladder.

Other uses: Urinary bladder infections (cystitis), rheumatism, as a diuretic. Has been used in the treatment of gonorrhoea.

Probable mode of action: Constituents include flavonoids and alkaloids, including boldine. Boldo essential oil contains the irritant and diuretic principle in juniper oil. Flavonoid and alkaloid constituents possibly produce effects on the gastrointestinal tract and liver and gallbladder. Animal experiments showed that boldine protected the liver against carbon tetrachloride-induced injury (carbon tetrachloride is a potent toxin of the liver). Boldine was also shown in animal experiments to have a dose-dependent relaxant effect on some parts of the gastrointestinal tract (ileum), acting as a competitive antagonist of acetylcholine – the chemical messenger that causes contraction of the bowel. Beneficial effects of boldo were increased when combined with rhubarb, cascara and gentian.

Adverse effects: Boldo volatile oil is one of the most toxic oils. In animal experiments application of the undiluted oil to the backs of mice had an irritant effect. Excessive doses have caused irritation of the kidney and genitourinary tract. A massive overdose can cause paralysis.

Precautions: Should not be used by patients with kidney disease. Treatment should always be under supervision of a physician for any disorder. Safety in pregnancy has not been established and in view of the potential irritant qualities, boldo should be avoided during pregnancy. Should not be used if there is an obstruction of the bile duct or in severe liver disease. The oil of boldo contains a high concentration of a toxin called ascaridiole and should never be used.

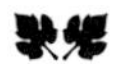

BONESET – COMMON BONESET

Eupatorium perfoliatum

Boneset leaves were used in bandages for broken bones since the joined leaves gave an impression that the plant would help in rejoining broken bones. Was used by Native Americans to treat malaria. Has been traditionally taken as a tea or tincture.

Medicinal parts: Aerial parts of the flowering plant.

Uses: To relieve the aches and pains that heralds the onset of flu. Reduces fever in flu and other fevers.

Other uses: Pain of rheumatism, muscular pains and to ease constipation.

Probable mode of action: Some constituents are known to increase the effectiveness of white blood cells in destroying bacteria (phagocytosis) and also to increase immunity. It is also a bitter and also a stimulant of the immune system. The flavones are considered to promote healthy functioning of cells.

Adverse effects: Sensitization may occur. Increased sweating and diarrhoea have also been reported. May cause dermatitis.

Precautions: Necessary to be aware that the herb has pyrrolizidine alkaloids which have the potential to cause liver toxicity. However, the content of these toxic alkaloids in boneset is considered to be very low. Some herbalists consider that boneset should not be used in patients with high fever (temperature in excess of 102°F). Others state that boneset should not be used continuously for more than six months. Should be considered as a potentially toxic plant and should not be used during breastfeeding.

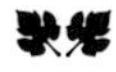

BORAGE

Borago officinalis

Originated in Syria. Leaves were used in salads and soups in Germany and are reported to taste like cucumber.

Medicinal parts: Dried flowers and dried or fresh foliage, stems and leaves.

Uses: For dermatitis, coughs and throat illnesses, rheumatism and depression; as an anti-inflammatory agent and diuretic for kidney diseases.

Other uses: Treatment of phlebitis (inflammation of the veins), menopausal complaints. **In folk medicine**, borage is used for coughs, throat illnesses and bronchial disorders. Also used as an anti-inflammatory agent in kidney and bladder disorders. Preparations containing borage have been used for blood purification, treatment of dehydration and as performance-enhancing agent.

Probable mode of action: Constituents include pyrrolizidine alkaloids, potassium and calcium, tannin, and mucin. Tannins contract cells (skin and other) following inflammation (astringent). The mucin constituent is considered useful in bronchial disorders. Constituents oleic and palmitic acid produce cholesterol lowering effects.

Adverse effects: Risk of hepatotoxicity (liver toxicity) and hepatocarcinogenicity (liver carcinoma) from the pyrrolizidine alkaloids.

Precautions: Even though the pyrrolizidine alkaloid content is small, the herb should not be administered medicinally.

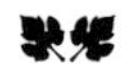

BOSWELLIA – FRANKINCENSE

Boswellia serrata – Indian frankincense

The Biblical incense frankincense was probably an extract from the resin of *Boswellia carteri*. Has been used in Ayurveda for centuries.

Medicinal part: The resin gum exuded when incisions are made in the bark.

Uses: As a carminative. The herb is considered obsolete for medicinal use as the mode of action has not been documented.

Other uses: Long history of use for a wide range of disorders including asthma, arthritis, diarrhoea and syphilis.

Probable mode of action: Constituents, of which there are several, have shown activity against bacteria (antibacterial). Local applications are beneficial possibly due to the essential oil and mucin constituents. A constituent is considered to inhibit production of some substances that cause narrowing of the small breathing tubes (bronchioles – bronchoconstriction).

Adverse effects: Irritant to the skin and may cause allergic contact dermatitis.

Precautions: Safety during pregnancy is not known. Best avoided during pregnancy and lactation.

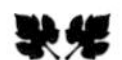

BROOM

Cytisus scoparius

Use as a medicinal herb dates back to the 15th century AD. Used in ancient Anglo-Saxon medicine and by Welsh physicians in early middle ages. Had a place in the London Pharmacopoeia of 1618. Twigs and branches are used for making brooms and for thatching of cottage roofs.

Medicinal parts: Flower, seeds, root and whole herb.

Uses: As a cathartic and diuretic and to induce labour.

Other uses: In folk medicine and homeopathy, broom has been used as a diuretic and to induce vomiting. Broom cigarettes are believed to cause euphoria and relaxation.

Probable mode of action: The active constituents include the alkaloids sparteine and scoparin. The exact actions of these are not certain as yet, but scoparin possibly induces diuresis.

Adverse effects: Nicotine-like poisoning has been reported. Has been an agent of abuse. Large doses may cause stomach discomfort and diarrhoea.

Precautions: Avoid during pregnancy as it can induce labour, and cause heart arrhythmias due to the oxysparteine constituent. Has an action similar to hemlock on the heart. Death may occur due to respiratory failure.

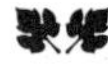

BUCHU

Barosma betulina

Traditional remedy of the Khoikhoin people of South Africa for treating urinary infections such as cystitis and urethritis. Has been used in Cape Town as a stimulant and remedy for stomach troubles, where the herb is infused in brandy – Buchu Brandy.

Medicinal part: Infusion made from dried leaves.

Uses: Used in urinary infections such as cystitis and urethritis.

Other uses: For prostate inflammation, fluid retention and vaginal thrush and as an insect repellant. Used for bloating caused by premenstrual syndrome. Also used to treat colds and flu.

Probable mode of action: Constituents include flavonoids, volatile oils including diosphenol, and mucilage. Diosphenol has antiseptic properties and may be responsible for diuretic and antiviral (effective against viruses) and vasodilator (dilates blood vessels) activity.

Adverse effects: Has been reported to cause abortion. Stomach upsets and or diarrhoea may occur.

Precautions: Not recommended during pregnancy or while breastfeeding. Because of the diuretic action of buchu, it is advisable to consume potassium-rich foods (e.g. bananas, fresh vegetables) while taking the herb. Avoid taking buchu on an empty stomach. Avoid in kidney disease.

BUCKTHORN – COMMON BUCKTHORN

Rhamnus catharticus

Has been used as a purgative though its toxicity makes it a harmful herbal medicine. It is rarely used at present. Used primarily as a dye.

Approved by Commission E for:
- constipation.

Medicinal parts: Whole ripe dried fruit and fresh ripe fruit.

Uses: Used internally as a laxative for constipation and for bowel movement in cases of anal fissures and haemorrhoids. It is used after ano-rectal surgery and in preparation for diagnostic procedures of the gastrointestinal tract and to achieve a softer stool. **In folk medicine**, it is used as a diuretic in blood purifying remedies.

Probable mode of action: Constituents include anthraquinones and frangulin. The anthranoid constituents produce a more liquid stool and increase the volume of the bowel contents; they also increase contractions of the bowel (peristalsis).

Adverse effects: Diarrhoea, weakness. May turn the urine dark yellow or red, which is harmless. If used for more than 10 days consecutively, potassium loss from the body may occur.

Precautions: Contraindicated in intestinal obstruction, acute inflammatory bowel disease, appendicitis and abdominal pain of unknown origin. Should not be used during pregnancy or nursing unless prescribed by a physician. Not to be administered to children under the age of 12 years.

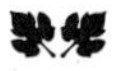

BUGLE WEED

Lycopus virginicus/Lycopus europaeus

Was considered to 'drive away' many forms of disease during the 17th century. Has been used to cure hangovers.

Approved by Commission E for:
- nervousness
- premenstrual syndrome.

Medicinal parts: Aerial parts collected just before the buds open.

Uses: As a sedative, and to contract cells (skin and other) following inflammation (astringent), as a diuretic, as a cardioactive agent used for nervous tachycardia (to prevent increase in heart rate due to nervousness), as a peripheral vasoconstrictor (constricts peripheral blood vessels causing an increase in blood pressure), an antitussive (cough suppressant) and an antihaemorrhagic (especially used to treat pulmonary haemorrhage – bleeding). Also used to treat thyroid disorders.

Lycopus extracts have been used empirically in the treatment of Graves' disease, characterized by hyperactivity of the thyroid gland or thyrotoxicosis with cardiac (heart) involvement where the symptoms include tightness of breathing, palpitations and shaking (tremors). Current uses are predominantly for increased activity of the thyroid gland and for premenstrual syndrome symptoms such as breast pain.

Other uses: Historically has been used to treat tuberculosis. Used in the treatment of nosebleeds, for heavy bleeding during menstruation and as a sedative. *Lycopus europaeus* yields a black dye which was used by gypsies to stain the skin.

Probable mode of action: Constituents include flavone glycosides, volatile oils, phenols and tannins. Tannins are attributed with effects on hormones (the hormone associated with reproduction – antigonadotropic hormone – affects reproduction) and the thyroid hormone. The antigonadotropic effect is also attributed to the phenolic constituents. Active constituents increase the force of contraction of the heart muscle and reduce heart rate; in Graves' disease the plant extract has been shown to bind and inhibit a thyroid-stimulating antibody found in the blood. Also inhibits the de-iodinization of a thyroid hormone.

Adverse effects: Has been known to cause enlargement of the thyroid gland.

Precautions: Should not be used by patients with thyroid disease or given concomitantly with thyroid therapy. Avoid use during pregnancy.

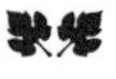

BURDOCK – GREATER BURDOCK

Arctium lappa

Japanese term: Gobo
Has been a favourite medicinal herb for centuries. The Swiss inventor George de Mestral developed Velcro after observing the seeds of the burdock plant.

Medicinal parts: Ripe seed and the fresh or dried roots.

Uses: For ailments of the gastrointestinal tract, and to induce perspiration (diaphoretic) and as a diuretic. Also for purifying the blood. Externally, burdock root is used for skin disorders such as ichthyosis, psoriasis and dandruff.

Other uses: In Chinese medicine, burdock is used to treat carbuncles, ulcers and erythema (redness) of the skin, and sore throats. Believed to increase production of breast milk.

Probable mode of action: Constituents have been shown to have mild antimicrobial activity (effective against bacteria). It is also considered to be a diuretic, to increase the formation and flow of bile and to reduce fever by inducing sweating. Also reported to cause contraction of uterine muscle. Root oil extract is rich in phytosterols and essential fatty acids, nutrients required to maintain a healthy scalp and promote natural hair growth.

Adverse effects: Can cause allergic reactions.

Precautions: Contraindicated during pregnancy.

BURNET – GREATER BURNET

Sanguisorba officinalis

Has been used in Traditional Chinese Medicine for thousands of years, particularly to treat bleeding.

Medicinal parts: The aerial parts, root. The root has been specifically used to treat bloody dysentery.

Uses: Ulcerative colitis and acute diarrhoea, treatment of peptic ulcers and the passage of blood in the urine (haematuria).

Other uses: For haemorrhoids, menstrual disturbances and to decrease bleeding (to slow or arrest blood flow). For nosebleeds. Used topically to treat eczema, burns and insect bites.

Probable mode of action: Insufficient information about the constituents of the herb. The roots have been found to contain tannins, which decrease bleeding.

Adverse effects: None documented.

Precautions: Best avoided during pregnancy in view of the lack of information about toxicity.

Suggested that the herb may interact with the group of allopathic medications known as fluoroquinolones.

BUTCHER'S BROOM – KNEE HOLLY

Ruscus aculeatus

Roman scholar Pliny reported the use of butcher's broom for the treatment of varicose veins in 60 AD. Was recommended by Dioscorides and other ancient physicians for dropsy (swelling, usually of the ankles). Butchers in Europe used the leaves and twigs to scrub chopping blocks clean.

Approved by Commission E for:

- haemorrhoids (piles)
- venous conditions.

Medicinal parts: Leaves, rhizomes and roots.

Uses: To treat symptoms of chronic venous insufficiency, such as pain and heaviness, as well as for cramps in the legs, itching and swelling, (oedema). Used for itching and burning associated with haemorrhoids. Considered to be useful in preventing eye changes that may occur in diabetes mellitus.

Probable mode of action: The primary active ingredients are the steroidal saponins. They possess activity on veins, increasing the tone of the veins, and have an effect on walls of blood capillaries and a diuretic effect. They reduce vascular permeability. The mechanism by which narrowing (constriction) of blood vessels occur is uncertain, but possibly calcium ions have a role.

Adverse effects: No adverse effects have been reported following administration of recommended doses. The berries may cause diarrhoea.

Precautions: Contraindicated during pregnancy and breastfeeding. Caution required if used in patients on treatment for high blood pressure. An increase in tone of veins (similar to constriction of the veins) can influence blood pressure by increasing the amount of blood returned to the heart.

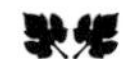

BUTTERNUT – WHITE WALNUT

Juglans cinerea

The Latin name *juglans* derives from Jovis glans – 'Jupiter's nuts', the nut fit for a god.

Medicinal part: Dried inner bark collected in early summer.

Uses: Constipation, liver disease (hepatic dysfunction) skin lesions associated with oozing (exudative skin eruptions). Specifically indicated in constipation associated with stomach complaints (dyspepsia). The quills or inner bark are one of the few potent laxatives that are safe to use in pregnancy. It is also of use in chronic or acute skin conditions associated with bowel and/or liver dysfunction. It will expel worms and has been used for colds with fever and flu-like illnesses.

Other uses: Syphilis, old (chronic) ulcers. Preparations of the bark are also used for gallbladder disease and haemorrhoids and in the treatment of skin disease (usually combined with dandelion). Considered particularly useful for skin disorders associated with diseases of the intestine.

Probable mode of action: The constituents have been shown to possess effects against bacteria (antimicrobial), against malignant or cancer cells (antineoplastic) and effects against intestinal parasites/worms (vermifuge). Constituents have a gentle laxative action and are considered to act as a tonic.

Adverse effects: The naphthoquinone constituents may cause gastric (stomach) irritation.

Precautions: To be avoided in patients with gallstones.

CAJUPUT – WHITE WOOD

Melaleuca leucadendra

Inhabitants of the islands in the Indian Ocean use the herb for rheumatism, epilepsy and many other disorders.

Recommended by Commission E for:

- rheumatism
- neurogenic pain
- temporary relief of muscular pain
- tendency to infection
- wounds and burns.

Medicinal part: Oil distilled from fresh leaves and twigs.

Uses: For painful muscles and joints in rheumatic disorders, sciatica, lumbago, slipped disk and low back pain. Also used for muscular tension and pain following sports injuries such as sprains, bruising and pulled muscles and ligaments. Applied to a cavity of a carious tooth to relieve discomfort.

Probable mode of action: The constituents have been shown in the laboratory to relieve muscle pains and to be active against bacteria.

Adverse effects: If applied locally to the face, life-threatening swelling of the upper respiratory passages (glottic oedema, asthma) may occur, particularly in children.

Precautions: Not to be applied to the face of infants or children. Should not be taken internally in the presence of inflammatory disease of the gastrointestinal tract, bile duct disease or liver disease. Avoid self-administration.

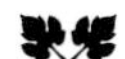

CALAMUS – COMMON SWEET FLAG

Acorus calamus

Has long been a symbol of male love and has been an item of trade in many cultures for thousands of years. Considered to be a powerful aphrodisiac.

Medicinal part: Rhizome after the removal of all other material.

Uses: As a carminative for acute and chronic dyspepsia, gastritis (spasmolytic, intestinal colic) and to induce perspiration (diaphoretic). Used externally for skin eruptions.

Other uses: Used orally for anorexia and externally for rheumatism, gum disease and tonsillitis. **In Indian medicine**, calamus is used for stomach (dyspeptic) complaints, worms, pain syndromes and toothache. **In Chinese medicine**, calamus is used to stimulate gastric and intestinal secretions in the treatment of diseases of the gastrointestinal tract. Used externally for fungal infestations. **In Ayurveda**, the herb is considered to be a rejuvenator of the brain.

Probable mode of action: Papaverine is a relaxant of smooth muscles and a constituent of calamus has a similar action. Has been found to inhibit monoamine oxidase activity (an enzyme which is involved in the breakdown of substances like adrenaline). Small-animal experiments have shown a sedative action potentiating the effect of barbiturates (a sleeping tablet). Calamus is an aromatic bitter which stimulates appetite and digestion. Thus the herb has spasmolytic, carminative and sedative effects.

Adverse effects: Bath oils containing calamus have caused redness of the skin (erythema) and dermatitis, particularly in hypersensitive individuals. Toxic effects have been associated with calamus oil, probably due to the beta asarone content. Tumours appeared in rats that received Indian calamus oils over a prolonged period.

Precautions: Use of the oil is not recommended. Only roots free from or with a low content of beta asarone should be used in human herb therapy. In foods and beverages, the level of beta asarone permitted in the final product is restricted. Should be avoided in patients taking monoamine oxidase inhibitor antidepressants because the effect of the antidepressant could be potentiated and dangerous side-effects of the antidepressant may occur. Should not be used during pregnancy and lactation. Long-term use is not recommended.

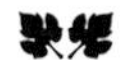

CALENDULA – MARIGOLD

Calendula officinalis

Calendula has been mentioned in medical texts dating back to 1373.

Marigold flowers are approved by Commission E for:

- inflammation of the mouth and pharynx (throat)
- wounds and burns.

Medicinal parts: Flowers collected and dried. Calendula herb consists of the fresh or dried above-ground parts harvested during the flowering season. Harvest begins in July. Drying takes place in the shade at a maximum temperature of 45°C.

Uses: Marigold has been extensively used as a folk medicine. Externally it is used for varicose disorders, vascular disease (diseases of blood vessels), wounds, inflammatory skin disease and eczema. It is used internally for inflammatory conditions of internal organs, gastrointestinal ulcers, constipation and worm infestations. During the 19th century, marigold was used as treatment for cancer.

The herb is used to improve the circulation, to treat ulcers, swelling of the glands, jaundice, wounds and eczema. The herb is used in **Russia** for streptococcal throat infections and in the **Canary Islands** for coughs and cramps. In **China**, it is used for irregular menstruation.

Other uses: For menstrual (period) pains, gastric and duodenal ulcers, colds, coughs and viral illnesses. Applied externally for skin problems including nappy rash, varicose veins, cuts and grazes (wounds), chilblains, fungal infections and insect stings. Also used for mouth ulcers. It is a constituent of treatment used for sore dry skin, bee stings and frostbite.

Probable mode of action: Constituents include flavonoids, the essential oil saponin and others. Effects attributed to the essential oil constituent are contraction of cells (skin and other) following inflammation (astringent) and granulation tissue promoting effects (promoting healing of wounds), anti-inflammatory, antifungal, stimulant and diuretic effects. A recent study suggests that calendula may stimulate the immune system.

Adverse effects: No adverse effects have been associated with the use of the herb in recommended doses. Low potential for sensitization and contact dermatitis. Allergies may occur in those allergic to plants of the daisy family. Topical use may cause a rash.

Precautions: Not recommended during pregnancy. If applied to a wound and there has been no improvement in 5–7 days, medical advice should be sought. To be used with great caution in children under 10 years of age.

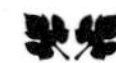

CALUMBA

The dried root of *Jateorhiza palmata*

Indigenous to Mozambique where it is used for dysentery. Calumba is included in nearly all pharmacopoeias.

Medicinal parts: The root.

Uses: To treat dyspepsia, diarrhoea and anorexia. A mild bitter which is free of astringent effects. Rarely used even though the bitter is compatible with iron preparations (e.g. iron salts).

Probable mode of action: Contains alkaloids that have narcotic (induce sleep) properties and side-effects similar to morphine.

Adverse effects: Large doses cause vomiting and abdominal pain. Overdoses would be expected to cause coma.

Precautions: Use in pregnancy should be avoided because safety has not been established.

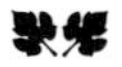

CANADIAN GOLDENROD

Solidago canadensis

Inventor Thomas Edison experimented with goldenrod to produce rubber.

Approved by Commission E for:
- infections of the urinary tract
- kidney and bladder stones.

Medicinal parts: Dried aerial parts collected during the flowering season, flowers, flowering twigs.

Uses: The herb is used as flushing-out therapy for inflammatory diseases of the lower urinary tract. The root has been used as a poultice for burns. Has been used as a mouthwash for thrush. A tea from the flowers is used for diarrhoea and body pains.

Probable mode of action: Canadian goldenrod is a diuretic, weak spasmolytic and an antiphlogistic (countering inflammation and fever). Contains saponins that are antifungal.

Adverse effects: Weak potential for sensitization.

Precautions: Irrigation therapy is contraindicated in cases of oedema (swelling, usually of the ankles) due to heart or renal disease. Care must be taken in patients with chronic kidney disease for whom it should be used only under the supervision of a physician.

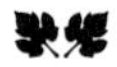

CAPSICUM

Capsicum annum
Capsicum baccatum
Capsicum frutescens
Capsicum pubescens

Has been a part of the human diet since about 7500 BC and is one of the oldest cultivated crops. Columbus is credited for introducing chillies to Europe and subsequently to Africa and Asia.

Approved by Commission E for:
- muscular tension
- rheumatism.

Medicinal parts: The fresh or dried fruits of different *Capsicum* species.

Uses: Applied externally for painful muscle spasms of the shoulder, arm and spine.

Other uses: Externally for neuralgia, rheumatic pains, unbroken chilblains. In the UK, creams containing capsaicin 0.025% and 0.075% are licensed for topical use in treating pain associated with osteoarthritis, diabetic neuropathy and post-herpetic neuralgia. Has been used for prophylactic therapy for arteriosclerosis, stroke and heart disease. Has also been used as an aid in female sexual dysfunction.

In folk medicine, the herb is used externally for frostbite and chronic lumbago, and orally for colic and flatulent dyspepsia when there is no inflammation. Also as a gargle for chronic laryngitis.

In Indian medicine, it is used for gout, arthritis, sciatica, coughs and hoarseness. It has been used for lowering the temperature in malaria, yellow fever, scarlet fever and typhus. Has been used to treat cholera, oedema, anorexia nervosa (a serious disease where there is severe loss of appetite) and to reduce the desire for alcohol, along with sugar and cinnamon.

Probable mode of action: Capsaicin is a major constituent and intravenous injection of capsaicin has been reported to cause a dose-dependent increase in the secretion of hormones from the adrenal medulla (noradrenaline and adrenaline – catecholamines). Also considered to mobilize fat from fat tissues and reduce triglyceride levels (one of the fat components) in the blood.

The effects on acid secretion in the stomach and of gastric enzymes are uncertain.

Adverse effects: May cause gastrointestinal irritation, and excessive intake could cause gastroenteritis. May also cause liver and kidney damage. Capsaicinoids could be strongly irritant to mucosal membranes. Inhalation of paprika can induce a form of allergic alveolitis (allergic response in the alveoli in the lung). Has caused loss of protective corneal reflexes in animals.

Precautions: Avoid in patients taking monoamine oxidase inhibitor antidepressants and antihypertensive drugs (as it causes increased release of catecholamines – substances like adrenaline). Avoid excessive intake. Use minimal amounts if required during pregnancy. It is not known if capsicum is secreted in breast milk. Topical creams should not be used for more than two days at a time, and should not be used again for two weeks.

CARAWAY – PERSIAN CUMIN

Carum carvi

Indian name: Siya jeera

Caraway was considered useful by ancient Egyptians, Greeks and Romans. It was an considered to prevent lovers from straying and was an essential ingredient of 'love portions'. The seeds of caraway were prescribed to bring bloom to the cheeks of pale-faced young maidens. Often recognized as the most typical spice of the German speaking countries.

Approved by Commission E for:

- dyspeptic complaints.

Medicinal parts: Fruit and the oil obtained from the squashed fruit when ripe.

Uses: Gastrointestinal cramps, flatulence, and stomach complaints thought to be the result of nervousness.

Other uses: In folk medicine, to improve breast-feeding, as an emmenagogue (to regulate menstruation) and as a mouthwash to remove bad breath.

Probable mode of action: In animal experiments, antispasmodic effects have been observed. Effects against several bacteria (antimicrobial) have also been documented.

Adverse effects: Not known.

Precautions: Excessive intake can lead to kidney and liver damage.

CARDAMOM

Elettaria cardamomum
Amomum cardamomum

One of the most valued spices in the world. Has been mentioned by Theophrastus in 4th century BC and five centuries later by Dioscorides. By 1000 AD, cardamoms were an article of trade from India to Western countries. Cardamom is used as an ingredient in traditional systems of medicine in China, India, Korea and Vietnam.

Vikings came across cardamoms in Constantinople about 1000 years ago. The Arabs considered cardamoms as an aphrodisiac while the Indians used it as a cure for obesity.

Approved by Commission E for:

- common cold
- cough/bronchitis

- fevers and colds
- inflammation of the mouth and pharynx
- liver and gallbladder complaints
- loss of appetite
- tendency to infections.

Medicinal part: The oil extracted from the seeds and the fruits and seeds harvested shortly after ripening.

Uses: Stomach and digestive complaints (dyspepsia, vomiting and diarrhoea, morning sickness during pregnancy, loss of appetite).

Other uses: In Chinese medicine, cardamom is used for stomachache, nausea, vomiting and flatulence. **In Indian medicine**, cardamoms are used for disorders of the kidney and bladder. Green cardamoms (*Elettaria subulatum*) or 'Eliachi' are used in **India** to treat infections of the teeth and gums, pulmonary tuberculosis and digestive disorders. Has also been used as an antidote for snake and scorpion venom.

Probable mode of action: The constituents in the oil are effective against bacteria and fungi (essential oil is antibacterial and antimycotic). In animal experiments, the essential oil caused an increase in bile secretion and a reduction of gastric secretion.

Adverse effects: Can cause colic due to gallstones due to its ability to increase movements of the stones within the bile duct. People with sensitive skins should use the oil carefully. The oil may cause diarrhoea, nausea and vomiting.

Precautions: Avoid in patients with gallstones. Ayurveda advises avoidance during pregnancy.

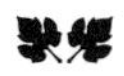

CASCARA SAGRADA

Rhamnus purshiana

Has a long history of traditional use by Native Americans. At present, it is one of the most common herbal laxatives.

Approved by Commission E for:

- constipation.

Medicinal part: Dried bark.

Uses: Constipation, relief of defaecation (passage of faeces) in patients with anal fissures, haemorrhoids and after recto-anal surgery. The herb is also used to prepare subjects for gastrointestinal procedures and to obtain a soft stool.

Other uses: In folk medicine, cascara is used as a tonic and for cleaning wounds.

Probable mode of action: One of the constituents – anthraglycoside – stimulates the lining of the lower intestine to normalize bowel function and cause a mild laxative effect.

Adverse effects: Abdominal cramps and dark pigmentation of the colon (melanosis coli) may follow use, the latter particularly after prolonged use. Can cause a shift of body fluids and electrolytes, particularly potassium. There is a report of cholestatic hepatitis (hepatitis following obstruction to flow of bile within the liver) complicated by portal hypertension following the use of cascara. Long-term use may also be associated with colorectal growths (adenomas and carcinoma). Cascara and senna may cause the passage of yellow-brown urine, which is harmless.

Precautions: Excessive use can cause cramps and diarrhoea. Do not use if intestinal obstruction is likely or in spastic bowel conditions, diverticulitis, heart failure, gastrointestinal cancers and after recent surgery on the large bowel (colon). Avoid during pregnancy and lactation. Limit treatment to 8–10 days. Long-term use can be habit forming. Fresh cascara can cause a bloody diarrhoea and vomiting. It should be aged for at least one year or treated with heat. Should not be used in children. May interact with digitalis therapy.

CASSIA – SENNA

Cassia senna
Cassia acutifolia

First record of use is by Arabic physicians in the 9th century. All ancient cultures (Aztecs, Asians, Africans) have used infusions of the cascara species as a laxative. Continues to be an ingredient of several over-the-counter laxatives. In Guatemala, Mexico, Venezuela and the Dominican Republic, the juice is one of the several remedies used for urinary ailments. Has been used as an abortifacient in South American traditional medicine.

Medicinal parts: The leaves, fruit and flowers.

Uses: Constipation.

Other uses: In Indian medicine, it is used for liver disease, jaundice, enlargement of the spleen (splenomegaly), anaemia and typhoid fever. Externally is used as suntan lotion, nasal spray, mouthwash, and as a counter-irritant.

In Chinese medicine, cassia bark was used for impotence, diarrhoea, enuresis, rheumatic conditions, menopause syndrome and amenorrhoea. **In folk medicine**, cassia has been used for heart pains, kidney troubles, hypertension, cramps and cancer. **In Ayurveda**, senna is used for skin ailments, jaundice, liver disease and typhoid infections.

Probable mode of action: Senna is an anthranoid-type stimulating laxative. Sennosides and their active metabolite rhein inhibit the absorption of water and electrolytes from the large intestine. This increases the bulk of the stool which stimulates peristalsis or contractions of the large bowel (colon). The laxative action of senna is also partially due to stimulation of colonic fluid and electrolyte secretion which is mediated by stimulation of endogenous prostaglandin E2 (a hormone) formation. Acts as a bulk laxative, i.e. by increasing the bulk of the stools. May also irritate the bowel and induce contraction.

Adverse reactions: May cause abdominal pain. Long-term use leads to loss of electrolytes, in particular potassium loss (hypokalaemia), which may result in hyperaldosteronism (aldosterone is a hormone that regulates loss of sodium and potassium from the body), albuminuria, haematuria, inhibition of intestinal motility and muscle weakness. Senna abuse has resulted in finger clubbing which was reversible upon discontinuation of the herb. In rare cases prolonged use may lead to cardiac arrhythmias (disturbances in the heart rhythm), nephropathies (kidney diseases), oedema and marked weakness of bones. Senna abuse has also resulted in tetany (symptoms associated with low body calcium) and hypogammaglobuminaemia (low gamma globulins – important for body defence in the blood).

Precautions: Limit treatment to 10 days. Do not use for treatment of intestinal obstruction, colitis, appendicitis or spastic conditions of the colon. Use under supervision during pregnancy and breastfeeding. Prolonged use of senna may lead to melanosis coli. Precursors of the melanic substance in melanosis coli may be derived from anthranoid laxatives. Anatomical alterations of the colon have occurred as a result of chronic use of senna (more than three times weekly for one year or longer).

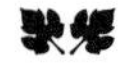

CASSIA ABSUS

Chamaecrista absus

In Pakistan, the seeds are considered to strengthen the eyes and the powdered form is used in the treatment of eye disorders such as conjunctivitis.

Medicinal parts: Leaves and seeds.

Uses: Eye conditions and dry skin conditions. In India, a plaster prepared from the leaves is used on sores on the penis and for purulent conjunctivitis. The seeds are prepared by enveloping them in a dough and placing in an onion and baking.

Other uses: Sterility, syphilis and gonorrhoea, pain, piles, upper gastrointestinal ailments (heartburn, dyspepsia), as an antiseptic/wound healing agent, to rid the body of internal parasites, and skin conditions such as carbuncles, boils, ulcers, abscess, pimples and pruritus.

Probable mode of action: To contract cells (skin and other) following inflammation (astringent). Contains an alkaloid that is reported to have effects against bacteria (antibacterial properties).

Adverse effects: Unknown.

Precautions: Safety unknown at present.

CASTOR OIL

Ricinus communis

Indian name: Arandi

Castor seeds were an important item of commerce in ancient Egypt and have been found in tombs dating from 4000 BC. The Indian script Susrutha Atharvaveda refers to castor seeds in 2000 BC as an oil used for lamps. The oil was used extensively as a laxative and to soften dry coarse skin. The Chinese used castor oil for centuries. Ayurvedic and Unani scriptures indicate that chewing of a single seed daily for a period of seven days after menstruation would prevent conception; however, chewing whole seeds would be extremely dangerous because the seeds of the castor oil plant contain ricin which is a deadly poison.

Castor oil is a vegetable oil obtained from the castor bean. US FDA recognizes castor oil as Generally Safe and Effective (GRASE) for over-the-counter use as a laxative. One of the derivatives, undecylenic acid, is also approved by the FDA for over-the-counter use for skin disorders.

Castor oil in the form of Cremophor EL is added to many allopathic medicines such as miconazole, paclitaxel, ciclosporin injections, nelfinavir mesylate and Emla cream.

Medicinal parts: Oil extracted from seeds, roots. Hulled seeds with the outer coat removed have been used but this is not recommended.

Uses: Castor oil is used orally as a laxative and to stimulate labour. It is used externally for rheumatic and skin disorders. A poultice of castor seeds was applied locally for gouty and rheumatic swellings, boils and swellings.

Other uses: In India, castor oil was massaged over the breasts after childbirth to increase the flow of milk. It was also applied locally to promote growth of hair and prevent dandruff. Cold pressed castor oil has been used for centuries throughout the world for its antibacterial and antimicrobial properties.

Probable mode of action: Castor oil does not contain the poisonous constituent ricin that is present in the whole seed. It contains ricinoleic acid which produces a laxative effect by stimulating the intestine and by increasing fluid secretion. Ricinoleic acid also has pain relieving (analgesic) and anti-inflammatory effects.

Adverse effects: Abdominal discomfort, cramping, nausea, loss of fluid and electrolytes. Studies have suggested the presence of allergens in *Ricinus communis*. Cases of asthma have been reported from the oil industry workers using *Ricinus communis*. Presence of castor oil in lipstick has allegedly caused allergic contact dermatitis.

Precautions: May be unsafe when used in high doses or for extended periods. Should not be used during pregnancy because it may induce premature labour and induce miscarriage. Should not be used to induce labour except under the supervision of a clinician.

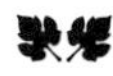

CAT'S CLAW

Uncaria tomentosa

Traditional Peruvian remedy for boosting the immune system to treat and prevent infection.

Some cultures refer to the plant as the 'sacred herb of the rain forest'.

Medicinal part: Root bark.

Uses: Cat's claw has been used **in folk medicine** for rheumatic complaints, diarrhoea, gastritis, treatment of wounds, as an adjunct in the treatment of cancer, asthma, menstrual irregularities and as a contraceptive.

Other uses: As an antiviral agent and for stimulation of the immune system and as an anti-inflammatory agent. In Peru it has been used as a contraceptive for centuries. The dose used is considered to be very high. Some herbalists use it to treat HIV infections.

Probable mode of action: The sterol constituents have been found to have an anti-inflammatory effect. Rhynchophylline has been found to inhibit venous and cerebral thrombosis (formation of blood clots in veins and vessels to the brain) in rabbits, and to increase dopamine (a chemical messenger found in the brain) release from certain parts of the brain. Hirsutine has potent ganglion blocking activity and has also been demonstrated to have antihypertensive effects (blockage of the sympathetic nervous system ganglia causing dilatation of the blood vessels).

Adverse effects: Serum oestradiol and progesterone (female hormones) levels may be reduced after prolonged use. A case of acute renal failure has been reported following the use of cat's claw. The tannins may cause some abdominal pain and/or diarrhoea.

Precautions: Although no serious adverse reactions have been reported, it is best avoided by pregnant and breastfeeding women. There are no known scientific reports on its use in children (paediatric use). As such the herb is best avoided in children. Should not be used by patients who have had skin grafts or suffering from tuberculosis or by those who have received organ transplants. Should not be used with immunosuppressants.

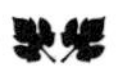

CAT'S FOOT

Antennaria dioica

Medicinal part: The flower.

Uses: For chronic problems of the bile ducts. For treatment of bladder stones, diarrhoea and respiratory and intestinal diseases, and as a diuretic. Considered to stimulate the flow of gastric juices and pancreatic secretions.

Probable mode of action: Has a spasmolytic action and increases flow of bile (choleric).

Adverse effects: Allergic reactions may occur in subjects sensitive to rag weed, chrysanthemums, marigold and daisies. May increase blood pressure.

Precautions: Safety during pregnancy is not known.

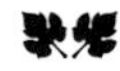

CATNIP

Nepeta cataria

Used for the treatment of nervousness, colds, influenza and fevers during the Middle Ages.

Medicinal parts: Aerial parts of the plant.

Uses: Folk medicine uses include treatment of colds, colic and fevers. It is also used for nervous disorders and migraine. In **England** and **France** there is a long tradition of using *Nepeta cataria* as a kitchen and medicinal herb and occasionally as a stimulating drink before the introduction of black tea. Considered to have astringent properties and is applied externally to cuts and scrapes to stop bleeding and promote healing.

Other uses: Indigestion, colic, headaches (migraine), insomnia, anxiety and as an emmenagogue (to regulate menstruation). Promotes sweating when used as a herbal tea. Used to promote and speed up growth of hair. Rarely used as an enema.

Probable mode of action: Constituents include nepetalactone, bitters, tannins and essential oils.

Considered to have antipyretic (lowers body temperature), antispasmodic (relieves spasms) and sedative properties and induces perspiration (diaphoretic). The tea has a diuretic effect and increases gallbladder activity. Constituents repel insects including mosquitoes.

Adverse effects: Catnip has diuretic properties and may increase the amount and frequency of urination. This may cause discomfort. Smoking catnip can produce euphoria and visual hallucinations. Sedation.

Precautions: Should not be taken by women who have inflammatory diseases of the pelvis or are pregnant. Subjects taking the herbal medicine should be careful when using machinery or driving motor vehicles.

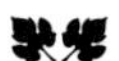

CELANDINE – GREATER CELANDINE

Chelidonium majus

Greater celandine was used to treat warts during the 17th century. Was used by French herbalists as hand and foot baths and teas, the latter particularly for diseases of the liver.

Medicinal parts: Aerial parts that have been collected during the flowering season and dried. The root which has been collected in late autumn and dried and the fresh rhizome are also used medicinally.

Approved by Commission E for:

- liver and gallbladder complaints.

Uses: Biliary colic and gastrointestinal colic, gallbladder disease (cholecystitis), intestinal polyps and breast lumps. Treatment of indigestion.

Other uses: In folk medicine, it is used for rashes, scabies, warts, chest pain (angina), cramps, asthma, arteriosclerosis, high blood pressure, stomach cancer, gout, oedema. **In Chinese medicine**, celandine is used for inflammation of the rim of the eyelid, febrile and ulcerating dermatitis, warts, oedema, ascites, jaundice and stomach carcinoma. Fresh roots are chewed to alleviate toothache. The root is used in Chinese medicine to regulate menstruation.

Probable mode of action: Alkaloids are the major constituents. Has mild pain relieving and central sedating properties. Increases flow of bile and acts as a spasmolytic (relieves or prevents spasms) on smooth muscle. In animal experiments, it has been shown to stop cell division (cytostatic). Also considered to have a non-specific stimulating effect on the immune systems. Extracts have been shown to increase the production of bile and increase pancreatic secretions.

Adverse effects: May cause burning sensation in the mouth, nausea and vomiting. Use of the fresh plant may cause stomach upsets. Topical use has been reported to cause intense itching.

Precautions: Avoid contact with eyes. Not to be used during pregnancy. At present there are concerns regarding liver toxicity and thus it is best avoided in those with liver disease. Should not be used in children under the age of 12 years.

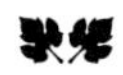

CELERY

Apium graveolens

Indian names: Ajmod, Ajwain-ka-patta

In Homer's *Iliad*, the horses graze on wild celery that grows in the marshes of Troy. Known to ancient Greeks, celery has been found in deposits dating back to the 9th century BC.

Root and seeds have been used in Ayurveda and Unani medicine and the beneficial effects have been known to the Chinese since the 5th century BC. In England, where it grew wild, it was known as smallage and was grown in gardens in the 16th and 17th centuries as a medicinal plant and for flavouring of soups and stews. Use of celery as a food was recorded in France in 1623.

Medicinal parts: The dried ripe fruits, roots and leaves.

Uses: Rheumatism, gout, headaches, loss of appetite and as a sedative and mild diuretic. Other traditional uses include prophylaxis of nervous agitation, treatment for loss of appetite and exhaustion. The seeds are attributed with anti-rheumatic, anti-inflammatory, diuretic, carminative and antispasmodic and sedative properties.

Other uses: For treatment of cough and as an antihelminthic. The plant has been used as an appetizer, diuretic and emmenagogue.

Probable mode of action: An irritant volatile oil in celery fruit is likely to contain the active constituents. The traditional view is that diuresis may result from irritation of the epithelial tissues of the kidneys. Phthalides, a volatile oil which give celery its distinctive smell, have been shown to have diuretic, antispasmodic, anticonvulsant and antitumour activity. A flavonoid constituent, apigenin, has been demonstrated to have antiplatelet activity (prevents normal action of platelets). Celery oil has bacteriostatic (prevents multiplication of bacteria) activity. Plant extracts have hypoglycaemic (blood sugar lowering) effects. The expressed juice of the plant has been considered effective for dropsy (swelling), rheumatic tendencies, gout, obesity and catarrh and is also considered to promote menstruation.

Adverse effects: Dermatitis has been reported in those handling or processing celery and may be caused by psolarens, which may be found in the vegetable stems or stalks. Allergic responses include anaphylaxis in sensitive individuals and cross-allergenicity can occur between celery, cucumber, carrot, watermelon and possibly apples. CNS depression has been documented following large doses of the oil, but the syndrome is not well characterized.

Precautions: Avoid during pregnancy, because emmenagogue, abortifacient and uterine stimulant activity has been reported. There is insufficient evidence to support safe use during lactation. Traditional texts caution the use of the herb in renal disorders because of the irritant effects of the volatile oil.

CENTAURY – FEVERWORT

Centaurium erythraea

Greek legend has it that Chiron (whom early Greeks considered to be the founder of medicine) used the herb to heal a wound caused by a poisoned arrow.

A magical herb during the mediaeval era, used by witches to increase their psychic powers. Considered a patron herb by the herbalists who used it to repel anger and other 'harmful energies'.

Listed by the Council of Europe as a natural source of food flavouring. In the US, the bitter principles of centaury are utilized in alcoholic and non-alcoholic beverages with maximum permitted doses between 0.0002% and 0.0008%.

Approved by Commission E for:
- dyspeptic complaints
- loss of appetite.

Medicinal parts: The dried aerial parts of the flowering plant.

Uses: Because it is an aromatic bitter, it is used in the treatment of anorexia (loss of appetite), dyspepsia and heartburn.

Other uses: In folk medicine, it is used to treat fever, worm infestations and to lower blood pressure. In **Mallorca** it is used for diabetes, and in **Egypt** for expelling kidney stones. It is used externally to treat wounds. **Saxon herbalists** used the herb for snake bites and other poisonings. Has also been used in the treatment of intermittent fevers, hence the name feverwort.

Probable mode of action: Constituents include acids (e.g. caffeic, vanillic), alkaloids, flavonoids, fatty acids and waxes. Has bitter and sedative properties and antipyretic (fever lowering effect) activity that is attributed to phenolic acids. Dose-dependent anticholinesterase activity (inhibition of the enzyme which metabolizes the chemical messenger acetylcholine) has been demonstrated in rats. This may be the basis for use in dyspepsia. Bitter constituents stimulate appetite and increase stomach secretions and causes salivation.

Adverse effects: May cause mild abdominal discomfort and cramps.

Precautions: Contraindicated in patients with peptic ulcers. Safety during pregnancy and lactation has not been established, so it is best avoided.

CEREUS – NIGHT–BLOOMING CEREUS

Selenicereus grandiflora
Cereus grandiflorus

The Death Valley Shoshone called this plant 'pain in the heart', and used it to treat angina-like pains. Several groups of Native Americans use the stem to treat diabetes. The Neapolitan homeopath Rubini used Cereus as a specific remedy in heart disease. In Mexico and Central America, folk medicine uses include haemoptysis (coughing of blood), menorrhagia (increased menstruation), dysmenorrhoea (painful menstruation), haemorrhage, cardiac complaints, urinary bladder infections (cystitis), shortness of breath and dropsy. Externally it is also used in these countries as a skin stimulant for rheumatism.

Used mainly in homeopathy. The plant was grown in the garden at Hampton Court during the 18th century. Considered by some to be an aphrodisiac.

Medicinal parts: The flower, stem and young shoots.

Uses: Angina pectoris (pain in the chest due to decreased blood supply to the heart muscle). It is used in the treatment of palpitations. Dropsy (swelling – oedema) and various heart diseases ('when the heart is enfeebled') where it is considered to increase the muscular energy of the heart. This effect is unconfirmed.

Other uses: Has been used for 'hot flushes' in women and for other post menopausal symptoms. Haemoptysis (coughing up of blood) and incipient apoplexy (stroke). Has been used for rheumatism in **Cuba**.

Probable mode of action: Reportedly contains a cardiotonic amine (hordenine), which increases the force of contraction of the heart (cardiac) muscle (inotropic). Considered to stimulate the nerve tone through improved nutrition of the entire nervous and muscular structure of the heart. Also reported to act on the brain centres controlling heart and blood vessel activity (vasomotor centre). The herb may act topically as an antiphlogistic (prevent inflammation).The constituents are considered to improve capillary stability by preventing leakage of fluid from capillaries. This may be the basis for use in swellings.

Adverse effects: In large doses cereus produces gastric irritation, slight delirium, hallucinations and general mental confusion. Fresh juice may cause itching and pustules on the skin, burning of the mouth, queasiness, vomiting and diarrhoea.

Precautions: Excessive doses will cause adverse effects in patients who are also taking monoamine oxidase antidepressants. This is probably due to the tyramine content which gives rise to adverse reactions in patients on monoamine oxidase inhibitor treatment. It is best avoided in patients with existing cardiac disease unless prescribed by a physician. Cardiac complaints are not suited for self-medication. May also interfere with the action of allopathic medicines used in the treatment of heart disease such as beta adrenegic blockers (beta-blockers), angiotensin-converting enzyme inhibitors (ACE inhibitors) and calcium channel blockers. Best avoided during pregnancy and lactation since safety has not been established.

❧

CHAMOMILE

Matricaria recutita
Chamaemelum nobile
Chamaelum nobile

Three varieties of chamomile plants are described in the herbal literature. They are German chamomile (*Matricaria recutita*), English chamomile (*Chamaemelum nobile*) and Roman chamomile (*Chamaemelum nobile*). True chamomile is often used as another name for Roman (English) chamomile. German chamomile and Roman chamomile are botanically unrelated. The term Roman chamomile has its origin in the 19th century as it was found growing in the Coliseum. It is apparent that English and Roman chamomile are likely to be the same herb. However, the most extensively studied variety has been German chamomile for which the German Commission E has approved uses. Many herbalists believe that the German chamomile volatile oil is the more potent and has been more widely used whilst the Roman (English) volatile oil is less potent. The uses/mode of action and adverse effects of German chamomile have by and large been extrapolated to Roman (English) chamomile.

In Egypt, chamomile was a religious plant consecrated to the God of the Sun. Anglo-Saxons believed it was one of the nine sacred herbs given to humans by the god Woden. Romans used chamomile as an incense and also for brewing. In contemporary Germany, it is considered a 'cure-all'. A Czechokoslovakian saying is ' one should always bow before curative powers of the chamomile plant'.

Chamomile is considered safe by the FDA, with no known adverse effects in pregnancy, lactation (breast feeding) or childhood.

German chamomile is approved by Commission E for:

- coughs and bronchitis
- fevers and colds
- inflammations of the skin
- inflammation of the mouth and pharynx
- tendency to infection – improve immunity
- wounds and burns

Medicinal parts: Dried flowers or entire flowering herb for the German chamomile and the green leaves for Roman chamomile.

Uses: German chamomile is used for insomnia, as a sedative, a spasmolytic to relieve intestinal cramps and as an anti-inflammatory agent. Widely used for disorders of the digestive tract such as indigestion, peptic ulcers, gastrointestinal tract (gut) spasms (colic), nervous diarrhoea, and travel sickness. Roman chamomile is also used as a carminative for dyspepsia (flatulent dyspepsia) and to prevent vomiting (anti-emetic); also to prevent nausea and treat heart burn. Chamomile, particularly Roman chamomile, is used also to treat vomiting during early pregnancy. Both German and Roman chamomile are popular as sedatives for mental stress including premenstrual tension.

Other uses: German chamomile is used externally for skin conditions such as eczema, mastitis (inflammation and redness of breasts), psoriasis and leg ulcers. It is also used for inflammation of the gums and mouth (usually as a mouth wash), to relieve toothache and for teething problems in babies. German chamomile has been prescribed for hay fever, bronchitis, catarrh, and asthma. Teas/infusions have been used to treat worm infestations.

Probable mode of action: The flavonoid constituent apigenin in German chamomile exhibits a dose-dependent reversible inhibition of skin inflammation caused by irritants and protects against gastric ulcers which may be caused by medications (e.g. aspirin), stress and alcohol. Apigenin also binds to the same receptors as does Valium (a benzodiazepine) and probably exerts its anxiolytic and mild sedative actions by this binding. Laboratory experiments have shown that the volatile oil from German chamomile can act as an anti-oxidant and kill some pathogens (e.g. Staphylococci, Candida). The volatile oil in Roman chamomile is azulene, which has been found to possess anti-allergic and anti-inflammatory properties in laboratory experiments. Azulene has also been shown to protect the liver and increase its activity.

Adverse effects: Allergic reactions (tongue thickening, tightness in the throat, swelling of the lips, throat and eyes, itching over the body) have been reported with German chamomile but are infrequent. Roman chamomile can also cause allergic and even anaphylactic reactions. Both German and Roman chamomile contain anthemic acid, which may give rise to vomiting.

Precautions: Patients with severe allergic responses to ragweed (ragwort) should be warned about the possible cross-sensitivity to chamomile and other members of the Asteraceae/ Compositae family (e.g. echinacea, feverfew, milk thistle). Best avoided by patients with bronchial asthma.

The constituent (-) alpha bisabolol has been shown to have teratogenic effects (that is, cause abnormalities during the development of organs in the fetus) in some animal species. Extracts of chamomile herbs have been reported to increase the tone of the uterus and Roman chamomile has sometimes been classified as an abortifacient (induces miscarriage). Thus the chamomiles are best avoided during pregnancy. Though German chamomile has been used for teething problems in babies, some herbalists do not recommend the use of Roman chamomile for this disorder. As with all essential oils, the oil of the chamomile should only be used under medical supervision. Reports suggest that it would be dangerous to use Roman chamomile in patients who are receiving warfarin treatment.

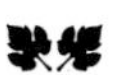

CHEBULIC MYROBALAN

Terminalia chebula

Indian name: Harad, Haritaki

Indigenous to India where ancient physicians used the plant to treat diarrhoea, heartburn and dyspepsia. An old Indian proverb says 'If one bites a piece of haritaki everyday after meals and swallows its juice, he will remain free from all diseases'. A decoction is used by Indian women to blacken grey hair.

Medicinal parts: Unripe fruit, ripe fruit, outer dried parts surrounding the seed.

Uses: Orally, as a laxative, and for relief of stomach acidity and heartburn. Has been used topically as a mouthwash.

Other uses: Treatment of haemorrhoids, as a gargle for inflammation of the mouth, as a dilute decoction for eye disorders, for vaginal disorders and to treat skin diseases. The herb is one of the ingredients of the well known Ayurvedic preparation 'Triphala' which is used to treat an enlarged liver, stomach disorders and pain in the eyes.

Probable mode of action: Constituents include tannins and nearly 18 amino acids. Also present are resins and the purgative principal of anthraquinone and sennoside.

Adverse effects: Has been reported to cause liver and kidney damage.

Precautions: There is insufficient information about safety. Avoid use during pregnancy as it may induce abortion.

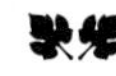

CHICKWEED

Stellaria media

Was recommended in the 17th century for mange. Has a long history of use externally for itching associated with skin disorders.

Medicinal parts: The fresh flowering or dried herb.

Uses: For rheumatism, gout, stiffness of joints, tuberculosis and diseases of the blood.

Other uses: Externally for poorly healing wounds, haemorrhoids, inflammation of the eyes,

herbs

eczema and other skin diseases. Added to bath water to relieve inflammation.

Probable mode of action: Constituents include flavonoids, vitamin C and alkaloids. The specific effects of the constituents are not known with any certainty.

Adverse effects: None has been reported following the proper administration and use of recommended doses. However, there has been a report of paralysis that has been attributed to excessive intake of chickweed. Adverse effects are considered to be due to the nitrate content of the herb.

Precautions: Should not be used during pregnancy or during breastfeeding.

CHICORY

Cichorium intybus

Chicory was used as a substitute for coffee when coffee became unavailable or too expensive. Was known to the Romans who used it as a vegetable or in salads. Has been mentioned in the scripts by Horace, Virgil, Ovid and Pliny.

Approved by Commission E for:
- loss of appetite
- dyspepsia.

Medicinal parts: Dried leaves and roots, the fresh plant.

Uses: Treatment of loss of appetite and dyspepsia (stomach ailments). Was used internally for sore throat, tuberculosis, haemorrhoids, abdominal cramps, melancholia, deafness and rashes. The juice of the chicory plant was also used as a laxative for children.

Other uses: In Indian medicine, it is used for headaches, dyspeptic symptoms (stomach complaints), skin allergies, vomiting and diarrhoea. In **folk medicine**, the herb is used externally for liver complaints and as a gargle. The bruised leaves have been used as a poultice for swellings and inflammations and inflamed eyes.

Probable mode of action: An important constituent is inulin. The constituents have been stated to have anti-exudative (preventing loss of fluid following or during inflammation from affected small blood vessels); to stimulate the formation of bile (chloretic); and to be negatively inotropic on the heart (decreases the force of contraction of the heart muscle). Animal studies have noted a definite reduction in pulse rate and contractility of the heart. Other effects reported from animal experiments include a cholesterol lowering effect and relief of the symptoms of dyspepsia. Some herbalists consider it similar to dandelion with actions as a tonic, laxative and as a diuretic.

Adverse effects: Slight potential for sensitization. It is stated that when chicory is taken habitually, it causes passive venous congestion in the digestive organs within the abdomen and a 'fullness of the blood' in the head. Also can affect vision.

Precautions: None known.

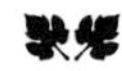

CHINESE CUCUMBER – CHINESE SNAKE GOURD

Trichosanthes kirilowii

Has been used in Chinese medicine for several thousands of years.

Medicinal parts: The fruit and root.

Uses: Chinese cucumber fruit is used to reduce fevers, swelling and coughing. The root has been used in the treatment of HIV infections. **In Chinese medicine**, the root is used to treat coughs, fever, swelling, tumours and diabetes.

Other uses: The fruit is used orally to treat diabetes and to induce abortions. The root has also been used by injection to induce abortions. The plant has been used for centuries to treat tumours.

Has also been used for amenorrhoea, jaundice and polyuria.

Probable mode of action: The root constituents can prevent the spread of HIV in white blood cells and destroy the white blood cells (macrophages) that have ingested the HIV. Is under investigation for the treatment of AIDS.

Adverse effects: Extracts of the root are extremely toxic; parenteral (intravenous) administration has been reported to cause pulmonary oedema (fluid in the lungs), cerebral oedema (fluid in the brain cells), cerebral (brain) haemorrhage and myocardial (heart muscle cells) damage. Parenteral administration may cause seizures and fever in HIV patients. The fruit may cause gastric discomfort and diarrhoea. Allergic reactions may also occur.

Precautions: Both the root and the fruit should be avoided during pregnancy. The root is not safe for self-medication.

CHINESE RHUBARB – DA HUANG

Rheum palmatum

Was mentioned in the 1st century AD. Described by Marco Polo following his travels to China. One of the most widely used herbs in Chinese Medicine and was mentioned in the Chinese herbal text *Pen-King* in 2700 BC.

Medicinal parts: The dried underground parts and most of the root bark in the dried form.

Approved by Commission E for:

- constipation.

Uses: As an appetite stimulant and for digestive problems and painful teething. Used externally for burns and skin disorders.

Other uses: In Chinese medicine, rhubarb is used in complex formulae for delirium, tenesmus (pain in the anal region during passage of faeces), oedema, amenorrhoea (absence of menstrual periods) and abdominal pain. Externally the root is used to treat burns.

Probable mode of action: The laxative effect is due to the constituents being able to absorb water into the intestinal lumen and also to prevent the reabsorption of fluid from the intestinal lumen. This causes an increase in the volume of intestinal contents which stimulates bowel movements (peristalisis).

Adverse effects: May cause abdominal pain. As a side-effect of the laxative action, long-term use can lead to electrolyte imbalances within the body, particularly loss of potassium (hypokalaemia) which may lead to muscle weakness and also increase the toxicity of drugs acting on the heart muscle such as digoxin. Other effects include an increase in the secretion of aldosterone (a hormone that regulates sodium and potassium balance in the body), passage of albumin and blood in the urine (albuminuria and haematuria) and a decrease or loss of intestinal movement (ileus).

Precautions: Contraindicated in cases of intestinal obstruction, acute intestinal inflammatory disease, appendicitis and abdominal pain of uncertain origin. Following long-term use the resulting electrolyte imbalances could seriously affect the toxicity of allopathic medications especially digoxin. Use in pregnancy should be only under medical supervision. Because of the oxalic acid content, subjects suffering from rheumatism, arthritis, gout and kidney stones should be cautious when using Chinese rhubarb.

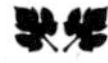

CINNAMON

Cinnamomum zelanicum (Ceylonese cinnamon)
Cinnamomum verum

Cinnamon was highly prized by ancient nations and considered as a gift fit for monarchs. Cinnamon tree was known to ancient physicians before 2700 BC. The physicians Galen, Dioscorides and Sasaferes described various uses of cinnamon. One of the oldest records available is in the Torah, the Jewish religious text. The medicinal uses were described in some detail by Khizvenee during the 13th century. Was imported to Egypt from China in 2000 BC and is also mentioned in the Bible.

Cinnamon is listed by the Council of Europe as a natural source of food flavouring. It has been commonly used as a spice for centuries. In the US, cinnamon is categorized as Generally Recognized as Safe.

Approved by Commission E for:

- loss of appetite
- dyspepsia.

Medicinal parts: Cinnamon oil extracted from the bark, oil extract from the leaves, and the dried bark of younger branches.

Uses: For anorexia (loss of appetite), intestinal colic especially flatulent colic, dyspepsia (stomach disorders) with nausea, for infantile diarrhoea and as an antimicrobial (antibacterial agent).

Other uses: As an antihelminthic (treatment of worm infestations), and for the common cold and influenza. Used externally for cleaning wounds. **In Indian medicine**, used to treat toothache, nausea and vomiting. Also used as an insect repellent.

Probable mode of action: The constituents are reported to be effective against bacterial, viral and fungal infections (bactericidal, antifungal, antiviral) and effective against the larvae of insects. One of the constituents, eugenol, has antiseptic and anaesthetic properties. Cinnamon has a mildly positive oestrogenic (an effect similar to the female hormone oestrogen) effect on the genitals of animals tested. It increases gastric secretions and has insecticidal properties due to some constituents.

Adverse effects: Contact with the bark or oil may cause an allergic reaction. Cinnamon oil contains cinnamaldehyde which is an irritant and sensitising agent. The daily intake of eugenol should not exceed 2.5 mg/kg.

Precautions: The acceptable daily intake of cinnamaldehyde has been temporarily estimated as 700 μg/kg body weight. Cinnamon oil should not be used on the skin or taken internally. Doses below the accepted daily intake may be taken during pregnancy, though some workers state that cinnamon should not be consumed during pregnancy.

CLEAVERS – COACHWEED – CATCHWEED – GOOSEGRASS

Galium aparine

Has a long history of domestic medicinal use.

Medicinal parts: Aerial parts collected during the flowering season and dried. Also the fresh flowering herb and the fresh or dried whole plant.

Uses: For treatment of painful urination (dysuria), enlarged and festering lymph nodes (lymphadenitis) and psoriasis.

Other uses: As a diuretic for dropsy (oedema or swelling due to fluid), bladder problems and retention of urine. May be used for calculi (stones) of the urinary tract. Also used for skin disorders such as psoriasis and other skin eruptions. Has been used as a tonic.

Probable mode of action: Not known. Contains constituents which are reported to produce a mild laxative action in mice.

Adverse effects: Can cause severe skin irritation.

Precautions: It is recommended that diabetics should not take the juice though there is no evidence of pharmacological activity to affect diabetics. Because of the lack of information on toxicity, this herb is best avoided during pregnancy and lactation. *Galium aparine* is a noxious weed.

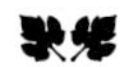

CLOVE

Syzgium aromaticum

Clove has been used in India and China for over 2000 years as a spice, to prevent tooth decay and to prevent halitosis (bad breath). Used by the Persians as an aphrodisiac. The oil was used to promote removal of secretions from the lung and upper airways (expectorant). The effect against vomiting was inconsistent with clinical results. Clove tea was used to relieve nausea. Use of the oil in dentistry as an analgesic and local antiseptic continues to date.

Approved by Commission E for:

- dental analgesia
- inflammation of the mouth and pharynx.

Medicinal parts: Oil extracted from the whole or macerated flower buds, the pedicles and leaves, the dried flower buds and the 'not-quite-ripe' fruit.

Uses: Clove oil is used for abdominal pain, as a carminative and for toothache. Used externally for colds and headaches. Has been used to relieve pain locally (as a local anaesthetic) and as an antiseptic in dental care. Also used to reduce fever (antipyretic).

Other uses: In Indian medicine, clove is used for halitosis (bad breath), toothache, eye disease, flatulence, colic, stomach discomfort and the treatment of anorexia (loss of appetite). It is used topically for ringworm. A clove stub rubbed in water and applied to a stye was considered very effective in India.

Probable mode of action: The constituents are reported to possess antiseptic, antibacterial, antifungal, antiviral, antihelminthic (effective against bacteria, fungi, viruses, worms) activity and also to prevent spasms (spasmolytic). Eugenol constituents may cause relief from pain (analgesic) and have local anaesthetic properties. Eugenol can depress sensory receptors due to inhibition of prostaglandin (a hormone associated with inflammatory processes). It is reported to have anticarcinogenic (effective against cancer cells) properties.

Adverse effects: Clove oil is a skin and mucous membrane irritant and sensitizer. Clove oil ingestion caused disseminated intravascular coagulation (a serious disorder where there is consumption and hence depletion of the factors in the blood that cause clotting, which leads to bleeding in the whole body) and liver failure in a 2-year-old child. A 7-month-old child developed electrolyte imbalance (i.e. disturbances usually of sodium and potassium contents in the blood) after accidental ingestion. Clove cigarettes called 'kreteks', generally containing about 60% tobacco and 40% ground cloves, are popular in Asian countries. More than a dozen cases of pulmonary (lung) toxicity (coughing of blood – haemoptysis) have been reported in smokers of kreteks.

Precautions: Clove and clove oils are used safely in foods, beverages and toothpaste. The concentrations should not exceed 0.25% for cloves and 0.06% for the oil. Avoid using clove oil during pregnancy and lactation.

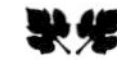

COLA NUT – KOLA

Cola nitida
Cola acuminata

Cola nut trees have been important in Africa for centuries. Africans used the pods to ease labour pains, the seeds to relieve diarrhoea, nausea and 'hangover', the bark to heal wounds and the wood to build houses, boats and images. The nuts were chewed as a stimulant and the roots were used to clean teeth.

Approved by Commission E for:

- lack of stamina.

Medicinal part: Seeds.

Uses: For depression (especially depressive states with muscle weakness), exhaustion, mental and physical fatigue, anorexia and migraine.

herbs

Other uses: It is used for dysentery and atonic diarrhoea (diarrhoea due to poor muscular activity of the bowel). **In folk medicine**, it is chewed to treat diarrhoea, morning sickness and migraine, to suppress hunger and thirst, and to promote digestion. It is also ground and made into poultices for wounds and inflammations. Cola is also an indigenous cult drug.

Probable mode of action: Constituents include caffeine, theobromine and xanthines which stimulate the central nervous system. They also cause relaxation of the smooth muscle and diuresis (passage of urine). Also contains tannins.

Adverse effects: Sleeplessness, anxiety, tremor and palpitations due to excessive stimulation of the central nervous system (including respiratory and cardiac centres within the brain). People who consume cola products frequently may experience withdrawal symptoms such as headache if they reduce their intake abruptly.

Precautions: Best avoided by patients with high blood pressure or heart disease. It is generally recommended that the caffeine consumption should be restricted during pregnancy, although the reports are conflicting. Though caffeine is excreted in the breast milk, the concentrations are considered to be too low to cause effects in the infant. On the basis of the information available at present, it is possibly best to avoid excessive consumption during pregnancy and lactation.

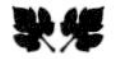

COLEUS

Coleus forskohlii

Recorded in the Sanskrit scripts as a 'power herb' and was used in Ayurveda to treat heart and lung disease, insomnia and intestinal spasms. Coleus is a member of the mint family of plants and has been cultivated in India, Thailand and parts of South East Asia as a spice and as a condiment for heart ailments and stomach cramps.

Medicinal part: Root.

Uses: To treat hypertension (high blood pressure), congestive heart failure (heart failure due usually to weakness of the heart muscle), as an anti-ageing agent, for relaxation of smooth muscle in the walls of arteries and for the relief of intestinal colic and uterine cramps.

Other uses: As an antiasthmatic, antiglaucoma agent, antiplatelet agent, for the treatment of eczema and psoriasis and to promote digestion. Extract of *Coleus barbatus* B has been used in **folk medicine in Brazil** to interrupt pregnancy.

Probable mode of action: The effectiveness of *Colteus forskohlii* is considered to be due to its effect on one of the most important molecules that regulate cell activity and function – cyclic adenosine monophosphate (cyclic AMP). Cyclic AMP is important for many of the biological processes that occur in cells. It is responsible for transferring the effects of hormones that cannot pass through the cell membrane such as adrenaline. Cyclic AMP also activates protein kinase, an enzyme which catalyses many reactions within a cell. The basic mechanism of action of *Coleus forskohlii* is to increase the amount of cyclic AMP in the cells. The chief alkaloid of *Coleus forskohlii*, is considered to increase the force of contraction of heart muscle and relax the arteries and other smooth muscles to produce vasodilatation. The alkaloids have been found to inhibit platelet activation and granulation tissue formation and to increase insulin secretion. Extracts have been found to stimulate the secretion of saliva, hydrochloric acid, pepsin and pancreatic enzymes. Direct application of an ophthalmic preparation to the eyes lowers pressure in the eye, hence its use in patients with glaucoma.

Adverse effects: May increase gastric acidity and cause heartburn. May cause transitory tearing, burning and itching when applied directly to the eyes.

Precautions: Could cause adverse effects in individuals taking anticoagulants and in individuals taking antihypertensive medication. Children and pregnant or lactating women should avoid supplements containing *Coleus forskohlii*. Preparations should be avoided by individuals with stomach ulcers because they can cause an increase in gastric acidity. Not recommended for use as a dietary supplement except under direct supervision of a physician.

COLTSFOOT

Tussilago farfara (L)

The Greek physician Dioscorides recommended smoking coltsfoot for the relief of coughs and asthma and it remains an ingredient of some herbal cigarettes.

Medicinal parts: Dried flowers and leaves.

Uses: To treat bronchitis, laryngitis, pertussis (whooping cough) and asthma. Specifically indicated for spasmodic cough in bronchitis.

Other uses: In China, the flowers (kuan dong hua) are used specifically for chronic coughs with profuse phlegm and 'to force rising lung qi (energy) to descend'.

Probable mode of action: The constituents are reported to possess smooth muscle relaxing properties and to promote removal of secretions from the lung and upper airways (expectorant) and to prevent cough (antitussive). Other effects attributed to the constituents are an ability to relieve inflammation or irritation (demulcent), to prevent catarrh (anticatarrhal) and to promote the flow of urine (diuretic). The flowers contain mucilage, flavonoids and tannin, and essential oil. The leaves contain mucilage, more tannin and zinc. The mucilage coats mucous membranes with a layer that protects the throat from chemical and physical irritation.

Adverse effects: Risk of liver toxicity.

Precautions: Contains pyrrolizidine alkaloids, so there is a risk of liver toxicity. Contraindicated during pregnancy and lactation. The herb is restricted in Australia and New Zealand because of the risk of liver damage caused by the pyrrolizidine alkaloid constituents. Coltsfoot leaf was originally approved for the treatment of sore throat in the German Commission E monograph but has since been banned in Germany.

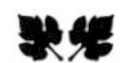

COMFREY

Symphytum officinale

In the past comfrey baths were popular to repair the hymen and thus restore virginity.

Approved by Commission E for:
- blunt injuries.

Medicinal parts: Root and rhizome, leaf.

Uses: The leaf has been used in the treatment of gastric and duodenal ulcer, rheumatic pain and arthritis. Specifically indicated in gastric ulceration and for gastric and duodenal ulcers, haematemesis (vomiting of blood) and colitis. The fresh root preparation is only used for topical application for ulcers, varicose ulcers, wounds, fractures and hernia.

Other uses: Used topically with some success in the treatment of psoriasis. Also used topically as a poultice or fomentation for bruises, sprains, athlete's foot, crural ulcers and mastitis. The root has been used externally as a gargle for gum disease, pharyngitis and streptococcal throat infections.

Probable mode of action: The leaf and root are documented to have several constituents with properties to reduce inflammation and bleeding, bring relief in arthritis and promote removal of secretions from the lung and upper airways (expectorant). Comfrey stimulates healing by promoting activity of fibroblasts which are involved in the repair of damaged tissue and also stimulates bone and cartilage formation. The wound healing properties are partially due to the presence of allantoin which stimulates cell multiplication, thereby accelerating wound healing both internally and externally. The mucilage content was reported to have a protective effect by forming a thin film to prevent irritation and inflammation.

Adverse effects: Comfrey contains pyrrolizidine alkaloids which are absorbed through broken skin and hence there is a risk of hepatitis. Hepatic veno-occlusive disease and severe portal hypertension has been reported, and in one case death resulted due to liver failure. May cause loss of appetite, abdominal pain, vomiting. On the skin, an inflammatory reaction (dermatitis) may occur.

Precautions: Comfrey is contraindicated during pregnancy and lactation. Comfrey should only be used topically on unbroken skin. Symphytine, one of the pyrrolizidine alkaloids in comfrey, caused cancer in rat experiments. Should not be used with eucalyptus. Do not combine with any other herbs known to contain pyrrolizidine alkaloids (e.g. agrimony, alpine ragwort, help, tansy ragwort).

CONDURANGO

Marsdenia condurango

Found in the high mountain jungles in Peru, Ecuador and Colombia where it has been used by the indigenous population to treat nausea and vomiting and to relieve stomach pain and cramps. Was included in the US Pharmacopeia in the 1900s.

Approved by Commission E for:

- dyspeptic complaints
- loss of appetite.

Medicinal parts: Dried bark of the branches and trunk.

Uses: For loss of appetite and atonia of the stomach, and for stomach cancer to alleviate nausea. Has been used to relieve flatulence.

Other uses: For nutritional disorders. Herbal medical systems in **Peru** consider it as an analgesic, carminative and tonic. Also used to stop bleeding (haemostatic). In **Brazil**, it is used for loss of appetite, neuralgia and stomach cancer.

Probable mode of action: Constituents include the bitter condurango glycosides which cause an increase in the secretion of saliva and gastric juices. Has an antitumour effect in animals. Other constituents are flavonoids and coumarin derivatives. In animal experiments, it was found to be effective against the bacteria that cause tuberculosis.

Adverse effects: An anaphylactic reaction has been reported due to condurango bark in a patient allergic to natural rubber.

Precautions: To be avoided by those allergic to latex.

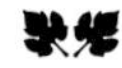

CORIANDER

Coriandrum sativum

Indian name: Dhania

A belief is that the use of coriander originated in 5000 BC and there is evidence of its use by Egyptians. Coriander has been used as a folk medicine for the relief of anxiety and insomnia in Iranian folk medicine. Introduced to Britain by the Romans as a meat preserver.

Approved by Commission E for:

- dyspepsia
- loss of appetite.

Medicinal parts: Oil and dried ripe fruit.

Uses: For dyspepsia (stomach ailments), loss of appetite and to kill bacteria (as a bactericidal). Seeds are roasted to produce a brew to treat flu and the common cold.

Other uses: Has been used as a fungicide and a larvicide. **In folk medicine**, coriander is used for digestive and gastric complaints, worms, rheumatism and joint pains. In other cultures, coriander has been used for coughs, chest pains, bladder complaints, leprosy, rash, fever, and dysentery. Externally coriander has been used for headache, oral and pharyngeal disorders, halitosis and complications after child birth (postpartum complications).

In Chinese medicine, coriander is used for loss of appetite, the pre-eruptive phase of chicken pox and measles, haemorrhoids and rectal prolapse, dysentery, haemorrhoids and toothache. **In Indian medicine**, coriander is used to treat nosebleeds, coughs, haemorrhoids, painful micturition (passage of urine), oedema, bladder complaints, vomiting, amoebic dysentery and dizziness.

In Sri Lanka, coriander is used to treat flu-like illnesses and the common cold.

Probable mode of action: Coriander is a rich source of vitamin C, calcium, iron and magnesium. The essential oil in laboratory experiments delayed the growth of the organism *Escherichia coli.*

Adverse effects: Powdered coriander and the oil can cause allergic reactions and photosensitivity.

Precautions: Dry coriander should be used sparingly by persons suffering from bronchial asthma and chronic bronchitis. Avoid in allergy.

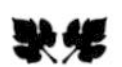

COUCH GRASS

Agropyron repens

Couch grass has been used for medicinal purposes for centuries. In early 20th century, couch grass was used in France as a home remedy to soothe sore throats and to help 'sweat out' illnesses. Couch grass is listed by the Council of Europe as a natural source of food flavouring.

Medicinal parts: The herb and fleshy underground stem.

Uses: Urinary tract infections (cystitis, urethritis, prostatitis), benign prostatic hypertrophy and kidney stones (renal calculi).

Other uses: Flavouring food.

Probable mode of action: Has diuretic and sedative properties in experimental animals. The constituent agropyrene is considered to possess antibiotic activity. The flavonoid constituents may cause phytotoxicity.

Adverse effects: Prolonged use may result in loss of potassium from the body due to the diuretic action. No other documented adverse effects.

Precautions: Avoid in patients who are likely to have depleted body stores of potassium. Needs to be used with caution by patients taking medication that may be affected by blood potassium levels (e.g. digoxin). Since there is limited toxicological data, use in pregnancy and during lactation should be avoided. Be cautious in patients with heart and kidney disease. Take plenty of fluids when used in the treatment of urinary tract disease.

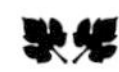

COWSLIP

Primula veris

Cowslip is not commonly used in foods. A related species *Primula elatior* is listed by the Council of Europe as a natural source of food flavouring.

Approved by Commission E for:
- cough/bronchitis.

Medicinal parts: The roots and flowers.

Uses: For insomnia (difficulty in falling asleep), nervous excitability, hysteria, anxiety states associated with restlessness and irritability.

Other uses: Catarrh. As a cardiac tonic for feelings of dizziness and heart failure. Also used as a nerve tonic for shaking limbs, headaches (externally) and neuralgia.

Probable mode of action: Constituents include saponins, phenols, flavonoids, quinones and silicic acid. The component responsible for the central nervous system effects is not known. Saponins are attributed with the effect of promoting removal of secretions from the lung and upper airways (expectorant) and diuretic effect. Effects are postulated to be due to stimulation of the vagus nerve.

Adverse effects: Saponins may cause hypotension (fall in blood pressure) initially and prolonged hypertension (rise in blood pressure). Also causes gastrointestinal irritation. Allergic reactions are likely to be due to the quinine constituents, of which primin is considered to be a strong contact allergen.

Precautions: Should be avoided by individuals with allergies. Excessive or prolonged use may interfere with the treatment of high blood pressure (hypertension) or may cause irritation of the gastrointestinal tract. In view of the lack of toxicological data, cowslip is best avoided during pregnancy and lactation.

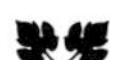

CRAMP BARK – GUELDER ROSE

Viburnum opulus

Used by Native Americans for mumps and other swellings.

Used in North America as a diuretic and sedative.

The 'Gaitre-Berries' of which Chaucer makes mention among plants that 'shal be for your hele to picke hem right as they grow aned ete hem in' are the deep red clusters of berries of the wild Guelder rose. This fruit is used in Canada as a substitute for cranberries.

The name Guelder comes from Gueldersland, a Dutch province where the tree was first cultivated.

The berries turn black on drying and have been used for making ink.

The bark, known as cramp bark, was included in the US Pharmacopeia. It is now omitted though it has been introduced into the UK's National Formulary in the form of fluid extract, compound tincture and compound elixir for use as a nerve sedative and antispasmodic in asthma and hysteria.

Medicinal part: Bark.

Uses: To relieve muscle cramps including menstrual cramps and cramps occurring during pregnancy. Considered to help prevent miscarriages.

Other uses: For complaints of the nervous system and for debility. Treating convulsions, fits and tetanus (lockjaw). Also has been used for heart complaints such as palpitations. Also used in rheumatism. Has been used as a diuretic, emetic, purgative and sedative.

Probable mode of action: The active constituent is a bitter glucoside – viopudial – which is thought to relax muscles. Also contains tannins and resins. The exact action of the constituents is not known with certainty. The constituents are identical with the species *Viburnum* that is more widely used and is an official drug in the US – *Viburnum prunifolium* or black haw.

Adverse effects: May have side-effects which are not known with certainty as yet as reports of such effects are scarce in the literature.

Precautions: Should not be used during pregnancy.

CRANBERRY

Vaccinium oxycoccos

The Pilgrim Fathers learned about cranberries from the Native Americans who knew of the preservative power (benzoic acid) in the berries. Cranberry sauce was ordered to be served to the troops during the siege of Petersburg in 1864.

Medicinal part: The berry.

Uses: Has been used to treat urinary infections, such as cystitis, and scurvy (disease due to lack of vitamin C). Also to treat nausea.

Probable mode of action: Cranberry is thought to interfere with the adhesion of micro-organisms, particularly *Escherichia coli*, to epithelial cells lining the urinary tract and to cause acidification of the urine.

Adverse effects: Diarrhoea and other gastrointestinal disturbances can occur when large amounts of the juice are ingested.

Precautions: Not recommended for those suffering from kidney disease without professional advice. There is insufficient evidence on safety during pregnancy and lactation. May interact with warfarin.

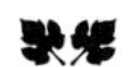

CREOSOTE BUSH – CHAPARRAL

Larrea tridentata

The word chaparral is from the Spanish word *chaparro* (small and dwarf evergreen oak). Creosote bush was widely used by various North American Indian tribes. A decoction was used to treat diarrhoea and stomach troubles and the young twigs were used for toothache.

Medicinal part: The herb.

Uses: To treat bronchitis, cancer, venereal diseases, tuberculosis and chronic skin disorders. Also used to relieve pain (as an analgesic) and to delay the ageing process.

Probable mode of action: An active constituent is documented to possess antioxidant properties. Other constituents may bring about relief from pain and also promote removal of secretions from the lung and upper airways (expectorant). Other properties attributed to constituents are emetic, diuretic and anti-inflammatory effects.

Adverse effect: Acute hepatitis has been associated with oral use, and contact dermatitis has also been reported.

Precautions: Not considered safe for use as a herbal remedy. Sale is banned in North America because of the potential toxic effects on the liver.

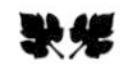

CUMIN

Cuminum cyminum

Indian name: Jeera

Cumin was known to the Egyptians five millennia ago. Originally cultivated in Iran and the Mediterranean region. Mentioned in the Bible. During the Middle Ages, cumin was believed to keep chickens and lovers from wandering and it was believed that a happy life awaited the bride and groom who carried cumin seed throughout the wedding ceremony.

Medicinal parts: Cumin oil extracted from the ripe fruit and ripe dried fruit.

Uses: Cumin is used as an antiflatulent.

Other uses: Traditionally cumin was used as a stimulant, antispasmodic, diuretic and aphrodisiac. **In folk medicine**, cumin is used as a carminative for stomach disorders, diarrhoea and colic. **In America, Africa and India**, the herb is used as an abortive and as an emmenagogue (to regulate menstruation). **In Indonesia**, cumin is used for bloody diarrhoea and headache (as a paste applied to the forehead). It is also taken for rheumatic ailments. **In Indian medicine**, in addition to being used as an abortifacient, it is used for kidney and bladder stones, chronic diarrhoea, leprosy and eye diseases. Also very commonly used in veterinary medicine.

Probable mode of action: Cumin is a rich source of iron and one of the constituents is cuminaldehyde. Cumin has been reported to have larvicidal (activity against larvae) and antibacterial actions due to the fatty oil content. The constituents have also been reported to have carminative, antispasmodic, diuretic and stimulant effects. Some constituents are considered to have an analgesic effect while others have a galactogenic (increase lactation) effect.

Adverse effect: May cause hypoglycaemia.

Precautions: Should be used with caution by diabetics. Best avoided by individuals taking barbiturates (a sleeping tablet).

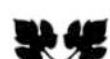

CURCUMA – JAVANESE TURMERIC

Curcuma xanthorrhiza

Originates from Indonesia.

Approved by Commission E for:
- liver and gallbladder complaints
- treatment of loss of appetite.

Medicinal part: Rhizome.

Uses: In the treatment of dyspepsia, flatulence and acne. In **Indonesia**, curcuma has been traditionally used for liver and gall bladder complaints. Considered to lower blood cholesterol levels and increase the production of breast milk.

Probable mode of action: Curcuma acts in a manner similar to turmeric root but its main effect is as a chloretic (on bile system). Has been shown to have antitumour properties in animal experiments. Also contains essential oils.

Adverse effects: Excessive use or overdosage may result in stomach complaints. Patients with gallstones may get colicky abdominal pain.

Precautions: Because of the stimulating actions on the bile tract, it should not be administered if there is bile duct blockade, e.g. bile stones. Information on safety during pregnancy is not available.

DAMIANA – MEXICAN HOLLY

Turnera diffusa

Recorded to have been used as an aphrodisiac in ancient Mayan civilization and also to treat giddiness and loss of balance. A Spanish missionary observed Mexican Indians making a drink from damiana leaves, adding sugar and drinking it to enhance love making. Leaves were smoked for relaxation and the effects were considered somewhat similar to that of cannabis.

Medicinal parts: Aerial parts and leaves.

Uses: Headache, for treating depression and for constipation due to poor intestinal contractions (atony). Also used as an aphrodisiac and in disorders of sexual function (e.g. impotence, infertility).

Other uses: To stimulate digestion and increase urination.

Probable mode of action: Hypoglycaemic (lowering of blood sugar) and antibacterial activities have been reported. Contains arbutin which is said to have urinary antiseptic properties. Leaves contain volatile oils, tannins, flavonoids and a bitter. Studies suggest that the hypoglycaemic constituents may be lost or inactivated when alcohol is used for extraction.

Adverse effects: Tetanus-like rigidity and genitourinary irritation was associated with ingestion of damiana in one patient. Has been reported to cause hallucinations. Some animal data suggest the possibility of a blood sugar lowering effect.

Precautions: Theoretically may affect the control of blood sugar in diabetic patients.

DANDELION

Taraxacum officinale

Indian name: Kukraundha, Kanphool.
Derived from the French word *dent-de-lion* (lion's tooth). Dandelion is a registered drug in Canada and is sold as a diuretic. The medicinal values of dandelion have been mentioned in the Arabian writings of the 10th century, Welsh

manuscripts of the 13th century and the English herbal literature of the 16th and 17th centuries. Planted in India as a remedy for liver complaints.

Approved by Commission E for:

- dyspepsia (indigestion)
- infections of the urinary tract
- liver and gallbladder complaints
- loss of appetite.

Medicinal parts: Roots, leaves, latex.

Uses: As a diuretic, a laxative and to improve the appetite and to relieve stomach complaints (dyspepsia). Also used in liver and gallbladder disorders.

Other uses: Gout, rheumatic disorders, eczema, skin disorders. **In Chinese medicine**, dandelion is used in complex formulae for acute mastitis (pain due to inflammation of the breasts) and urinary disorders and when there is decreased production of breast milk (lactation). **In Indian medicine**, dandelion is used for chronic ulcers, tuberculosis, flatulence, colic, kidney disease, gout, jaundice and biliary disease. The milky latex is used as an insect repellent.

Probable mode of action: Reported to have anti-inflammatory and antioxidant activity (attributed to luteolin). Contains lactones which are considered to be natural diuretics. Also enhances liver and gallbladder function. Also contains amaroids which increase bile and intestinal secretions. **Indian physicians** consider dandelion to contain almost as much iron as spinach and four times the vitamin A content of lettuce and to be a very rich source of magnesium, vitamin C and potassium. Dandelion leaves contain possibly the highest vitamin A content of all greens.

Adverse effects: Diarrhoea; rashes have been reported following repeated contact with the raw herb. May cause symptoms due to increased acidity in the stomach and gastrointestinal tract. One advantage of dandelion as a diuretic is that it contains potassium.

Precautions: Generally considered safe even in large quantities. Do not use in the presence of bile duct or gallbladder obstruction. Avoid dandelion if on lithium therapy as the diuretic properties of dandelion may lower sodium levels leading to lithium toxicity. Caution also with some blood pressure lowering tablets.

DANG GUI – DONG QUAI – CHINESE ANGELICA

Angelica sinensis

A highly respected Traditional Chinese Medicine, second only to ginseng.

For centuries, Chinese women have used dang gui to regulate menstrual cycles and reduce painful cramps associated with menstruation. It has been used for thousands of years in China as a tonic and spice.

Medicinal part: The root.

Uses: Used in a variety of gynaecological ailments, to regulate menstruation, for painful menstruation (dysmenorrhoea), absence of menstruation (amenorrhoea) and menopausal symptoms (hot flushes).

Other uses: For insomnia, anaemia, constipation (as a laxative), injuries following trauma, swellings, ulcers, rheumatism, malaria and hypertension. Has been used to treat pulmonary hypertension (increased pressure in the blood vessels to the lung) in combination with the allopathic medication nifedipine.

Probable mode of action: Reported to have effects similar to that of the female hormone oestrogen (phytoestrogenic activity). The volatile oil constituent causes relaxation of the uterus and decreases rhythmic contractions of the uterus. The non-volatile constituent produces an excitatory action on the uterus causing stronger contractions. The combined effect appears to depend on the functional state of the uterus. Also has an anti-

herbs

inflammatory effect and antiplatelet effect and is believed to prevent the release of serotonin (a chemical messenger) by blood platelets. Contains vitamin B_{12} which promotes the formation of blood cells. Lubrication of the bowel produces the laxative effect. Shown to relax smooth muscles of the arteries.

Adverse effects: Diarrhoea, photosensitivity (sensitivity to sunlight), some suggestion that the oil may be carcinogenic (may cause cancers).

Precautions: Not recommended during pregnancy. Not to be used if menstrual flow is heavy or during menstruation. High doses (over 500 mg a day) may cause abdominal bloating and changes in menstrual timing or flow. Be aware of an unproven but possible effect on heart rhythm and a lowering of blood pressure. Should be used with caution by diabetics and by those with acute viral infections such as influenza. Caution necessary if on treatment with anticoagulants (e.g. warfarin).

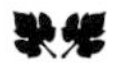

DEVIL'S CLAW

Harpagophytum procumbens

Native to South Africa. Has been used by native Africans as a folk remedy for kidney and liver disease, allergies, headaches and rheumatism.

Conservation issue: Only reputable products from sustainably produced resources should be used.

Approved by Commission E for:
- dyspeptic complaints (indigestion)
- loss of appetite
- rheumatism.

Medicinal parts: The dried tubular secondary roots and the thick lateral tubers.

Uses: The dried root of devil's claw is used for osteoarthritis, gout, rheumatoid arthritis and to improve appetite. The dried root is used for pain relief. Also used to relieve discomfort during pregnancy.

Other uses: For heartburn and digestive problems, liver, kidney and bladder disease and for degenerative disorders of the central nervous system. Used as an ointment for skin injuries. In **South Africa**, it is used for fevers and digestive disorders. Traditional South African remedy for digestive problems, especially gallbladder or stomach. In **Europe**, it is used as an appetite stimulant.

Probable mode of action: Primarily used as an anti-inflammatory agent and painkiller. Exact effects of the constituents are not known as yet.

Adverse effects: May cause gastric symptoms due to increased secretion of acid in the stomach. Considered to be a sensitizing agent. Also reported to have caused headaches, ringing in ears, loss of appetite and loss of taste.

Precautions: Not recommended during pregnancy or for use by patients with gastric or duodenal ulcers as it stimulates the secretion of gastric juice. Caution also in patients with diabetes mellitus, high blood pressure and heart disease. There is little or no evidence of the safety and use of devil's claw in children.

DIGITALIS – FOXGLOVE

Digitalis purpurea

The scientific use of this herb was investigated by the British physician William Withering in the late 1700. The use of this drug in folk medicine originated in Ireland, then spread to Scotland and England and finally to central Europe. In South America, preparations of powdered leaves were used to treat asthma, while in India, an ointment was used to treat wounds and burns.

Medicinal parts: The dried leaves (in powder form), the ripe dried seeds, the fresh leaves of the one year old plant or the leaves of the two-year-old plant collected at the beginning of flowering season.

Uses: It was used to treat ulcers in the lower abdomen, boils, headaches, abscesses and paralysis. Externally it was used to promote granulation of poorly healing wounds and to cure ulcers. Digitalis was also used for 'cardiac insufficiency' and high blood pressure. Use of the raw product is now obsolete, since the pure glycoside digitoxin has become available.

Probable mode of action: The glycosides increase the force of contraction of the heart muscle (inotropic) and decrease the rate at which the heart beats (negatively chronotropic). Overall, it improves the contraction and function of heart muscle.

Adverse effects: It can be difficult to determine the dose that will produce the desired effects in an individual without unwanted toxic effects. Toxic effects may sometimes occur with therapeutic doses, such as loss of appetite, diarrhoea, headache, vomiting. Acute overdose can have life-threatening effects on the heart (arrhythmias including potentially fatal ventricular tachycardia). Other effects include visual disorders, depression, confusion, hallucinations, psychoses. Administration over a prolonged period has caused gynaecomastia (enlargement of the breasts in males).

Precautions: Unsafe for self-medication. Use requires monitoring by a physician to determine the correct dose for each individual. Avoid use of the herb as standardized dosing is very difficult; use the pure glycoside (digitoxin). In case of overdose, give activated charcoal. Always monitor the potassium status in the body. Do not allow children to come into contact with this potentially lethal plant. Ingestion of very small amounts of the plant may be fatal to humans, particularly children.

DIGITALIS LANATA – GRECIAN FOXGLOVE

Digitalis lanata has three times the physiological effects of *Digitalis purpurea* and is now preferred because of the quick onset of effects.

Medicinal part: The leaves.

Uses: Because of the unsatisfactory reproducibility of effects during herbal use, the administration of the pure glycoside is strongly recommended.

It is rapidly absorbed following oral intake and produces wide ranging effects.

Probable mode of action: Same as for *Digitalis purpurea*. All parts of the plant are poisonous and there are no edible uses.

Adverse effects: Same as for *Digitalis purpurea.*

Precautions: Same as for *Digitalis purpurea.*

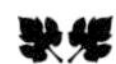

DILL

Anethum graveolens

An ancient Egyptian remedy in the Eber papyrus (1500 BC) recommends dill as one of the ingredients in a painkilling mixture. Used by Babylonian and Syrian herbalists. Romans considered dill to be an effective stimulant for gladiators.

The name is derived from the Old Norse *dylla*, meaning 'to lull', or 'soothe', alluding to its carminative properties. Dill was used as a charm against witchcraft during the Middle Ages and was burned to clear thunderclouds. Dill seed is a popular pickling spice, and the leaves are commonly used to flavour fish dishes. The stems and flowers are also used for flavouring. Also used as an antidote to witchcraft and sorcery.

Approved by Commission E for:

- dyspepsia.

Medicinal parts: Leaves, seeds and oil.

Uses: Flatulent dyspepsia (stomach ailment due to excess wind); specifically indicated for flatulent pain in infants. Anethum is a common ingredient in gripe water, given to relieve wind and colic in babies.

Other uses: Chewing the seeds is helpful in cases of halitosis (bad breath). Also used for sleep disorders and for spasms.

Probable mode of action: Constituents include volatile oil, flavonoids, coumarins, protein, and fixed oil. Dill has carminative, aromatic, stomach-soothing and antispasmodic effects and is a galactagogue (promotes lactation). Anethum stimulates milk flow in lactating mothers, and is often given to cattle for this reason.

Adverse effects: Photodermatitis may occur after contact with the juice of the freshly harvested plant. May show cross allergies with other plants.

Precautions: Dill oil should be avoided during pregnancy. Some herbalists recommend that dill should be avoided by those required to take a diet low in salt because of the high content of salt in dill.

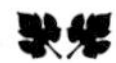

DROSERA – SUNDEW

Drosera ramentacea

Used as medicinal herbs in the 12th century. An Italian doctor described the plant as a herbal remedy for coughs, calling it 'herb sole'.

Approved by Commission E for:
cough/bronchitis.

Medicinal parts: The whole herb.

Uses: For diseases of the respiratory tract (e.g. bronchitis, asthma, tracheitis, pertussis – whooping cough).

Other uses: Warts, gastric ulcers.

Probable mode of action: The herb has effects such as causing increase in secretions (secretolytic), relieving spasms of the small airways or bronchi and preventing cough (antitussive). The constituents are considered to prevent the spasm of the small airways caused by chemical messengers such as acetylcholine or histamine and to relax the spasm of the bowel caused by such messengers. It is also stated that coughing due to stimulation of the laryngeal nerve is inhibited. The naphthaquinone constituents are also considered to possess antibacterial activity.

Adverse effects: None documented for *Drosera*.

Precautions: The safety of *Drosera* has not been established for use during pregnancy and lactation, hence it is best avoided.

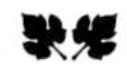

ECHINACEA – PURPLE CONE FLOWER

Echinacea purpurea
Echinacea angustifolia
Echinacea pallida

Native plains Indians valued this member of the daisy (Asteraceae) family for its medicinal properties and introduced it to European settlers after using it for over 400 years to treat infections and wounds and as a general 'cure-all'. In Germany, Echinacea is approved by the Federal Health Agency as supportive therapy for upper respiratory tract infections, urogenital infections and wounds. It is the most popular herb in the US, generating more than $300 million in sales annually. Has been used historically to treat syphilis, scarlet fever, malaria, diphtheria and blood poisoning.

Approved by Commission E for:
- common cold
- cough and bronchitis
- fevers and colds
- infections of the urinary tract
- inflammation of the mouth and pharynx (throat)
- tendency to infection – to increase resistance to infection
- wounds and burns.

Medicinal parts: Depending on varieties – the roots, leaves or the whole plant in various stages of development. Chemicals contained in the root differ considerably from those found in the upper part of the plant.

Uses: Prevention and treatment of colds, supportive role in treating infections (stimulating or enhancing the immunity), wound healing.

Other uses: Can be helpful for chronic fatigue syndrome, allergic conditions such as asthma and hay fever, shingles, herpes and mouth ulcers, or applied topically for eczema, boils or acne. Also used to treat psoriasis.

Probable mode of action: In animal studies, echinacea affects several aspects of the immune system. Constituents of echinacea increase the number of circulating white blood cells, enhance phagocytosis (engulfing of foreign particles by white blood cells), stimulate the formation of protective compounds (cytokine production) and promote the pathway that forms antibodies. In the laboratory, antibacterial and antiviral activity was observed. Based on its stimulation of cytokine production, echinacea is being investigated as a possible antineoplastic agent (to treat cancers) in preliminary human trials.

Topical echinacea has shown anti-infective activity against *Candida*, a fungal infection. In rodents, echinacea also decreases inflammation, protects against radiation-induced skin damage, and hastens wound healing.

Adverse effects: The most common side-effect reported is an unpleasant taste. Possible suppression of immunity with habitual use, high doses (over 1000 mg) can sometimes cause dizziness or nausea. May cause liver toxicity (hepatitis). A rash may occur in children. In rare instances, echinacea may cause allergic reactions ranging from a mild rash to life-threatening anaphylaxis. There is report of a patient developing erythema nodosum (a painful skin condition) after taking echinacea to treat flu.

Precautions: German guidelines discourage use of echinacea in place of antibiotics for more than 8 weeks at a time (one study suggests that long-term use may suppress immunity). The guideline recommends that the herb is used for 10–14 days and then stopped for a few days. Echinacea should not be used except under supervision of a healthcare professional by individuals with immune system dysfunction, autoimmune conditions and progressive systemic conditions such as multiple sclerosis, HIV, tuberculosis and diabetes mellitus. It should be used with caution by individuals taking medications that have liver toxicity. Best avoided in patients with active infections and wounds and in individuals who have recently had, or are awaiting, surgery.

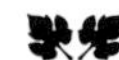

ELDER – EUROPEAN ELDER

Sambucus nigra

Various parts of the elder have long been used in traditional medicine as a diaphoretic (promotes sweating), diuretic, astringent, laxative and emetic. Has been referred to as the 'medicine chest of country people'. Elder is listed by the Council of Europe as a source of natural food flavouring.

Elder is approved by Commission E for:

- cough and bronchitis
- fevers and colds.

Medicinal parts: Inner bark, flowers, leaves.

Uses: For influenza, colds, chronic nasal catarrh with deafness and sinusitis.

Other uses: As a diuretic, laxative and an anti-inflammatory agent. **In folk medicine**, elder flowers are used internally as a tea for colds and other feverish conditions. Elder is also used as a gargle/mouthwash and for respiratory disorders such as coughs, head colds, laryngitis, flu and shortness of breath. Elder has been used occasionally by nursing mothers to increase production of breast milk (lactation). Externally herbal pillows are used for swelling and inflammation. An ointment made from the leaves has been used on bruises, sprains, chilblains and wounds.

Probable mode of action: The lectin constituents may exert an antispasmodic effect. An infusion made from flowers of elder, St John's wort and root of soapwort (*Saponaria officinalis*) has exhibited antiviral activity against type A and type B influenza virus. The flavonoid constituent, quercetin, has been found to possess antiviral activity against influenza type A virus in laboratory studies. Constituents include vitamins A and C.

Adverse effects: Nausea, vomiting and diarrhoea has followed poisoning with *Sambucus* species. However, no specific adverse effects have been reported for elder. Excessive or prolonged use may result in hypokalaemia (lowering of blood potassium levels) due to the diuretic effect.

Precautions: Parts of the plant other than the flowers are considered to be poisonous and should not be ingested. Should be used cautiously by patients who may have low levels of potassium due to drug therapy or disease or who are taking drugs that may be affected by potassium levels. Lectins isolated from elder bark are reported to have caused teratogenicity (abnormalities during organ formation) when administered to pregnant mice. Elder is best avoided during pregnancy and lactation. The root is no longer recommended for use as a herbal medicine

ELECAMPANE

Inula helenium

The herb is supposed to have got its name from Helen of Troy. She was thought to be in a garden when she was abducted by Paris and the plant grew where her tears fell.

Roman poets mention *Inula* as a medicine and condiment. Was described by Dioscorides and Pliny and Galen recommended it for the treatment of sciatica.

Before the advent of antibiotics, elecampane was often used to treat pneumonia and tuberculosis.

Elecampane is listed by the Council of Europe as a natural source of food flavouring.

Medicinal parts: Dried or fresh rhizome.

Uses: Bronchial and tracheal infections: catarrh, cough and whooping cough.

Other uses: As an antihelminthic to treat roundworm, thread worm, hookworm and whip worm infestations. **In folk medicine**, elecampane was used to relieve stomach ailments, as a diuretic, as a carminative and to stimulate bile production. Also used for menstrual complaints. Hot elecampane tea has been used to bring down a fever while the cooled tea has been used as an antiseptic wash for wounds and cuts and for skin infections such as scabies and herpes. In **Spain**, it has been used as a surgical dressing.

Probable mode of action: The constituents have been documented to possess bactericidal and fungicidal (antibacterial and antifungal) properties. The volatile oil constituents are reported to relax the smooth muscle of the trachea; and to be responsible for the effectiveness of elecampane in treating cough and tracheo-bronchial disease. A related plant *Inula racemosa* is stated to prevent electrocardiographic changes that follow heart attacks (proven ischaemic heart disease) and to have a beneficial effect on the chest pain (angina) in such patients.

Adverse effects: Allergic reactions, particularly in those who are allergic to plants belonging to the family Asteraceae. Has the potential to interfere with the treatment of diabetes mellitus and high blood pressure.

Precautions: Best avoided by patients who are on treatment for diabetes mellitus and high blood pressure (hypertension). Avoid in patients with a history of allergy. Safety in pregnancy and during lactation has not been established, hence it is best avoided.

EMBELIA RIBES – FALSE BLACK PEPPER

Susrutha, the ancient Indian physician, described the fruit as an antihelminthic, alternative and tonic and recommended its use along with liquorice root for strengthening the body and preventing the effects of ageing. Also has a reputation as an antifertility herb.

Indian/Tamil/Sri Lankan names: Vidanga, Viranga, Walangasal

A traditional Ayurvedic medicine from a climbing herb found in the Himalayas, Singapore, Sri Lanka and India.

Medicinal part: Fruit.

Uses: As an antihelminthic, a laxative, to treat flatulence.

Other uses: Powdered berries were administered on an empty stomach in the mornings to expel dead worms. A paste has been applied for ringworm infestations and as a 'butter' to relieve headaches. As a decoction for fevers and diseases of the skin and chest. One of the active constituents, embelin, has been shown in experimental work to have anti-implantation activity (prevents the fertilized ovum from embedding in the mucosa of the uterus) in rats.

Probable mode of action: Dried berries act as a carminative, antihelminthic and a stimulant. An active constituent is considered to be effective against tape worms. The pulp is a purgative and the fresh juice is considered to be cooling and act as a diuretic and as a laxative. The dark-coloured fatty oil is reported to be similar to linseed oil in its properties.

Adverse effects: The compound embelin isolated from the berries has been shown to cause anti-implantation and post-coital antifertility effects. Considered to impair the production of sperms (spermatogenesis).

Precautions: Aqueous extracts of the berries have shown antifertility effects. Should not be used during pregnancy and by those who wish to have children.

EMBLICA OFFICINALIS – INDIAN GOOSEBERRY

Phyllanthus embelia

Indian name – Amalaki, Amla
Tamil name: Nelli
Regarded as sacred by many Hindus and the Hindu religion prescribes the ripe fruits to be eaten for 40 days after a fast to restore health and vitality. This is one tree left standing when forests are cleared in Thailand. It is common practice in Indian homes to cook the fruits with sugar and saffron and give one or two to a child every morning. Was issued to Indian military personnel as a vitamin C ration. The fruit was used successfully in the treatment of human scurvy.

Medicinal part: The dried fruit.

Uses: In the treatment of dysentery and diarrhoea. It is used in combination with iron in the treatment of anaemia.

Other uses: In the treatment of jaundice and stomach ailments (dyspepsia). Has been used in the treatment of atherosclerosis.

Probable mode of action: The constituents have been attributed with varying properties including the ability to restore body strength (anabolic), effects on the heart, ability to prevent vomiting (antiemetic) and with activity against viruses. Amla, as it is known in India, is a very important dietary source of vitamin C and minerals. Considered to contain more minerals and amino acids than apples.

Adverse effects: Nausea, headache, vomiting.

Precautions: None documented.

ENGLISH IVY

Hedera helix

The Greeks and Romans used its leaves in poets' laurels. Ivy was dedicated to Bacchus, the god of wine, and was often tied to the brow to prevent intoxication. English taverns displayed the sign of an ivy bush over the door.

Approved by Commission E for:

- cough
- bronchitis.

Medicinal parts: The leaves and berries.

Uses: Symptomatic treatment of chronic inflammatory disease of the bronchi.

Other uses: For treatment of gout, rheumatism. Externally it is used in the treatment of burn wounds, calluses, cellulitis, neuralgia, parasitic disorders, ulcers, rheumatic complaints and phlebitis. **In folk medicine**, English ivy is used internally for liver, spleen and gallbladder disorders.

Probable mode of action: English ivy constituents promote removal of secretions from the lung and upper airways (expectorant) and are an antispasmodic. In animal experiments, English ivy has been shown to be antiexudative (prevent movement of fluid from inside the blood vessels) and cytotoxic (kills cells). One of the constituents has been shown to possess antiviral, antibacterial, antimycotic (antifungal), antihelminthic (effective against worms) as well as an antiflagellate (there are organisms with flagella which help them to move) effects.

Adverse effects: The fresh leaves are irritant to the skin and mucosa and can cause allergic reactions.

Precautions: No adverse effects have been recorded following the administration of recommended doses. No information is available on safety during pregnancy.

ENGLISH LAVENDER

Lavandula angustifolia

Use has been documented for 2500 years. Was used as a perfume and for mummification by Egyptians, Phoenicians and people of Arabia. Romans used lavender for bathing and scenting the air. During the great plague in London in the 17th century, it was suggested that a bunch of lavender fastened to each wrist would protect the wearer against the disease

Approved by Commission E for:

- loss of appetite
- nervousness and insomnia
- circulatory disorders
- dyspeptic complaints.

Medicinal parts: The essential oil extracted from the fresh flowers.

Uses: For mood disturbances (restlessness, insomnia) and abdominal complaints considered to be functional (not due to disease of organs).

Other uses: Externally English lavender has been used in the treatment of disorders of the circulation. **In folk medicine**, English lavender is used for migraine, cramps and bronchial asthma. Externally it is used for rheumatic conditions, as a sedative and for poorly healing wounds (lavender baths) and to promote sleep in aromatherapy (herb pillow).

Probable mode of action: The main active constituents are linalyl acetate and linalool. As early as 1936 an effect on bile secretion was demonstrated. In animal experiments the constituents, including the essential oil, showed depressant effects on the nervous system, shortening the time taken to fall asleep, lengthening the duration of sleep and reducing motor activity. In humans, inhalation produced an effect on the limbic system (a part of the brain associated with wakefulness and sleep) similar to that produced by some Valium-like drugs (benzodiazepines).

Adverse effects: None documented. The volatile oil may rarely cause sensitization.

Precautions: No health hazards or side-effects have been reported following the proper administration of recommended doses.

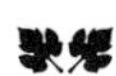

EPHEDRA – MA HUANG

Ephedra sinica

In Chinese medicine, the herb has been used for over 4000 years for severe febrile illnesses, bronchial asthma, joint symptoms, inability to perspire, coughing with shortness of breath (dyspnoea), oedema (swelling) and pain in bones. As of February 2007, sale of ephedra-containing supplements remains illegal in the US. The FDA has stated that 'no dosage of dietary supplements containing ephedrine alkaloids is safe and the sale of these products in the United States is illegal and subject to FDA enforcement action'.

Approved by Commission E for:

- cough and bronchitis.

Medicinal parts: The young cones collected in autumn and the dried rhizome with roots.

Uses: Bronchial asthma, upper respiratory tract infections (stuffy nose, watery eyes, hay fever).

Other uses: As a stimulant (stimulates the central nervous system and the cardiovascular system), to cause weight loss. Used by bodybuilders. May be abused. **In Chinese medicine**, the herb has been used for severe febrile illness, bronchial asthma, joint symptoms, inability to perspire, coughing with shortness of breath (dyspnoea), oedema (swelling) and pain in the bones.

Probable mode of action: Contains ephedrine and pseudoephedrine which are responsible for the stimulant, antiasthmatic and cough suppressant effects. These substances are very similar in action to adrenaline and noradrenaline. The level of active principles may change considerably. It is generally considered that *Ephedra sinica* has a total alkaloid content of 1–3% by dry weight. Ephedrine constitutes 40–90% of this alkaloid content with the remainder consisting of pseudoephedrine and the demethylated forms of each compound. The herb has been found to be bacteriostatic (prevents the multiplication of bacteria).

Adverse effects: Headache, irritability, restlessness, nausea, sleeplessness, rapid beating of the heart (tachycardia), hyperthermia (increase in body temperature), loss of appetite, insomnia, restlessness and increased blood pressure. May lead to heart attacks and strokes and even death.

Precautions: Not recommended for use by individuals with high blood pressure, heart disease, diabetes, thyroid disease or inflammation of the prostate gland. Should be avoided in anxiety states and when there is restlessness. Not to be used in patients with glaucoma. Avoid in patients with over-activity of the thyroid gland (thyrotoxicosis). Administer for only short periods. Dependence may develop after prolonged use. May also cause tachyphylaxis (the requirement of larger doses for similar effect).

ESPINHEIRA SANTA

Maytenus ilicifolia

Has been used by native groups in Paraguay as a contraceptive and a 'fertility regulator'.

The Argentinian name is cangorosa.

Medicinal parts: Leaves are brewed into a tea.

Uses: To treat indigestion, chronic gastritis, dyspepsia, gastric ulcers. Also used to increase libido and as a laxative.

Other uses: Leaf tea is also applied topically to wounds, skin rashes and skin cancer. To regulate menstruation, and to detoxify skin, blood, kidney and stomach. Widely used in **South America, e.g. in Argentina, Brazil and Paraguay**, for abortions, asthma, as an antiseptic to treat cancer, diarrhoea, menstrual difficulties, ulcers and wounds and as an aphrodisiac. In **Brazilian** pharmacies, a topical ointment is sold for skin cancer.

Probable mode of action: Constituents include maytansinoids, a class of substances that have been studied since 1970 for their effects on tumour cells and cancer cells (antitumour and anticancerous activity). Another constituent, cangorin, has also shown to have significant antitumour, antileukaemic and anticancerous properties.

Adverse effects: May increase secretion of saliva. May increase the actions of barbiturates (sleeping tablets). Many adverse effects are possibly not reported in the literature.

Precautions: Water extracts may have anti-oestrogenic (effects opposed to female hormone oestrogen) effects and reduces fertility in women. Should be avoided by individuals who have oestrogen hormone-dependent malignancies, e.g. cancer of the breast, and by those planning to have children.

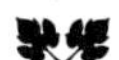

EUCALYPTUS – TASMANIAN BLUE GUM

Eucalyptus globulus

Floral emblem of Tasmania; *Eucalyptus* leaves are a traditional Aboriginal remedy.

Approved by Commission E for:

- cough and bronchitis.

Medicinal parts: Oil extracted from fresh leaves and branch tips as well as the dried leaves.

Uses: Leaves and oil have been used as an antiseptic and febrifuge (reduce fevers) and to promote removal of secretions from the lung and upper airways (expectorant).

Other uses: As a rubefacient, and for ear infections. **In folk medicine**, eucalyptus is used internally for the treatment of bladder diseases, asthma, fever, flu, whooping cough, liver and gallbladder complaints, loss of appetite and diabetes. It is used externally for wounds, acne, poorly healing ulcers, stomatitis, bleeding gums, pain and rheumatism, neuralgia, gonorrhoea and as a gastrointestinal remedy.

Probable mode of action: Various *Eucalyptus* species have been shown to possess antibacterial activity against both Gram-positive and Gram-negative organisms. Gram-positive organisms such as *Bacillus subtilis* and *Micrococcus glutamicus* have been found to be the most sensitive. The flavonoid constituents quercitrin and hyperoside have been shown in experiments to possess antiviral activity against influenza type A. The essential oil is a very powerful antiseptic, especially when it is old, because ozone is formed on exposure to air.

Adverse effects: Externally, eucalyptus oil is considered to be non-toxic, non-sensitizing and not phototoxic. If taken internally, very small amounts may be fatal. Symptoms of poisoning include epigastric (upper abdomen) burning, nausea, vomiting, dizziness, muscular weakness, small pupils (miosis), a feeling of suffocation, delirium and convulsions. Sensitive individuals may develop urticaria from handling the leaves and other parts of the plant.

Precautions: The oil should not be taken orally. Eucalyptus oil should be diluted before external use. It should be avoided by patients who are on treatment for diabetes mellitus. Infants and small children should not have preparations containing the oil applied to their faces as this practice can lead to dangerous life-threatening spasm of the upper airway (spasm of the glottis, bronchi) and asthma-like attacks. Citronella, an essential oil found in most eucalyptus species is reported to be mutagenic when used in isolation. In large doses, oil of eucalyptus has caused deaths. Death is reported from ingestion of 4–24 ml of the essential oil.

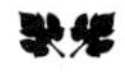

EUPHORBIA – PILL-BEARING SPURGE

Euphorbia hirta

Indian names: Dugadhika, Dudhi

Euphorbia plants were named in honour of the Greek physician Euphorbus. The leaf is used in Anglo-American traditional medicine to treat intestinal amoebiasis.

Medicinal parts: Aerial (above ground) parts.

Uses: Diseases of the respiratory tract such as asthma, bronchitis, catarrh and laryngeal (the larynx is at the entrance to the lungs) spasm and to promote removal of secretions from the lung and upper airways (expectorant). Laryngeal spasm is a serious and life-threatening disorder.

Other uses: Intestinal amoebiasis (due to infestation with amoebae – *Entamoeba histolytica*). Juice of the plant has been used for dysentery and colds. Latex of the plant is used for warts. In **Mexico**, the plant is used to treat scorpion stings, snake bites, vaginitis, sores and wounds.

Probable mode of action: One of the constituents, shikimic acid, is considered to have muscle relaxing properties, and another constituent is choline, which can cause contraction of smooth muscle. Experimentally, it has been shown to have antibacterial properties against both Gram-positive and Gram-negative bacteria. Laboratory work has also shown that euphorbia decoction has ameobicidal activity against *Entamoeba histolytica* which causes amoebiaisis.

Adverse effects: Nausea, vomiting, allergic reactions. The herb relaxes the small breathing tubes (bronchioles) but apparently depresses the heart and respiration.

Precautions: Safety in pregnancy has not been established. The shikimic constituent may possess carcinogenic (ability to cause cancers) activity. The sap contains a latex which is toxic on ingestion and highly irritant externally causing photosensitive skin reactions and severe inflammation, especially on contact with eyes or open wounds (cuts).

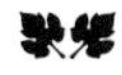

EVENING PRIMROSE – TREE PRIMROSE – SUN DROP

Oenothera biennis

The native people of North America as well as the Pilgrim Fathers were aware of the healing properties of the leaves and bark and the astringent and sedative properties. Also used for stomach and liver complaints, coughs and female disorders. The roots were eaten as vegetables.

Medicinal parts: The fatty oil extracted from the ripe seeds; the fresh plants gathered at the beginning of the flowering season.

Uses: To treat bronchial asthma, allergies, symptoms of irritability, headaches, breast tenderness associated with premenstrual syndrome and eczema, and to lower blood cholesterol.

Other uses: Rheumatoid arthritis, multiple sclerosis, diabetes mellitus and obesity and hyperactivity in children. In **America**, the herb was originally used for the treatment of asthma, stomach and digestive disorders and bruises.

Probable mode of action: Active ingredients have been found to affect chemical messengers involved in inflammation and thus have a powerful anti-inflammatory action and stabilizing effect on cell membranes. A constituent has been considered to be beneficial to the development of the nervous system of infants, as it is a constituent of normal breast milk. However, this substance is not added to infant formulae. Evening primrose oil is an omega-6 rich oil containing linoleic acid and gamma linoleic acid which is a polyunsaturated fatty acid.

Adverse effects: Few have been reported. May cause headache and nausea if taken on an empty stomach. High doses may cause diarrhoea. There are reports of seizures in schizophrenic patients who were being treated with evening primrose oil along with phenothiazines (a group of drugs popularly used as antihistamines to relieve allergy).

Precautions: Should not be used in patients with epilepsy as evening primrose oil has a potential to lower the threshold for fits. There is some evidence that people with temporal lobe epilepsy (a type of epilepsy) in particular should avoid evening primrose oil. Should be used cautiously by patients on anticoagulants. Should also be used with caution in people on allopathic medications called phenothiazines as the combination can trigger seizures even in an individual without a past history of epilepsy.

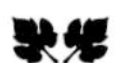

EYEBRIGHT

Euphrasia species:
Euphrasia brevipila
Euphrasia officinalis
Euphrasia rostkoviana

Was first used in the 14th century when it was considered to cure 'all evils of the eye'.

Eyebright is listed by the Council of Europe as a natural source of food flavouring.

Medicinal parts: Fluid extract from plant in fresh state gathered when in flower.

Uses: Nasal catarrh, sinusitis, as an eye lotion for conjunctivitis.

Other uses: Also used as a poultice. Used for disorders considered to be due to inflammation of the blood vessels. As a preventive measure against mucus and catarrh of the eyes. **In folk medicine**, eyebright is used for blepharitis, conjunctivitis, styes, eye fatigue symptoms, functional eye disorders of muscles and of nervous origin, cough and hoarseness. As a bitter tonic, eyebright has been used to aid digestion. In **Iceland**, the expressed juice is used for most eye ailments, and in **Scotland**, highlanders make an infusion in milk and anoint weak or inflamed eyes with a feather dipped in it.

Probable mode of action: One of the constituents, caffeic acid, is considered to be bacteriostatic (prevents the multiplication of bacteria). The tannins are known to contract cells (skin and other) following inflammation (astringent).

Adverse effects: Mental confusion, headache, raised pressure in the eye, redness and swelling of the eye if 10–60 drops of the lotion are used. These eye symptoms may be followed by increased sensitivity to light (photophobia), sneezing, nausea, constipation, cough, shortness of breath and increased passing of urine.

Precautions: Use of eyebright for eye conditions is not recommended at present. Due to the lack of data, use during pregnancy and lactation is best avoided.

FENNEL

Foeniculum vulgare

One of the oldest cultivated plants. Roman warriors used fennel to maintain good health. One of the nine sacred herbs of the Anglo-Saxons. In medieval times, the seeds were chewed to stop gastric rumbling during church services. For centuries, people wanting to lose weight and stay young ate fennel seeds. In **Mexico**, fennel is used to treat colic in babies and to relieve menstrual cramps.

Approved by Commission E for:

- cough
- bronchitis
- dyspeptic complaints.

Medicinal parts: Fennel oil extracted from the ripe fruit, the dried ripe fruit and fennel seeds.

Uses: Stomach (peptic) discomfort, flatulence, catarrh of the upper respiratory tract. Fennel honey is used for catarrh of the upper respiratory tract in children.

Other uses: As an antispasmodic for pain during menstruation and as a diuretic. The cooled tea was applied to the skin to reduce wrinkles. Also used to increase milk production during breastfeeding. Often combined with uva-ursi to treat cystitis. In **Chinese medicine**, the seeds (hui xiang) are considered to tone the spleen and kidneys.

Probable mode of action: The fennel seed promotes intestinal peristalisis – contractions of the bowel. The constituents anethole and fenchone have been shown to increase secretions in the respiratory tract and extracts are also known to increase the ciliary activity in the cells of the respiratory tract. Fennel seed extracts could reduce muscle spasms.

Adverse effects: Allergic reactions may occur rarely. May cause contact dermatitis and/or photosensitivity. Cross-sensitivity with celery is a possibility. Ingestion of even small amounts of undiluted fennel oil can cause nausea, vomiting and fits.

Precautions: No preparations except the drug itself or the tea should be used during pregnancy. Should not be administered to small children. Diabetics should check the sugar content of the preparations in the market. Seeds are potentially toxic in excessive amounts. Best avoided by patients with cirrhosis or other liver disorders.

FENUGREEK – TRIGONELLA

Trigonella foenum-graecum

The Egyptian Ebers papyrus (1500 BC) records a prescription for burns that included fenugreek seeds. Hippocrates (5th century BC) considered fenugreek a valuable soothing herb. Dioscorides recommended fenugreek for gynaecological disorders. It was also used to induce childbirth. One of the oldest cultivated medicinal plants, fenugreek is widely grown today in the Mediterranean countries, Argentina, France, India, North Africa and the US as a food, condiment, medicinal, dye and forage plant.

Approved by Commission E for:

- loss of appetite
- inflammation of the skin.

Medicinal parts: Ripe dried seeds, aerial parts.

Uses: Fenugreek is used as a carminative, to reduce inflammation and irritation (demulcent), to promote removal of secretions from the lung and upper airways (expectorant) and as a laxative. Also used in bronchitis, fevers, sore throats, wounds, skin irritations, diabetes, ulcers and in the treatment of cancer. The herb is used as a poultice for local inflammation, ulcers and eczema.

Other uses: Known to promote breastfeeding (lactation). Used as an aphrodisiac. Fenugreek seeds have been used as an oral insulin substitute. **In Chinese medicine**, fenugreek is used to treat pain in the lower abdomen, impotence and hernia. **In Indian medicine**, fenugreek is used for fever, vomiting, anorexia (loss of appetite), coughs, bronchitis and colitis (inflammatory disease of the large bowel). In the **Middle-East** and **Balkans**, aerial parts are a folk remedy for abdominal cramps associated with menstruation, diarrhoea or gastroenteritis and is used to ease labour pains.

Probable mode of action: The exact mode of action of the constituents is not known with any certainty. The aerial parts are considered to have an antispasmodic effect. Constituents include vitamins A, B_1 and C, flavonoids, minerals, saponins, alkaloids and steroids. The saponins (diosgenin and tigogenin) are chemically similar to the female hormone oestrogen and are considered useful in postmenopausal complaints.

Adverse effects: Allergic reactions (uncommon) have been reported. May change the colour and smell of urine, which is harmless. However, this change in urine may be mistaken for 'maple syrup urine disease'. Sensitization may occur.

Precautions: Should not be used during pregnancy. Diabetic individuals taking antidiabetic allopathic medications need to be careful as fenugreek may lower the blood sugar due to the fibre content. Constituents can alter the effects of monoamine oxidase inhibitors (e.g. isocarboxazid, tranylcypromine, phenelzine) and of blood thinning agents. Can affect the absorption of drugs taken simultaneously due to the high fibre content.

❦

FEVERFEW

Tanacetum parthenium

The name stems from the Latin *febrifugia*, 'fever reducer.' The first century Greek physician Dioscorides prescribed feverfew for 'all hot inflammations' due to the fibre content. Constituents can alter the effects of monoamine oxidase inhibitors (e.g. isocarboxazid, tranylcypromine, phenelzine) and of blood thinning agents. Can affect the absorption of drugs taken simultaneously due to the high fibre content. Canadian Health Officials recently approved encapsulated feverfew leaves as an over-the-counter medication for migraine prophylaxis.

Medicinal part: The herb.

Uses: Migraine prophylactic and other headaches.

Other uses: Also used for arthritis, irregular or painful menstruation (promoting menstruation), fevers, childbirth, asthma, dermatitis and as an abortifacient. **In folk medicine**, feverfew is used for cramps, as a tonic, a stimulant, a digestive agent and a blood purifier. Other uses in folk medicine include migraine prophylaxis, digestive problems, intestinal parasites and gynaecological disorders. The herb is also used as a wash for inflammation and wounds, as a tranquillizer, an antiseptic and following tooth extraction as a mouthwash. The infusion is used for dysmenorrhoea (pain during periods) and in postnatal care (care after delivery). The herb is used externally as an antiseptic and for insect bites.

Probable mode of action: Feverfew inhibits the formation of a hormone involved in inflammation (prostaglandin) and reduces inflammation. Feverfew inhibits phagocytosis (engulfing of foreign bodies by white blood cells), platelet aggregation and secretion of inflammatory mediators (arachidonic acid and serotonin). Feverfew is thought to decrease (downregulate) the response of the blood vessels in the brain to substances that are attributed to cause headaches (amines), consistent with its ability to prevent but not abort headaches.

Adverse effects: Oral ulcers (aphthous ulcers in 5–15%) and/or gastrointestinal disturbances. Sudden discontinuation can precipitate rebound headaches – 'post-feverfew syndrome', anxiety and insomnia. The herb has a high potential for sensitization following skin contact. May cause allergic reactions in those who are allergic to other plants in the Compositae family. Symptoms of post-feverfew syndrome include headache, stiffness, joint pains, tiredness and nervousness.

Precautions: Feverfew should not be used during pregnancy (historically it has been used to induce menstrual bleeding) or in patients with coagulation problems (feverfew can alter platelet activity). Feverfew may need to be used for several months before migraine sufferers recognize any improvement. It has been suggested that other drugs used in the treatment of headache (e.g. non-steroidal anti-inflammatory drugs – ibuprofen, naproxen) may reduce the effect of feverfew. Caution when used in children. Some reports suggest that feverfew will interfere with the action of allopathic medications such as calcium channel blockers, aspirin, warfarin and ticlopidine.

FIGWORT

Scrophularia nodosa

Known in the past as 'scrofula plant' and was used to treat abscesses and purulent wounds. During the 16th and 17th centuries, figwort was esteemed as the best medicinal plant for relieving all kinds of swellings and tumours.

Medicinal parts: Dried herb harvested before flowering, the herb with the root and the root alone.

Uses: For skin diseases (e.g. eczema, psoariasis and itching) and as a diuretic.

Other uses: Venereal warts, haemorrhoids, lachrymation. Believed to be useful in heart disease. According to some English sources, the herb was used as a remedy for rabies.

Probable mode of action: Cardioactive properties and anti-inflammatory activity has been attributed to the constituents harpagide and other iridioids. The iridioid constituents have been shown to cause diarrhoea.

Adverse effects: None documented.

Precautions: Avoid in patients with ventricular tachycardia (increased heart rate). The lack of toxicological data excludes its use during pregnancy and lactation.

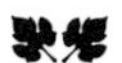

FLAX – LINSEED

Linum usitatissimum

The plant may be grown for the fibre or seed. Flax has been used as a source of fibre for weaving and clothing for more than 10,000 years. Linseed oil which is derived from flax is used in paints and varnishes.

Approved by Commission E for:

- constipation
- inflammation of the skin.

Medicinal parts: The stem as a sterile linen thread, the oil extracted from the seeds, the dry ripe seeds, linseed cakes and fresh flowering plant.

Uses: Internally flax is used for diverticulitis (a disease of the bowel where small sacs protrude from the bowel lumen and tend to get inflamed) and irritable colon and as a mucilage for gastritis and enteritis. A decoction was used for bladder disease and gastritis. Has been used externally as a poultice for local inflammatory lesions.

Other uses: Externally flax is used for removing foreign bodies from the eye. A single flax seed is moistened and placed under the eyelid, the foreign body should stick to the mucus secretion of the seed. **In Indian medicine**, flax seed is used as a tea for coughs, bronchial diseases, urethritis, diarrhoea and gonorrhoea. It is also used externally for skin infections. The seeds are also used in **Indian veterinary medicine**.

Probable mode of action: The bulk material and mucins are responsible for the laxative action. In animal experiments reduction of blood cholesterol levels was observed. A blood sugar lowering effect was also noted. The lignan constituents are considered to have an antitumour effect.

Adverse effects: The cyanogenic constituents may cause prussic acid poisoning in humans.

Nausea, bloating and diarrhoea may occur. A more serious adverse effect is stomach pain and failure to have a bowel movement.

Precautions: Flax seeds are contraindicated when there is a stricture of the oesophagus, in conditions where there is no bowel movement (ileus) and acute inflammatory diseases of the gut, including stomach. The absorption of other drugs taken simultaneously may be delayed. Flax is contraindicated in pregnancy due to the alleged content of substances which have properties similar to the female hormones. Some herbalist suggest that it should be avoided by patients with disease of the prostate gland.

FRANGULA

Rhamnus frangula

Frangula is listed by the Council of Europe as a natural source of food flavouring. The Committee on Proprietary Medicinal Products (CPMP) has adopted a core SPC (Summary of Product Characteristics) for frangula. The core SPC includes indications for short-term use of frangula in cases of occasional constipation.

Approved by Commission E for:

- constipation.

Medicinal parts: The dried bark of the trunk and branches and the fresh bark of the trunk and branches.

Uses: Constipation. To ease bowel movements in patients with haemorrhoids, anal fissures and after ano-rectal surgery.

Probable mode of action: The laxative action of Frangula can be attributed to the anthraquinone glycoside constituents such as emodin. These constituents are not absorbed from the gut and tend to absorb water. They also actively stimulate the secretion of electrolytes within the bowel.

Adverse effects: Chronic use may lead to pigmentation of the colon (pseudomelanosis coli) which is harmless and reversible after discontinuing the herb. Long-term use may also lead to dependence and the need for increased doses. Genotoxicity (a toxic effect on genes) has been reported with emodin in animal experiments.

Precautions: Not to be used in cases of intestinal obstruction, stenosis, atony, inflammatory colon diseases (e.g. Crohn's disease, ulcerative colitis), appendicitis, abdominal pain of unknown origin, severe dehydration with water and electrolyte depletion. Long-term use should be avoided. Can be used for periods in excess of two weeks only under medical supervision.

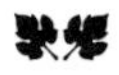

FUCUS – KELP

Fucus vesiculosus

Fucus is listed by the Council of Europe as a natural source of food flavouring. Seaweeds are commonly included in the diet of many population groups. They are also used in the dairy and baking industries to improve texture, body and smoothness of products.

Medicinal part: Seaweed.

Uses: Disorders of the thyroid gland (e.g. goitre, myxoedema).

Other uses: Obesity, arthritis, rheumatism.

Probable mode of action: Seaweeds are known to have a high iodine content, hence use in thyroid gland disorders.

Adverse effects: Hyperthyroidism (increased activity of the thyroid gland and thyroid hormones), which causes weight loss, sweating, palpitations, diarrhoea, heat intolerance and agitation, has been attributed to increased intake of kelp (fucus) at least in one report. A lady was reported to have developed hyperthyroidism after a daily intake of six 200 mg tablets of kelp. May make acne worse. Because marine plants are capable of accumulating heavy metals, there is a risk of toxicity from metals such as arsenic and mercury following excessive ingestion of fucus.

Precautions: Avoid in patients receiving medications for thyroid disease. Ingestion of kelp by children is not advised, not only due to the ability of kelp to cause or worsen acne, but also children, particularly girls, often have some enlargement of the thyroid gland during puberty. Ingestion of fucus can interfere with the absorption of iron tablets due to the binding properties of a constituent, fucoidan. There may be associated reduction in the absorption of potassium and sodium. It is necessary to monitor thyroid function and make frequent assessments to exclude toxicity due to heavy metals in subjects receiving treatment with fucus. Use of fucus during pregnancy and lactation is best avoided.

FUMITORY

Fumaria officinalis

Fumitory as a medicinal herb has been described from the Middle Ages. Was used in Turkish traditional medicine as a blood purifier and an anti-allergic agent.

Medicinal parts: Above-ground parts.

Uses: Used orally for spasms of the gastrointestinal tract and to stimulate the flow of bile.

Other uses: Historically fumitory has been used for skin diseases such as eczema and as a diuretic (to increase flow of urine), as a laxative and for heart disease.

Probable mode of action: The constituents are reported to possess an antispasmodic effect on intestinal muscle and bile duct. One of the major constituents, protopine, has been found to possess activity against histamine (antihistamine) and to cause a slowing of the heart rate and lowering of the blood pressure. Some constituents have been shown to be effective against *Bacillus anthracis* and staphylococcal infection. Some of the constituents are fumaric acid salts, mucilage and quercetin.

Adverse effects: May cause sedation in small doses, and excitation and even convulsions in large doses. Has been reported to cause a slowing of the heart rate and a fall in blood pressure. Gastrointestinal disturbances and flushing have also been reported as adverse effects.

Precautions: Best avoided in those with fits or epilepsy. Contraindicated in patients with glaucoma. Not to be used during pregnancy and breastfeeding. May increase the effects of allopathic medications used to treat high blood pressure and allopathic drugs that have the potential to slow the heart rate.

GARLIC

Allium sativum

Some records indicate that Khnoum Khoufouf the builder of one of the oldest pyramids (4500 BC) decreed that all his workers should take garlic every day to maintain their health and strength. Greeks and Romans used garlic both as a staple food and as a medicine for several ailments. Louis Pasteur was among the earliest medical celebrities to demonstrate garlic's antiseptic activity.

Garlic is considered safe by the FDA, based on the lack of known serious adverse outcomes. Has been a popular culinary and medicinal agent throughout human history (including daily use by pregnant or lactating women).

Medicinal parts: The whole fresh bulb, the dried bulb and oil of garlic.

Approved by Commission E for:
- arteriosclerosis
- hypertension
- raised levels of cholesterol.

Uses: Antiatherosclerosis, heart disease (lowering of cholesterol and other fats in the blood), antithrombotic (prevention of clot formation), fibrinolytic (dissolves the fibrin in the clot) and antihypertensive.

Other uses: Anticancer, colds, flu, coughs, sinusitis and chest infections, *Candida albicans* infections, high blood pressure and heart disease, circulatory problems, skin problems including acne and impetigo, blood sugar regulation, digestive disorders (flatulence) and bladder infections (cystitis).

Probable mode of action: One of the main active ingredients, allicin, is considered to lose its effectiveness by crushing, heat and contact with acid. Thus for garlic to be efficacious it should be consumed raw or as enteric-coated tablets. Both animal studies and epidemiological analyses suggest some effectiveness against cancers. However, it is best known to be effective as an antiatherosclerotic agent (via antithrombotic, antiplatelet, antihypertensive and especially antilipidaemic effects) i.e. preventing or reducing the formation of plaques of fat that narrow blood vessels and cause serious diseases like heart attacks and strokes. Some animal studies (in male rats) have shown that garlic may decrease the ability to make sperm cells.

Adverse effects: Bad breath is the most notorious result of consuming raw garlic. High doses may cause stomach upset, indigestion (heartburn), abdominal discomfort, nausea, vomiting.

Allergies and contact irritation may occur rarely, particularly after frequent contact. Burns may occur when the herb had remained in contact with the skin for at least 6–18 hours. The allicin may produce tearing when the garlic is crushed. Some reports state that heavy menstrual flow and uterine contractions may result from the use of garlic. There have been also reports of headache, myalgia (muscle pain), fatigue and vertigo with therapeutic doses of garlic.

Precautions: Not to be taken with anticlotting medication. If you're breastfeeding, you may find that garlic makes your baby's colic worse. Avoid for several weeks prior to surgery.

GENTIAN

Gentiana lutea

Gentian is named after Gentius, King of Illyria in the 1st century BC, who is said to have discovered the plant's ability to reduce fevers. Gentian root is used in many bitter liqueurs. Has been used for centuries as a bitter for mild to moderate digestive disorders.

Gentian is included in the European and British Pharmacopoeia.

Approved by Commission E:
- as a tonic.

Medicinal parts: Dried root and rhizome. They should be sliced and dried slowly, during which time the characteristic odour, colour and taste develop.

Uses: As a bitter, as a gastric stimulant and to increase salivary secretions and bile secretion.

Other uses: Tonic, antiemetic, anti-inflammatory and to decrease fever. Best known as a bitter that stimulates stomach activity.

Probable mode of action: Constituents include several bitter principles that stimulate digestion, and help in dyspepsia.

Adverse effects: May cause headaches and gastrointestinal irritation (nausea and vomiting with overdose).

Precautions: Contraindicated in patients with gastric or duodenal ulcers. Some herbalists recommend avoidance during pregnancy and in patients with high blood pressure.

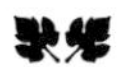

GINGER

Zingiber officinale

A long and well-documented history of culinary and medicinal use throughout Asia, during the Roman Empire and in Europe. Most widely used for nausea. The Chinese used ginger to expel cold and restore yang: 'By inducing sweating ginger expelled toxins'. For 2500 years, the Chinese have used this plant as a flavouring agent and antiemetic. Ancient Greeks wrapped ginger in bread and ate it after meals as a digestive aid. Was used in India to treat colds, nausea, cough, dyspepsia and rheumatism. Has been applied to the temples as a paste to relieve headache.

Medicinal part: The root.

Approved by Commission E for:
- loss of appetite
- travel sickness
- dyspepsia (indigestion).

Uses: Used as an antiemetic and in colic, in stomach ailments (dyspepsia) as a carminative, and for rheumatoid arthritis.

Other uses: Travel sickness, morning sickness or nausea, indigestion, colds and flu, bronchitis and productive coughs, chilblains and arthritis (osteoarthritis). Also helps to lower blood pressure.

In Chinese medicine, ginger is used to treat colds, nausea, vomiting and shortness of breath. **In Indian medicine**, ginger is used to treat anorexia, dyspepsia and pharyngitis.

Probable mode of action: Active constituents are gingerols and shogaol. Constituents cause an increase in the secretion of saliva, gastric juices and bile. Gingerols have pain relieving activity (analgesic), sedative, antipyretic, antibacterial and gastrointestinal tract motility effects (increase of tone and peristalsis). Anti-inflammatory effects are attributed to inhibition of an enzyme involved in the inflammatory process – cyclo-oxygenase. Some studies have shown that ginger increases the force of contraction of the heart muscle (inotropic). Some experiments have also demonstrated antioxidant effects and anti-migraine effects.

Adverse effects: Heartburn, allergic reaction (rare). May alter the clotting time of blood.

Precautions: Not to be taken by those suffering from peptic ulcers. Caution when used to treat nausea after surgery. The German Commission E contraindicates the use of ginger for morning sickness associated with pregnancy. The essential oil shouldn't be taken internally without professional supervision. Long-term use in pregnancy isn't recommended. Patients with gallstones should avoid using ginger, and ginger should not be taken by patients who have a risk of haemorrhage, e.g. awaiting surgery.

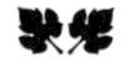

GINKGO BILOBA

Ginkgo biloba

One of the oldest surviving tree species, *Ginkgo biloba* has grown in China for more than 200 million years.

Standardized ginkgo biloba extracts are among the leading prescriptions in Germany and France and are available in the US as a dietary supplement. The Federal German Drug Law considered ginkgo effective for the treatment of peripheral arterial occlusive disease (disease due to narrowing or blockage of arteries particularly to the lower limbs).

Medicinal parts: Fresh or dried leaves. The seeds are used in **Traditional Chinese Medicine**.

Uses: Dementia, enhancing memory, improving concentration, intracerebral and peripheral vascular insufficiency, Alzheimer's disease, tinnitus (ringing in the ears) and vertigo (dizziness).

Other uses: Mountain sickness, high blood pressure, stroke, varicose veins, piles and asthma.

Probable mode of action: The mechanisms of ginkgo's therapeutic effects are not fully understood. They are attributed in part to synergistic effects of its constituents, particularly the flavonoid glycosides and terpene lactones. These act to varying degrees as scavengers of free-radicals and antioxidants that are considered to improve the tolerance to reduced supplies of oxygen to the brain either during disease or following head injury. Ginkgo is reported to improve peripheral circulation, through an effect on blood viscosity and/or affecting the smooth muscle of blood vessels. Ginkgolides are reported to inhibit platelet activation factor and thereby reduce thrombosis (clot formation within blood vessels) and dilate arteries and capillaries.

Adverse effects: Gastrointestinal tract disturbances (mild stomach upset), high doses (over 120 mg a day) can cause headaches, contact dermatitis (each is rare/mild). *Ginkgo biloba* seeds can cause fatal neurological and allergic reactions. Spontaneous bleeding – intracerebral haemorrhage, bilateral subdural haematomas, subarachnoid haemorrhage (bleeding within the different layers covering the brain) and bleeding from the iris into the anterior chamber of the eye – are known to occur due to inhibition of platelet aggregation (platelets form a plug by aggregating to stop bleeding).

Precautions: Do not use in those with known allergy to *Ginkgo* or species that cross-react (cashew, poison ivy). Not usually recommended for children and not to be taken by those on blood thinning medication such as warfarin. Can cause serious postoperative bleeding and should be discontinued prior to surgery. Severe circulatory disturbances (hypotension, shock, dizziness) have followed parenteral use which is not recommended. Excess ingestion of *gingko* seeds – a delicacy in Japan – can cause 'gin-man' food poisoning, particularly in children, which is characterized by convulsions and coma. May antagonize the effects of insulin and other allopathic medications taken to control blood sugar.

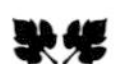

GINSENG

Panax ginseng

Panax ginseng was discovered over 5000 years ago in the Manchurian Mountains of China. The human shape of the plant became a symbol of divine harmony on earth. The English name is derived from the Chinese term 'ren-shen' literally meaning man-root, referring to the resemblance of the root to the legs of a man.

The botanical term *Panax* means 'all-heal' in Greek.

Ginseng is one of the most popular and expensive herbs in the world. As in ancient China, ginseng is still widely believed to be a panacea or cure-all. In the *Panax* family two descriptive terms based primarily on geographical locations are known.

American ginseng, which is found primarily in America, has been used by the American people of central and eastern North America for 300 years. It was discovered near Montreal by a Jesuit priest, searching the Canadian hardwood forest.

The *Panax* grown in Korea and China is referred to primarily as Korean ginseng. Cultivation of *Panax* began in Korea around 1,700 AD.

In this book we discuss American/Korean/Chinese *Panax ginseng* as one group. However, according to traditional Chinese medicine, American ginseng promotes 'yin' energy (shadow, cold, negative, female), cleanses excess 'yang' and calms the body. In contrast Korean or Chinese ginseng is considered to promote 'yang' (sunshine, hot, positive, male) energy, improve circulation, increase blood supply, and aid recovery after illness. The herbal literature lists differing uses and other details for American ginseng and Korean/Chinese/Asian ginseng.

Eleutherococcus senticosus, so-called Siberian ginseng, is not the *Panax* (true ginseng) genus, and is described separately in this book under the heading 'Ginseng – Siberian'.

American ginseng is approved by Commission E for

- lack of stamina

Uses: Primarily as an adaptogen to treat physical and mental stress and fatigue. Used as a tonic to enhance performance including sexual activity (as an aphrodisiac). Has also been used to treat male and female subfertility. Used as a general supplement to improve concentration and memory, as an anti-ageing herb, and to counter depression and anxiety. Some herbalists recommend its use for subjects who have been diagnosed as suffering from chronic fatigue syndrome.

Other uses: In Chinese Medicine, ginseng has been and is used to treat haemoptysis (coughing up of blood), gastric disturbances and vomiting. It has been used in the treatment of anaemia, diabetes mellitus and hot flushes due to menopause. Other uses have included the treatment of cancer, high blood pressure, to stimulate immunity and bleeding disorders.

Probable mode of action: Due to the wide variations in quality and sources of ginseng used in studies, it has been very difficult to establish with any precision using the modern methods of scientific investigation, the constituents that are considered responsible for the therapeutic effects.

The main active constituents in ginseng are the ginsenosides, a diverse group of substances with a structure similar to the hormones secreted by the cortex (outside layer) of the adrenal glands. There have been at least 25 ginsenosides that have been separated in laboratory experiments.

These ginsenosides have been found in laboratory experiments to produce a wide range of effects. Ginsenosides have been shown to stimulate the secretion of hormones from the adrenal gland and pancreas (insulin). However, there is no certainty as to whether such effects do occur in humans and the doses necessary for the production of these effects are not known. Some constituents have been found to influence production and motility of sperm. An American study in 2002 on laboratory animals showed that American and Korean (Asian) ginseng enhanced libido and copulatory performance. In males, ginsenosides facilitated penile erection by increasing the blood flow to the cavernous tissues in the penis (corpus cavernosum). This effect was considered to be related to the release of nitric oxide from the cells lining the blood vessels (endothelial cells) to the penis.

A non-ginsenoside component has been found to have an affinity for some receptors in nerve cells in the brain, which are considered to be important in maintaining mental acuity even in old age. Some constituents have been found to protect the liver against some liver toxins, while another effect that has been reported is the inhibition of the proliferation of lung cancer cells. Ginseng has been found to improve immunity against infections. The constituents have been considered by some workers to help in the prevention of heart disease by lowering blood cholesterol and concentrations of low density lipo-proteins. Another effect on the cardiovascular system is an anti-platelet (anti-clotting) effect – the prevention of aggregation of platelets to form clots or platelet plugs.

It needs to be stated that there is considerable variation in the degree and nature of effects produced by the constituents from the large body of laboratory work that is available.

Adverse effects: Amongst the commonest side-effects reported are inability to fall asleep, an increase in heart rate (tachycardia), an increase in blood pressure (hypertension – even though ginseng has been advocated by some to treat high blood pressure). A well documented adverse effect is the 'ginseng abuse syndrome'. Overuse or prolonged use may cause a general state of over stimulation (diarrhoea, nervousness, skin eruption). A rash or itching may follow abuse. As such, ginseng is best not prescribed with other stimulants (some specialists advise even against caffeine containing drinks). Some herbalists state that Korean ginseng is a stronger stimulant than American ginseng. Rare hormonal (endocrinological) effects have been reported following the use of ginseng and these include mastalgia (pain in breasts) and post-menopausal bleeding.

Precautions: Not recommended for use during pregnancy and breast feeding. It is best avoided in children until safety in relation to paediatric use is known with certainty. Subjects with high blood pressure and heart disease should take ginseng only under medical supervision if considered necessary. Ginseng is to be avoided when there is excessive bleeding (possibly due to its effects on platelets) such as nose bleeds or heavy menstruation. It should also not be used in patients with psychosis and manic disorders.

GINSENG – SIBERIAN

Eleutherococcus senticosus

In Chinese Traditional Medicine, Siberian ginseng has been valued for its beneficial effects on qi and its ability to treat yang deficiency of the spleen and kidney.

Siberian ginseng is not considered a true ginseng as instead of the fleshy root of *Panax ginseng*, *Eleutherococcus* has a woody root. More importantly, instead of ginsenosides, Siberian ginseng contains eleutherosides.

Has been used for centuries in Russia and China where it was renowned for its ability to restore vigour, increase longevity, enhance overall health, stimulate appetite and improve memory. Used in Russia primarily as an adaptogen and to enhance productivity.

Approved by Commission E for:
- tendency to infection
- lack of stamina.

Medicinal parts: The pulverized root rind, the pulverized root and an alcoholic fluid extract of the rhizome and the roots.

Uses: Used as a tonic for increasing strength and vitality in times of fatigue and debility, and for improving athletic performance. It is an adaptogen. Used to treat to normalize blood pressure, pyelonephritis, cranio-cerebral trauma (trauma to the brain and skull), rheumatic heart disease. Siberian ginseng isn't a member of the ginseng family.

Other uses: In Chinese medicine, Siberian ginseng is used for kidney pain, retention of urine, impotence, sleep disturbances, loss of appetite, pain and weakness in hip and knee joints, rheumatoid arthritis and as a stimulant for immune system. Also for high blood pressure, chronic inflammatory disease and infections (colds).

Probable mode of action: Eleutherosides are considered to increase stamina and stimulate the immune system. Most studies on eleutherosides have been on their effects on the immune system, mental performance, physical performance and male fertility. Effects on viral infections have also been studied. The liquid extract of the herb has been shown to possess antioxidant, immune-stimulating, immune-modulating and antiviral effects. Animal experiments have demonstrated an ability to withstand stress. Following the intake of the liquid extract, the lymphocyte count (a white blood cell involved in immunity) increased in human volunteers. Other effects reported is a blood sugar lowering effect and an antiplatelet-aggregating effect.

Adverse effects: High doses may cause drowsiness, anxiety, irritability, mastalgia (pain in the breast) and uterine bleeding. It may also increase blood pressure and cause irregular heart beats. May potentiate the effects of antidiabetic drugs, sedatives and anticoagulants.

Precautions: Use with caution in patients with high blood pressure. Not to be taken with coffee or for more than six weeks at a time. Avoid if pregnant. Unsuitable for children. May produce elevated blood digoxin levels.

GOLDENROD – SOLIDAGO

Solidago virgaurea

Was used in herbal medicine to mask the bitterness of other medicines. Has been popular in the treatment of bladder stones since the 13th century.

Approved by Commission E for:
- infections of the urinary tract
- kidney and bladder stones.

Medicinal parts: Flowers, leaves and roots.

Uses: Arthritis, allergies, colds and flu, inflammation of the bladder or urinary tract, kidney stones. Has been used as a tea, a gargle, a fluid extract and a tincture.

Other uses: Laryngitis, sore throats. Topical application is considered to aid wound healing and bring relief from skin conditions such as eczema. **In folk medicine**, goldenrod is used internally for rheumatism, gout, diabetes, haemorrhoids, prostatic hypertrophy, nervous bronchial asthma, internal bleeding, enlargement of the liver, acute exacerbation of pulmonary tuberculosis. Used externally for inflammations of the mouth and throat as well as for festering wounds.

Probable mode of action: The herb has a diuretic action due to some of the constituents. Goldenrod also inhibits the formation of urinary calculi. One of the constituents has been shown to have pain relieving effects while others (saponin constituents) are antimicrobial, weakly spasmolytic and antiexudative.

Adverse effects: Mild allergic reactions. May rarely cause asthma.

Precautions: Not to be used during pregnancy and breastfeeding. Irrigation therapy is contraindicated in cases of oedema (swelling usually of the ankles) resulting from reduced heart or kidney function. Care must be taken when used in patients with chronic kidney disease.

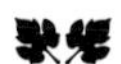

GOLDENSEAL

Hydrastis canadensis

Cherokee Indians used the herb for cancer, general debility, 'dyspepsy' and to improve appetite and as a tonic. Used by them topically for eye or skin irritation (wounds and ulcers) and orally for infections. The Irioquois used a decoction of roots to treat whooping cough, diarrhoea, liver disease, fevers and as an emetic for bile disorders.

Has been listed as an endangered species in the US since 1991.

Cherokee Indians used it topically for eye or skin irritation (wounds and ulcers), and orally for infections.

Medicinal parts: The air-dried rhizome with the root fibres.

Uses: Used as an antidiarrhoeal agent, as an antiseptic externally on wounds in treatment of herpes labialis, and for oral sores.

Other uses: Also used as an adjunct in the treatment of cancers. Has been used to treat HIV patients. Used also for cold and flu symptoms, vaginal infections and menstrual bleeding. Has been used to treat trachoma (a disease of the eye), stomach ulcers and gallbladder disease.

Probable mode of action: One of the main alkaloid constituents is an effective antidiarrhoeal agent which is thought to act inside the bowel lumen and is not considered to be absorbed to any significant extent. These effects have been confirmed by laboratory experiments. Another effect is that it has an antagonistic (antimicrobial) activity against numerous bacteria, fungi and protozoa. In addition, it blocks adhesion of bacteria to epithelial cells, inhibits the intestinal secretory response of cholera and *Escherichia coli* toxins, and normalizes mucosal cell structure after damage by the cholera toxin.

Adverse effects: Large doses can cause mucocutaneous irritation, gastrointestinal tract disturbances (vomiting, diarrhoea), cardiac and uterine contractility, vasoconstriction, central nervous system stimulation, neonatal (babies) jaundice (displaces bilirubin). Symptoms of goldenseal poisoning include stomach upset, nervous symptoms and depression. Long-term use may reduce vitamin B absorption. May cause a fall in white blood cells involved in protecting the body against infections.

Precautions: Large (unspecified) amounts of goldenseal may cause uterine contractions. Should be avoided in babies with jaundice. It may oppose heparin or coumarin anticoagulation. Goldenseal should not be used by pregnant or lactating women, babies or patients with cardiovascular disease (high blood pressure), epilepsy or coagulation problems. Goldenseal is contraindicated in subjects with glucose-6-phosphate-dehydrogenase (G6PD) deficiency.

GREEN TEA

Camellia sinensis

The tea plant is considered to be one of the 50 fundamental herbs in Chinese herbal medicine. Myanmar (Burma) and then China are considered to be the original places where tea was drunk. Tea has played a significant role in Asian culture for centuries as a beverage, a curative and a symbol of status.

According to Chinese legend, which spread along with Buddhism, the semi-legendary Buddhist monk Bodhidharma is credited with the discovery of tea. Another Chinese legend attributes the discovery of drinking tea to Shennong, the Emperor of China who invented agriculture and Chinese medicine 5000 years ago.

As a dried plant, tea which preserves some vitamins is believed to have kept Chinese sailors healthy.

The Han dynasty in China used tea as a medicine in the 1st millennium BC. The beverage and the ceremony surrounding it played an important part in feudal diplomacy.

All tea (black, green and oolong) originates from one bush, *Camellia sinensis.* Herbal tea usually refers to infusions of fruit or herbs that do not contain *Camellia sinensis*.

Medicinal parts: The very young leaves from which green or black tea is prepared according to the treatment to be given.

Uses: Green tea is used for stomach disorders, migraine, symptoms of fatigue, vomiting and diarrhoea when taken as a beverage. It has also been used to enhance performance (stimulant effect). Also used for the prevention of dental caries.

Other uses: In **Indian medicine**, tea preparations are used for diarrhoea, loss of appetite, hyperdipsia (thirst), migraine, chest pain, fever and fatigue.

In **Chinese medicine**, green tea is used to treat migraine, nausea, diarrhoea resulting from malaria and digestive problems. It is also used for the prevention of cancer. Externally very young tea leaves or buds are used as a poultice or wash to treat cuts, bruises, insect bites and swellings.

Probable mode of action: Tea is a natural source of compounds referred to as methylxanthines (e.g. caffeine, small amounts of theobromine and theophylline, thianine) and of the antioxidant catechin. Green tea also contains fluoride. The caffeine in tea has a stimulating effect on the nervous system and an antidepressant effect. The antagonism of a hormone which restricts the formation of urine leads to increased passing of urine (diuresis). Caffeine also increases the force of contraction of the heart muscle (inotropic) and promotes the secretion of gastric juice. Has also been shown to have an effect on small blood vessels and to minimize inflammatory reactions. The antidiarrhoeal effect can be attributed to a combination of tannins and to the fact that 400 mg of polyphenols administered three times daily promotes the growth of certain organisms useful in countering diarrhoea (e.g. *Lactobacillus*) and inhibits the growth of some organisms that cause diarrhoea (clostridia).

Green tea has also been shown to be useful in prevention of cancers of the pancreas, colon, small bowel, stomach, lung and breast. Green tea mouthwashes have been shown to inhibit the growth of bacteria that tend to thrive in body cavities (*Streptococcus salivarius*, *Escherichia coli*).

Adverse effects: Side-effects of tea consumption are possibly commoner in persons with sensitive stomachs, and are caused by some of the constituents (e.g. tannin content). Excessive consumption could lead to hyperacidity, gastric irritation, reduction of appetite as well as diarrhoea. These effects can be minimized by the addition of milk. With long-term intake of doses in excess of 1.5 g caffeine per day, restlessness, irritability, sleeplessness, palpitations, vertigo, headache, loss of appetite, vomiting and diarrhoea may occur. The tannins in tea have been considered as a cause of oesophageal cancer.

Precautions: Should be used with great care in patients with heart disease and in those with increased activity of the thyroid gland (hyperthyroidism). It has been documented that pregnant females should not exceed 300 mg per day (five cups of tea spread out over the course of a day). Children who take excessive amounts may develop anaemia due to interference with the absorption of iron. Products containing extracts of green tea, especially if taken in high doses, may be associated with hepatitis. Some herbalists do not recommend the use of green tea during pregnancy.

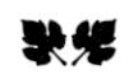

GROUND IVY

Glechoma hederacea

The medicinal properties have been described for millennia. Galen recommended the plant to treat inflammation. John Gerard, an English herbalist, recommended its use to treat tinnitus, as a diuretic, as an astringent and as a tonic.

Was the most common flavouring in beer by the Saxons prior to the use of hops in the 16th century.

Ground ivy is listed by the Council of Europe as a natural source of food flavouring.

Medicinal parts: The herb collected during the flowering season and dried, the fresh aerial parts collected during the flowering season and the whole plant. A herb tea is made from fresh leaves or dried leaves.

Uses: Bronchitis, symptomatic treatment of coughs, tinnitus (ringing in the ears), catarrh. **In folk medicine**, the herb is used internally for inflammation of the gastrointestinal mucous membranes and diarrhoea. Used to treat worm infestations.

Other uses: Haemorrhoids, as a diuretic in the treatment of bladder and kidney stones, cystitis, gastritis. Externally the drug is used for the treatment of poorly healing ulcers and skin diseases. In **Italy,** the herb is used for arthritis and rheumatism.

In Chinese medicine, ground ivy is used to treat carbuncles, erysipelas (a reddish rash of the skin), lower abdominal pain, scabies, irregular menstruation, coughs, dysentery and jaundice.

Probable mode of action: Considered safe and effective for disorders of the mucous membranes (the lining cells) of the ear, nose, throat and digestive tracts. An alcoholic extract of ground ivy has been shown to have anti-inflammatory properties. Some of the constituents have been shown experimentally to promote the healing of ulcers. Also reported is an ability to contract cells (skin and other) following inflammation (astringent). The anti-inflammatory properties are associated with the flavonoids and tannins.

Adverse effects: Poisoning has taken place in cattle and horses. The symptoms have been a weak pulse, difficulty in breathing, conjunctival haemorrhage, fever, dizziness and enlargement of the spleen and gastroenteritis. Ground ivy oil can be an irritant to the gastrointestinal tract and may cause stomach upsets.

Precautions: Considered to be an abortifacient and hence to be avoided during pregnancy. Contraindicated in epilepsy and best avoided by those with kidney disease.

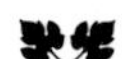

GUARANA

Paullinia cupana

The Tupi and Guarani Brazilian cultures believe guarana to be a magical cure for bowel complaints and to regain strength. Several brands of soft drinks are made from guarana extracts in **Brazil** and neighbouring countries where it is suggested that these drinks are more popular than drinks made from cola.

The FDA in the US has considered guarana as Generally Regarded As Safe (GRAS) and that the preparations must be labelled as not intended to diagnose, treat, cure or prevent any disease.

Medicinal parts: The peeled, dried roasted and pulverized seeds, formed into a thick paste with water.

Uses: Guarana is used as a tonic for fatigue and to quell hunger and thirst, for headaches and dysmenorrhoea.

Other uses: Digestive problems, fever, as a diuretic.

Probable mode of action: Guarana produces a stimulating effect due to the presence of caffeine, theobromine and theophylline. The caffeine causes stimulation of the central nervous system and also increases the force of contraction of the heart muscle (inotropic action). In high doses it also increases the heart rate (chronotropic) and works as short-term diuretic. Another effect attributed to caffeine is an increase in blood pressure due to release of catecholamines (chemical messengers of the sympathetic nervous system like adrenaline which constricts blood vessels) and also causes dilatation of the bronchi.

Adverse effects: May cause stimulation of the nervous system if taken in excessive amounts (restlessness, insomnia, agitation). The diuretic effect may lead to loss of potassium from the body.

Precautions: Should be avoided by those with disease of the cardiovascular system and by those with a tendency to develop panic attacks or anxiety states. Quantities corresponding to up to 400 mg of caffeine per day (7–11 g of herb) are considered toxicologically harmless to a healthy adult. May lead to habituation and withdrawal symptoms on discontinuing intake. Should not be taken with or mixed with ephedrine and ephedrine-like compounds.

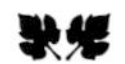

GYMNEMA

Gymnema sylvestre

Documented as a treatment for 'sweet urine' in Indian texts over 2000 years old.

The Hindu name, gurmar, 'destroyer of sugar', applies to the leaves (the medicinal parts of the plant), which when chewed interfere with the ability to taste sweetness.

Medicinal part: Leaves.

Uses: Has been used to lower sugar, cholesterol and triglyceride levels in the blood. Also used to reduce body weight.

Probable mode of action: Main constituent is gymnemic acid, a complex mixture of at least nine closely related acidic glycosides which are considered to increase activity of enzymes that are involved in the utilization of glucose which is produced by the action of insulin. The constituents are also thought to increase and also regenerate the cells that produce insulin in the pancreas (islets of Langerhans) and also to increase the levels of insulin that circulate in the blood. The blood sugar lowering effect of *Gymnema* leaves was first documented in the late 1920s.

Adverse effects: Used in recommended doses, there have been no adverse effects reported. However, when using allopathic medications for control of blood sugar, caution is necessary as gymnema can cause further reductions in blood sugar and produce symptoms such as sweating, confusion, shakiness and speech disorders.

Precautions: Safety during pregnancy and lactation has not been established as yet. Patients with diabetes mellitus should use gymnema only under clinical supervision. Gymnema cannot be used to replace insulin to control either type I or type II diabetes. Gymnema is likely to increase the blood sugar lowering effects of insulin and other medications used orally (by mouth) for lowering of blood sugar such as glipizide, metformin, glibenclamide. May also potentiate the cholesterol lowering effects of the group of drugs called statins (e.g. lovastatin, simvastatin, pravastatin, atorvastatin). Be cautious when using with other herbs with the potential to lower blood sugar (e.g. fenugreek, ginger, kudzu, *Panax ginseng*).

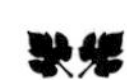

HAWTHORN

Crataegus oxyacantha

Hawthorn as a drug is said to have been first used as a secret remedy by a Dr Green of Ireland. A clinical résumé of crataegus is to be found in *New, Old and Forgotten Remedies* which quotes articles from the *New York Medical Journal* (1896) and the *Kansas City Medical Journal* (1898).

Medicinal parts: Berries, leaves, flowers.

Uses: In high blood pressure, pain of ischaemic (due to poor blood supply to heart muscle) heart disease (angina) and heart attacks, and heart failure.

Other uses: Prevention of disorders of heart rhythm (cardiac arrhythmias) and to promote the formation of urine (diuretic) to rid the body of excess salt and water. It is also used in diarrhoea and colic. Has been documented to improve poor memory, prevent nervous tension and promote sleep (treat insomnia). Has been considered as a 'food for the heart' to strengthen the heart and to 'balance the circulation'.

Probable mode of action: The active constituents (flavonoids and procyandins) have been shown to dilate the blood vessels to the heart (coronary vasodilators) and thus increase the blood flow to the heart muscle. This is believed to strengthen heart muscle tissue while also acting as a mild diuretic which would be the result of increased pumping of the heart muscle, thus increasing the blood flow to the kidneys. Some constituents are considered to increase the tone of the blood vessels and improve the elasticity of the arteries and veins. Animal studies have demonstrated a cholesterol lowering effect both by reducing the production of cholesterol and by increasing the breakdown of cholesterol by the body.

Adverse effects: May cause dizziness, headache, insomnia, nausea, sweating and stomach upsets. Local application may cause a rash. An important adverse effect is hypotension (lowering of blood pressure). May also cause sedation. May cause relaxation of the uterine muscle and thus cause miscarriages.

Precautions: It is suggested that the use of hawthorn be limited to appropriately trained health-care practitioners. Avoid use during pregnancy, and as its safety is not known in children, do not use in children or while breastfeeding. Co-administration with digoxin is best avoided. Likely to increase the side-effects of allopathic drugs such as clonidine, albuterol, theophylline and Viagra. Also do not co-administer with herbal medicines such as mistletoe (European), large doses of ginger, motherwort, *Panax ginseng* and squill. Caution in those with high blood pressure who are on medication.

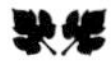

HIBISCUS ROSA-SINENSIS

Hibiscus rosa-sinensis

Hibiscus is the national flower of Malaysia, called the *bunga raya* in Malay and *sembaruthi* in Tamil. The flowers are used to shine shoes in parts of India as well as in worship.

Flowers have been reported in the ancient Indian literature as being useful to treat heart disease. Flowers of this plant are said to possess antifertility property by ancient Ayurvedic texts. The flowers are used in Kerala (Southern India) to promote menstruation (emmenagogue) and as a contraceptive.

Medicinal part: Flowers.

Uses: In disorders of the heart.

Probable mode of action: The herb's effect upon the male reproductive system may be due to the inhibition of synthesis or release of hormones involved in reproduction from the pituitary gland (gonadotrophins). The effects are considered to be transient. Some experimental work has shown that the flowers have some post-coital antifertility action dependent on the dose, duration of treatment and the stage of pregnancy. Flowers are considered to possess some antioestrogenic (anti-female hormone oestrogen) activity.

Adverse effects: No information available.

Precautions: Do not use during pregnancy or if planning to have children.

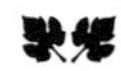

HIGH MALLOW

Malva sylvestris

One of the plants cited very early in the herbal literature. Horace mentions it in reference to his own

herbs

diet 'as for me olives, endives and mallows provide sustenance'. When planted on graves, it was thought that the dead could feed on it.

Approved by Commission E for:

- cough
- bronchitis
- inflammation of the mouth and pharynx.

Medicinal parts: Dried flowers.

Uses: In folk medicine, the herb is used internally for disorders of the small tubes in the lungs (bronchial disorders) and for the treatment of gastroenteritis and bladder complaints.

Other uses: Used externally for wounds and as a poultice and bath additive for treatment of wounds. To soothe the sore throat caused by coughs and colds. Poultices of flowers were used to disinfect wounds. Commonly used as a tea.

Probable mode of action: The main constituents in the leaf are polysaccharides, flavonoids and tannins. The herb has large amounts of mucilaginous substances which are believed to protect the mucous membranes of the body, particularly when irritant substances come into contact with such membranes. The flowers contain more mucilage than the leaf. Also contains antioxidants.

Adverse effects: No adverse effects have been reported following use in recommended doses.

Precautions: Not to be used by subjects with gallstones.

HOLLY

Ilex aquifolium

As the plant remains green in the winter, Celts and Anglo-Saxons associated holly with mystical power. Even at present, bringing a holly plant into the house is considered to bring good luck. To the Romans, the Christmas holly tree was sacred to Saturn and holly wreaths with bright red berries were given as gifts during his holiday, the Saturnalia, upon which the Christmas holiday was possibly modelled.

The leaves have been used as a substitute for tea, while the roasted fruit has been used as a substitute for coffee.

Medicinal parts: Dried and fresh leaves, fruit.

Uses: Not frequently used in herbal medicine at present. Leaves used as a diuretic, for coughs and digestive disorders. To bring down fevers (antipyretic). Has been used in the treatment of rheumatism and pleurisy. Fruit is used to stimulate the heart. The juice of the fresh leaves was used to treat jaundice.

Probable mode of action: The fruit and probably other parts of the herb contain saponins, which are thought to cause gastrointestinal irritation and vomiting. The beneficial effects of the constituents are not known with certainty.

Adverse effects: Gastrointestinal disturbances with nausea, vomiting and diarrhoea. Severe diarrhoea can cause muscle weakness due to electrolyte imbalance. The berries are poisonous and can cause vomiting, diarrhoea and stupor and may cause fatalities. The fruit has been known to cause severe diarrhoea and vomiting.

Precautions: Do not exceed recommended doses. Information about safety during pregnancy is not available. The fruits are particularly poisonous to children and should not be used. The herb is best used under supervision of a medical practitioner.

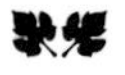

HOLY THISTLE – BLESSED THISTLE

Cnicus benedictus

Romans used the leaves and root as a vegetable 1500 years ago. During the Middle Ages, blessed thistle was considered to be useful in the treatment of bubonic plague and smallpox and was grown in the herbal gardens of monasteries.

Historically, was also taken to increase the flow of breast milk.

Medicinal part: Seeds.

Uses: Loss of appetite (anorexia), gastric discomfort due to gas or loss of tone of the stomach muscles (flatulent dyspepsia, atonic dyspepsia). Used when there are increased secretions in the small tubes of the lung (bronchial catarrh). Used as a bitter, taken by mouth to relieve indigestion and diarrhoea.

Other uses: Topically for gangrenous and indolent ulcers and to soothe the skin irritated by burns, scrapes, shaving or sunburn.

Probable mode of action: One of the constituents has been shown to have antibacterial effects in the laboratory. It is considered to be effective against many bacteria including *Staphylococcus aureus*, *Streptococcus faecalis* and *Brucella bronchoseptica*. This component has been shown to protect against inflammation similar to the allopathic medications, namely, non-steroidal anti-inflammatory agents such as indometacin. The tannins are also considered to contract cells (skin and other) following inflammation (astringent).

Adverse effects: May cause abdominal pain. Can irritate the lining of the gastrointestinal tract. Considered to cause allergy particularly to those allergic to plants of the Compositae family (e.g. ragwort, chamomile, tansy).

Precautions: Safety in pregnancy has not been established, and it has not been confirmed that it increases the production of breast milk. Best avoided during pregnancy and breastfeeding. As it can irritate the lining (mucous membranes) of the gut, avoid use in patients with Crohn's disease and irritable bowel syndrome.

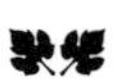

HONEYBUSH – HEUNINGBOS

Cyclopia intermedia

In *King's American Dispensatory* of 1898, under the heading of tea, honeybush is listed as a substitute, with reference to a report from 1881 indicating use of honeybush as a tea in the Cape Colony of South Africa. The Khoisan tribes of South Africa were known to use the tea for treatment of coughs and upper respiratory symptoms associated with infections. Since then it has become known as a substitute for ordinary tea and one of the recognized benefits is its lack of caffeine, which makes it especially suited for night-time consumption and for those who experience nervousness and want to avoid ordinary tea.

Medicinal part: Leaves.

Uses: As a tea, for coughs and inflammatory respiratory tract infections, treatment of constipation.

Other uses: Postmenopausal symptoms, as a mild relaxant.

Probable mode of action: The active constituents include pinitol which promotes the removal of secretions from the lung and upper airways (expectorant). It is also known to lower blood sugar. Other active constituents act as antioxidants and may help to lower the fat content (lipids) in the blood. Some constituents have been detected to have female hormonal properties and have been used to treat menopausal symptoms.

Adverse effects: No reported adverse effects.

Precautions: None reported.

HOPS

Humulus lupulus

Other than the use in beer, hops have a long history of use as a sedative and sleep aid (hypnotic). Hops are used in beer because of their bitter taste and preservative properties. Hops are usually taken as a tea and there are reports of the herb being smoked.

Approved by Commission E for:

- nervousness and insomnia.

Medicinal parts: Female flowering parts.

Uses: Has been used in insomnia, anxiety, excitability, nervousness, neuralgia and tuberculosis and for tension headaches.

Other uses: Priapism (persistent erection of the penis) and cystitis. Topically for ulcers.

Probable mode of action: The constituents of hops include more than 330 different chemicals. Some active constituents have been found experimentally to have sedative/narcotic properties in mice. The sedative effect depends strongly on the quality of the extract used. Other activities of the constituents reported are against bacteria while the bitter acids are reported to increase secretion of gastric juices and to have a spasm relieving (spasmolytic) effect on the smooth muscle of the gastrointestinal tract.

A constituent may have effects similar to female hormone oestrogen.

Adverse effects: Contact dermatitis and sensitizing effects. There have been concerns that herbs such as hops are considered to possess female hormone-like activity (oestrogenic activity) which may be a cause of breast cancer. Excess intake would cause sedation and a diminution of brain activity. Excessive intake may also cause indigestion and vomiting. Allergic reactions have also been reported.

Precautions: Hops should be avoided by patients suffering from depressive illness as the sedative effect may worsen the depression. The sedative effect can have an additive effect with other central nervous system depressants such as alcohol and opiates and concomitant use should be avoided. As hops are known to have an antispasmodic action on the uterus, use during pregnancy should be avoided. Should be avoided in patients with breast, uterine and cervical growths or cancers. May cause dangerous increases in body temperature with some drugs used for the treatment of psychiatric disorders. Known to have an effect on enzymes which metabolize allopathic medications and unexpected responses may follow the use of such medications.

HOREHOUND

Marrubium vulgare

Has a long history of use as a cough remedy and as a flavouring agent. Listed by the Council of Europe as a flavouring agent.

Approved by Commission E for:

- dyspepsia
- loss of appetite.

Medicinal parts: The dried flowering branches, the fresh aerial parts of the flowering plant and the whole plant.

Uses: Dyspepsia, loss of appetite, flatulence and respiratory inflammations. **In folk medicine**, the herb is used internally for acute and chronic bronchitis, whooping cough, asthma, tuberculosis, respiratory infections, diarrhoea, jaundice and debility.

Other uses: Painful menstruation, as a laxative. Externally for skin damage, ulcers and wounds and as a gargle for mouth and throat infections.

Probable mode of action: The bitter constituents act as a stimulant of gastric juice and some constituents stimulate the production and flow of bile. Has been shown to antagonize the effects of the chemical messenger serotonin. *Marrubium* has also been found experimentally to be an antispasmodic and to relieve pain (analgesic).

Adverse effects: Large doses can affect heart rhythm, blood pressure and blood glucose levels. No adverse effects have been reported with use in recommended doses.

Precautions: Not to be used in pregnancy and during breastfeeding. Avoid concomitant administration of allopathic medications that affect the release of the chemical messenger serotonin (e.g. some antidepressants, some antiemetics and some antimigraine medications). Should be used with caution in patients with diabetes mellitus who are on allopathic medications to lower the blood sugar.

HORSE CHESTNUT

Aesculus hippocastanum

Horse chestnut has been administered intravenously in Europe to treat postoperative oedema.

The seeds are used in the popular children's game conkers.

Has been used as a component for the use of ballistics during World War II.

Approved by Commission E for:

- chronic venous insufficiency in the legs.

Medicinal parts: The dried leaves and seeds (conkers). The oil is extracted from the peeled fruit seeds.

Uses: Treatment of varicose veins, inflammation of the veins (phlebitis) and haemorrhoids.

Other uses: Diarrhoea, fever, enlargement of the prostate. Seeds are used for swellings of soft tissues caused by injuries and after surgical operations. **In folk medicine**, the leaves are used as a remedy for cough and for arthritis and rheumatism.

Probable mode of action: One of the active constituents has been shown to cause narrowing of the veins (venoconstriction). The extracts have also been shown to decrease the loss of fluid from the small blood vessels, the capillaries (decrease of capillary permeability). Both factors may be important in the reduction of swelling that follows injury to small blood vessels in soft tissues of the body. Animal experiments have shown an effect against viruses (antiviral). These experiments have also shown that the constituents have an effect on the bowel, the small bowel in particular (ileum), and on substances that cause the spread of fluids in the tissues.

Adverse effects: A toxic nephropathy (kidney disease) has been attributed to the ingestion of high doses of one of the constituents. In **Japan**, horse chestnut has been used as an anti-inflammatory drug after surgery and trauma. Liver injury has been described in a male patient who received an intramuscular injection of a proprietary product containing horse chestnut. Other reported side-effects for the herb have been nausea, vomiting, urticaria and shock. One of the other constituents has been considered to cause irritation of the gastrointestinal tract.

Precautions: Avoid in patients with kidney or liver disease. Horse chestnut can interfere with anticoagulant therapy and should not be used in patients taking warfarin. One of the constituents has a protein binding capacity and thus could interfere or interact with other medications which also bind to proteins. Thus there is the need to monitor for drug interactions with a wide range of allopathic medications. Use during pregnancy and lactation is contraindicated. The fruit, leaves and older bark of the horse chestnut are poisonous.

HORSERADISH – PEPPEROOT

Armoracia rusticana

Horse radish has been acclaimed for its medicinal and gastronomic properties for centuries. Has been used as an aphrodisiac, as treatment for rheumatism and to add flavour to beef. Egyptians used horseradish in 1500 BC. The Greeks used horseradish as a rub for back pain. During the early 17th century, horseradish was consumed only by country folk and labourers. Later, it was grown at inns and coach stations to make cordials to revive exhausted travellers.

The FDA considers horseradish as generally safe.

Approved by Commission E for:

- internal and external use in catarrhs of the respiratory tract
- internally as supportive therapy for urinary tract infections
- externally for the hyperaemic (by improving blood flow) treatment of minor muscle aches.

Medicinal part: The fresh or dried root.

herbs

Uses: Has been used in urinary tract infections, urinary stones and chest conditions such as cough and bronchitis.

Probable mode of action: Active constituents are sulphur- and nitrogen-containing glycosides or glucosinates similar to mustard oil in composition. The active ingredients are converted by enzymes when the herb is crushed to corrosive isothiocyanates which are responsible for the pungent properties.

Effects probably include increased blood flow to the respiratory mucosa, a reflex irritation of the upper digestive mucosa and a decrease in the thickness of mucus (by altering the structures of its mucopolysaccharide constituents) thus giving the sensation of clearing congestion and catarrh. May cause reflex irritation of the upper gastric mucosa.

Adverse effects: Harmless in low doses. Excessive internal doses can cause gastrointestinal discomfort from irritation and inflammation of the stomach mucosa. Topical concentrated forms can cause blistering in sensitive individuals.

Precautions: A number of traditional texts suggest that the herb can depress thyroid function and that it should not be used in thyroid disease when thyroid hormone levels are low. Empirically the herb is contraindicated or inappropriate in some cases of chronic nephritis, hepatitis, gastro-oesophageal reflux or hyperacidity conditions and in inflammatory bowel conditions with diarrhoea due to its irritant properties and ability to stimulate gastrointestinal acid secretion. For similar reasons, horseradish is said to have potential abortifacient effects and its use should be avoided during pregnancy and lactation, although moderate amounts with food are acceptable. Traditional texts suggest that ingestion should be avoided in children under the age of four years.

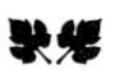

HORSETAIL

Equisetum arvense

Horsetail is considered to be the sole descendent of the giant fern-like plants that covered the earth about 200 million years ago. Was recommended by the Roman physician Galen as a remedy for kidney and bladder disease and also for tuberculosis. Topically horsetail was considered to stop bleeding from wounds and promote healing.

Approved by Commission E for:

- infections of the urinary tract
- kidney and bladder stones
- wounds and burns.

Medicinal parts: The dried green shoots and fresh shoots.

Uses: Swelling (oedema) following injury or stasis (post-traumatic and static oedema), inflammatory disease of the urinary tract, and for renal stones.

Other uses: Externally as supportive treatment for poorly healing wounds. **In folk medicine**, horsetail has been used for the treatment of tuberculosis, profuse menstruation, nasal, pulmonary and gastric haemorrhages. Other uses have been for brittle nails, loss of hair, rheumatic diseases, gout and frostbite.

Probable mode of action: Horsetail has mild diuretic and spasmolytic activity in animal experiments. The constituents contract cells (skin and other) following inflammation (astringent); this is attributed to the flavonoids and silicic acid. Because horsetail contains monosilicic acid which is considered a source of silicon, horsetail may be useful in strengthening broken bones, connective tissue and nails.

Adverse effects: Theoretically, excessive consumption of horsetail may lead to thiamine deficiency (deficiency of a vitamin), decrease of body potassium content and nicotine toxicity. Has been reported to cause dermatitis.

Precautions: To be avoided in patients with oedema (swelling usually of the ankles) due to heart failure or impaired kidney function. Treatment using Horsetail as a bath additive should be after consultation with a physician. No information on safety during pregnancy.

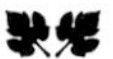

HYDRANGEA

Hydrangea arborescens

Has been used by the Cherokee Indians for diseases which lead to formation of calculi or stones (calculous disease). Was brought to England during the 18th century. It is native to Japan, and in Korea the herb is used as a popular tea (called sansugug). All parts of the plant contain the potentially toxic cyanogenic glycosides. The potted hydrangea is a symbol of Mothers' Day in France.

Medicinal parts: The dried rhizome and the roots.

Uses: As a diuretic, stimulant and carminative.

Other uses: Also used in cystitis, prostatitis, renal calculi, enlarged prostate and asthma.

Probable mode of action: The herb has a diuretic action. Active constituents include saponins, flavonoids and isocoumarin derivatives.

Adverse effects: Dizziness, chest pain, gastrointestinal distress. Weak potential for sensitization.

Precautions: Safety during pregnancy has not been established and should be avoided.

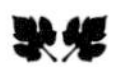

HYDROCOTYLE – GOTU KOLA

Centella asiatica

Has been an Ayurvedic medicine for thousands of years. Listed in the historic Susruta Samhila, the ancient Indian medical text, and also in the Shen Nong Herbal compiled in China over 2000 years ago. Has been called the 'miracle elixir of life' as legend states that a healer Li Ching Yun lived for 256 years by taking a tea brewed from gotu kola and other herbs. Was accepted as a drug in France in 1880.

Medicinal parts: The dried above-ground parts, the fresh and dried leaves and stem.

Uses: Gotu kola is used in venous insufficiency, to promote wound healing, to reduce fatigue and improve memory and intelligence, and for longevity.

Other uses: Diuretic, rheumatic conditions. Topical application for indolent wounds, ulcers caused by leprosy and scarring after surgery, to relieve itching, prevent balding and greying of the hair. Used in the treatment of psoriasis.

In Chinese medicine, the herb is used for dysentery and summer diarrhoea, vomiting, jaundice, urinary calculi, epistaxis (bleeding from the nose) and scabies. **In Indian medicine**, the herb is used for skin diseases, syphilis, rheumatism and leprosy. Gotu kola is also used for the treatment of mental illness, epilepsy, hysteria and for dehydration.

Probable mode of action: One of the active constituents has been shown experimentally to promote healing of wounds and the formation of keratin, the outer protective layer of the skin. In rats the active constituents prevented the formation of stomach ulcers that may follow stress, which was considered to be due to an effect on one of the chemical messengers (neurotransmitters) in the brain.

Adverse effects: A burning sensation may be associated with the use of an aerosol. Contact dermatitis as well as pruritus has been reported. Consumption of large amounts has been reported to cause dizziness, headache and passage of blood in stools.

Precautions: Can cause photosensitization and should be used with caution by sensitive subjects to avoid adverse effects of the sun. Best avoided in diabetics as hydrocotyle can interfere with drug treatment. Hydrocotyle is reported to be an abortifacient and hence should not be taken during pregnancy. Excessive use should be avoided during lactation.

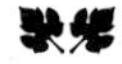

HYSSOP

Hyssopus officinalis

Derived from the Greek or Hebrew word *adobe* or *ezob*, meaning holy herb which is extensively mentioned in the Bible. In ancient times, hyssop was used to cleanse and purify humans both internally and externally. The herb was used to wash and polish sacred places. Hippocrates (460–377 BC) used hyssop to treat pleurisy and Diosocorides prescribed the tea for cough, wheezing and shortness of breath. It is stated that for nearly 2000 years people have bathed with or consumed hyssop for relief of arthritis and rheumatism.

Medicinal parts: The leaves, the flower tips and the essential oil.

Uses: Stimulation of the circulation, intestinal disorders, diseases of the respiratory tract – colds, chest and lung infections.

Other uses: For flatulence, absence seizures and anxiety. The volatile oil has been used externally for burns, cold sores and genital herpes. Used with sage as a gargle for sore throats.

Probable mode of action: The oil has been shown to have antibacterial and antihelminthic (effective against worms) activity. Extracts of the leaves have antiviral activity (against *Herpes simplex*) and are mildly spasmolytic. Hyssop contains terpenoids, flavonoids, tannins, resin and volatile oil. Reported to have anti-inflammatory, antiflatulent, antiseptic, antispasmodic, diaphoretic and expectorant properties. Claimed also to promote menstruation and to relax muscles. Crude extracts have been found to prevent replication of HIV.

Adverse effects: Rarely tonic–clonic spasms (patient goes rigid, then jerky) in adults after the intake of 10–30 drops of the volatile oil over a number of days. The volatile oil has been shown to contain chemicals that could cause convulsions. Rarely diarrhoea and indigestion may occur.

Precautions: Not to be used during pregnancy. Should not be used in patients with epilepsy or a tendency to fits. Some herbalists do not use hyssop in children under two years of age.

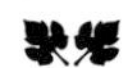

ICELAND MOSS

Cetraria islandica

Exported from Iceland to manufacture herbal medicines in Germany. Has been used in European medicine to treat asthma and gastrointestinal disorders. Many European pharmacies have preparations (usually drops) to be used for sore throats and as a laxative and also as a tonic. In Iceland, the plant has been used to bring relief from the symptoms of peptic ulcers (gastric and duodenal ulcers).

Approved by Commission E for:

- cough and bronchitis
- dyspepsia
- inflammation of mouth and pharynx
- loss of appetite.

Medicinal part: The dried thallus.

Uses: For irritation of oral and pharyngeal mucosa, loss of appetite, gastroenteritis.

Other uses: In folk medicine, Iceland moss has been used for lung disease, kidney and bladder complaints, nausea, vomiting (particularly with pregnancy and due to migraine), bronchitis, whooping cough and diarrhoea. Externally for poorly healing wounds.

Probable mode of action: The constituents can decrease discomfort caused by inflammation and irritation (demulcent effect). In animal tests, some of the constituents have been shown to have antitumour activity. Activity against the organism that causes tuberculosis (*Mycobacterium tuberculosis*) has also been demonstrated in some experiments.

Extracts of Iceland moss were found in experiments to inhibit the growth of the organism associated with peptic ulcers (*Helicobacter pylori*). Iceland moss has a high fibre content, probably accounting for its use as a laxative.

Adverse effects: Rarely sensitization. With large doses, indigestion and nausea may occur. Rarely liver damage may occur.

Precautions: The bitterness of the herb may be present in breast milk and best avoided during breastfeeding.

INDIGO – WILD INDIGO

Baptista tinctoria

All commercially available natural indigo is prepared synthetically. Indigo tinctoria is an active ingredient of a well-known traditional Chinese medicine. The Chinese have used indigo to bring about pain relief (as an analgesic), to lower temperature (antipyretic) and for purifying the liver.

Natural indigo has also been used to treat haemorrhoids and scorpion bites.

Note: Wild indigo is *Baptisia tinctoria* which is native to central and eastern US and Canada. Native American Indians have used the root to make a tea to treat fever, scarlet fever, typhoid and pharyngitis. Was used externally as an ointment for sores. Canadian Indians used the plant to treat gonorrhoea and diseases of the kidney and to promote removal of secretions from the lung and upper airways (expectorant). The constituent alkaloids in wild indigo are potentially toxic and the herb should not be used during pregnancy.

Medicinal parts: Leaves and branches

Uses: In the treatment of diabetes mellitus. The juice has been used to treat some cancers, infections and catarrh in the ear nose and throat – laryngitis and pharyngitis.

Wild indigo is known to heal mouth ulcers and gingivitis and help control of pyorrhoea (lesions causing the production of pus in the gums). Has been used to treat enlarged lymph glands and reduce fevers. Externally as an ointment it has helped in the healing of ulcers and to ease sore nipples. A douche has been recommended for white discharge from the vagina (leucorrhoea).

Other uses: Taken both internally and as a mouthwash.

Probable mode of action: The constituents of indigo have been shown to protect the liver against the damage caused by the potent liver toxin – carbon tetrachloride. Aqueous preparations of the indigo plant have been shown experimentally to lower blood sugar. The constituents are considered to stimulate the release of insulin by the pancreatic cells. Indirubin, which is also a constituent of indigo, has been shown in experiments to be effective against chronic myeloid leukaemia.

Wild indigo exhibits antimicrobial and anticatarrhal properties.

Adverse effects: Indigo can cause irritation of the eyes. May also cause dermatitis. Large doses of wild indigo may cause abdominal pain, vomiting, diarrhoea.

Precautions: Wild indigo should be avoided in inflammatory gastrointestinal diseases.

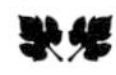

IRISH MOSS – CARRAGEEN

Chondrus crispus

It is known as carraigin in Ireland where it has been used since 400 AD. The name carraigin means ‘moss of the rock’ in Irish. Dried Irish moss was used during the famine of the 19th century. It is used by the pharmaceutical industry as an emulsifying agent.

Medicinal parts: Dried weed (carageenan).

Uses: Bronchitis, cystitis, and to treat stomach disorders (gastritis and dyspepsia). Used topically as a lotion for injured hands and dermatitis. Considered beneficial during convalescence following wasting in chronic diseases (cachexia).

Other uses: Has been used in the past to treat tuberculosis. Topically for dermatitis.

Probable mode of action: One of the constituents (carageenan) has been reported to reduce gastric secretions. Other effects attributed to constituents include demulcent (to relieve symptoms associated with inflammation and irritation), nutritive, relaxing properties, promoting removal of secretions from the lung and upper airways (expectorant), antitussive (prevent cough) and emollient activity. Irish moss contains a relatively large amount of mucilage, iodine and vitamins A and B. When injected into the paw of a cat, it produces inflammation which has been used as an animal model to test the efficacy of anti-inflammatory drugs.

Adverse effects: A degraded product of carageenan has been considered to be carcinogenic but is no longer used in food. May cause abdominal cramps and diarrhoea.

Precautions: May affect gastrointestinal absorption of drugs and thus decrease their effectiveness. However, a carrageen formulation of the antibiotic doxycycline has been shown to enhance the absorption of the antibiotic. May cause an increase in the tendency to bleed so be cautious when using anticoagulants. May increase the blood pressure lowering effects of some allopathic medications used in the treatment of high blood pressure. Considered by some herbalists to be contraindicated in patients with active peptic ulcer disease. As effects on pregnancy and during breastfeeding are not known with certainty, the herb is best avoided.

ISPAGHULA

Psyllium indian

Has been used in the traditional medical systems of China and India to treat diarrhoea, haemorrhoids, bladder problems and high blood pressure.

The European Medicine Evaluation Agency (EMEA) and Herbal Medicinal Products Working Group (HMPWG) have proposed the following uses:

- Treatment of habitual constipation; conditions in which easy defaecation with soft stools is desirable, e.g. after rectal or anal surgery.
- Adjuvant symptomatic therapy in cases of diarrhoea from various causes.
- Conditions which need an increased fibre intake, e.g. as an adjuvant in irritable bowel syndrome.

Approved by Commission E for:
- chronic constipation
- disorders in which bowel movements with loose stools are desirable, e.g. patients with anal fistula, haemorrhoids, pregnancy
- treatment of irritable bowel syndrome
- various forms of diarrhoea.

Medicinal part: Seeds.

Uses: Chronic constipation and as a bulk laxative mainly when easy bowel movement with loose stools is desirable as in patients with anal fissures, haemorrhoids, following anorectal surgery and during pregnancy. Also used to treat dysentery, diarrhoea, diverticular disease of the left colon and Crohn's disease.

Other uses: Cystitis. Topically as a poultice for furunculosis (furuncles in the skin). **In China**, the seeds of the related *Plantago* species have been used in the treatment of high blood pressure.

Probable mode of action: The constituents increase the bulk of the stool and are also considered to have a protective effect on the intestinal mucosa. The mucilage readily absorbs water in the gastrointestinal tract. This increases the volume and viscosity of the faeces and stimulates peristalsis (contractions of the bowel) of the gastrointestinal tract. It is also considered to possess a cholesterol lowering effect. Has been shown to reduce blood sugar (hypoglycaemic action) by delaying gastric absorption.

Adverse effects: May cause flatulence and abdominal distension. There is a possibility that ispaghula can cause intestinal obstruction. It must be taken with sufficient water because it can cause an obstruction in the oesophagus if it is swallowed dry. Rarely allergic reactions may occur (e.g. rhinitis, wheezing, skin irritations and in some cases anaphylaxis).

Precautions: Should not be given to patients with intestinal obstruction or for conditions that may lead to intestinal obstruction. As ispaghula causes an increase in the transit time of bowel contents, administration could interfere with the absorption of co-administered drugs. The absorption of coumarins (warfarin), calcium, iron, lithium, zinc, vitamins (B_{12}), and digoxin may be delayed. It is best to separate the intake of medications and ispaghula by at least 1 hour. As there is a tendency to hypoglycaemia, the dose of hypoglycaemic drugs, particularly insulin, may need to be reduced. Should not be used in patients who have had an alteration of bowel habits for over two weeks or in patients who have bleeding from the rectum. If chest pain, vomiting or difficulty in swallowing or breathing is experienced after taking ispaghula, immediate medical attention should be sought. Begin with small doses allowing the body to adapt to the high fibre content. Drink several glasses of water during the day to increase effectiveness of *Psyllium*.

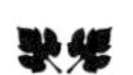

JAVA TEA

Orthosiphon spicatus

Java tea has been traditionally used in Java for the treatment of hypertension (high blood pressure) and diabetes.

Approved by Commission E for:

- infections of the urinary tract
- kidney and bladder stones.

Medicinal parts: The leaves and stem tips collected during the flowering season.

Uses: Treatment of hypertension and diabetes.

Other uses: Bladder and kidney disorders (including haematuria and albuminuria), gallstones, gout and rheumatism.

Probable mode of action: One of the active constituents produces an increase in the urinary volume (diuretic effect). An increase has been reported in the excretion of sodium, potassium and chloride ions in the urine. Another constituent produced a continuous reduction in systolic blood pressure and decrease in heart rate in rats. There are also reports of the constituents decreasing the contractile force of the aorta which may be useful in the treatment of high blood pressure.

Adverse effects: None documented.

Precautions: A fluid intake of at least 2 litres or more should be ensured in a patient taking Java tea. Due to the lack of toxicity data, Java tea is best avoided during pregnancy and lactation.

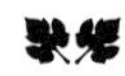

JUJUBE

Zizyphus jujube
Zizyphus vulgaris

Has been used in Chinese medicine for 4000 years. The ancient Chinese physician Shennong recorded the healing properties of the jujube fruit which he referred to as a miraculous health tonic. He prescribed it to nourish the blood, liver and spleen and also to calm the mind and cleanse the body through detoxification. The jujube fruit is considered to be as popular in Japan as is the apple in the US.

Medicinal parts: The fruit. The jujube berry is classed with raisins, dates and figs and can be eaten fresh or dried. Also roots.

Uses: Used to improve muscular strength, as a prophylaxis for liver diseases and stress ulcers, as a sedative and to neutralize drug toxicities.

Other uses: Used in the treatment of dry and itchy skin, lack of appetite, fatigue, diarrhoea, hysteria, anaemia, hypertension, purpura, fever, wounds, ulcers, inflammation, asthma and eye diseases. A decoction of the roots was used to treat fevers.

Probable mode of action: The constituents are mainly in the fruit. Animal data suggest that jujube increases body weight, increases endurance and protects against carbon tetrachloride (liver toxin) induced liver damage. Animal data have shown that an alcoholic extract may have anti-inflammatory effects and inhibit the growth of *Bacillus subtilis.*

Adverse effects: Works together with gymnema to reduce the strength of the taste of sugar. May have additive effects with drugs used to lower blood sugar.

Precautions: Caution in diabetics who are on allopathic medications for control of blood sugar.

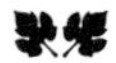

JUNIPER

Juniperus communis

Juniper has been a folk remedy for urinary tract disorders and an adjuvant (help) to diuretics in the treatment of oedema (swelling) due to kidney disease. Native Americans used the bruised inner bark to relieve the odour of foul smelling wounds. Has a tradition of use by the Carrier (Dakelh) people of British Columbia.

Medicinal parts: The berry, the essential oil from the dried ripe fruit. The heartwood and tops may also be used.

Uses: Ripe, dry juniper berry aids digestion, prevents cramps and eliminates gas. Applied to the skin as an oil, the herb helps relief of pain in rheumatism and arthritis.

Other uses: Used as a diuretic to rid the body of water and salt also used as an emmenagogue and an abortifacient. The oil has been used for flatulence and colic.

Probable mode of action: The active constituent increases the formation of urine by increasing filtering at the kidney tubule. Some constituents have been shown in experiments to lower blood sugar. Experimental work has also shown that extracts of the bark have antimicrobial activity similar to that of the antibiotic streptomycin.

Adverse effects: Diarrhoea with repeated use. Renal irritation. Use on the skin may cause a burning sensation, redness and vesicles.

Precautions: Do not use in kidney disease. Avoid if pregnant. Do not use internally for more than six weeks. Some herbalists do not advocate its use on open wounds or skin abrasions.

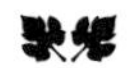

KAVA KAVA

Piper methysticum

Kava kava is widely used in the South Pacific as a ceremonial and welcoming drink.

Medicinal parts: The peeled dried cut rhizome which has normally been freed from the roots and the fresh rhizome with the roots.

Uses: Known for its relaxing effects and in the treatment of insomnia. Also reduces anxiety and nervousness.

Other uses: Also used in neuralgia, irritable bladder syndrome and rheumatic pain.

Probable mode of action: The active constituents, namely, kavalactones (e.g. kavain, dihydrokavain, methysticim) and kavapyrones are responsible for the effects on the central nervous system such as producing sleep and relieving anxiety. At low doses, kavapyrones have a pharmacological action that resembles the effect of drugs such as Valium by binding to the same receptors in the brain. The active constituents may also bind to receptors that increase activity in the brain and cause inhibition.

Adverse effects: A small percentage of users may develop gastrointestinal discomfort, nausea, vomiting, diarrhoea, dizziness, headache, allergic skin eruptions with skin discoloration. Dilated pupils, disturbances of balance, gait and vision (accommodation) can also occur.

Hepatitis and fulminant hepatic failure have recently been reported in Europe and the US with the use of herbal products containing kava kava. Excessive use as a beverage can cause dizziness and stupefaction and stimulation of the central nervous system. Consumption over a few months can lead to kava dermopathy, a reversible scaly skin disorder.

Precautions: Avoid during pregnancy as toxic pyrone constituents can cause loss of uterine tone. Constituents can pass to breast milk. May increase the sedative effect of alcohol and other depressants or sedatives on the central nervous system. Avoid if the patient has pre-existing history of liver disease. Liver function should be monitored if used regularly.

Excessive consumption may impair one's ability to drive or operate heavy equipment. Not recommended for use by persons under the age of 18 years.

KHELLA – BISHOP'S WEED

Ammi visnaga

One of the oldest of all known medicinal herbs.

The fruits were used in Egyptian folk medicine as diuretics and in the treatment of kidney and bladder stones. Was used traditionally in Israel for the treatment of diabetes.

Medicinal parts: Whole plant, fresh stalks.

Uses: Bronchial asthma. Bladder and kidney cramps.

Other uses: Used in the treatment of angina, possibly by improving blood flow to the heart muscle. Also found to be useful to dilate the small breathing tubes in the lung (bronchioles) and relieve gallbladder pain and painful menstruation.

Probable mode of action: Animal experiments have shown that the constituents of khella act at multiple sites to reduce contractions of the smooth muscle of the blood vessels. Thus a dilatation of blood vessels has been documented and it is considered to act on the blood vessels to the heart. Constituents are also reported to be effective against certain bacteria (antimicrobial activity). Interest in khellin as an adjunct to ultraviolet light therapy in vitiligo is based on the structural similarity between khellin and psoralens (photosensitizing substances).

Adverse effects: Allergic reactions (itching), mild sensitivity to sunlight, sleeplessness. Known to produce an increase of liver enzymes. Prolonged use or overdose can cause constipation, poor appetite, headache, vertigo, nausea and vomiting.

Precautions: Khella constituent's increases the skin's sensitivity to sunlight. Extreme care has to be taken with sun exposure while using any form of this herb. Avoid during pregnancy and lactation and if taking blood thinning tablets like warfarin (watch for bruising, bleeding gums or blood in the stools).

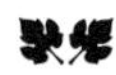

KUDZU

Pueraria lobata

The name kudzu appeared first in the *Kojiki* and *Nihon Shoki* as a type of vine or *kazura* used commonly by the people of Kudzu, the area around present day Yoshino, Nara prefecture, Japan. Kudzu has been in use for over 1300 years. In the Nara and Heian eras, records had been found reporting that the plants were collected and sent as a part of tax.

Kudzu is sometimes referred to as 'the plant that ate the South'. After being introduced into the US the vine spread rapidly and became an environmental menace.

Medicinal part: Root.

Uses: Migraine and cluster headache. To treat infections.

Other uses: To treat hangover with headache. Also to treat upset stomach, nausea and vomiting, menopause, hypertension, diabetes and psoriasis. In traditional **Chinese medicine**, where it is known as ge gen, kudzu is considered one of the 50 fundamental herbs and used in the treatment of tinnitus (ringing in the ears) and vertigo (dizziness).

Probable mode of action: Some constituents have been found to possess anti-inflammatory and antimicrobial activities. Kudzu root compounds can affect chemical messengers or neurotransmitters in the brain such as serotonin, gamma aminobutyric acid and glutamate which probably accounts for its use in the treatment of headaches and dizziness. Constituents of kudzu have been found to prevent the breakdown of serotonin in animal experiments. Kudzu is also considered to affect calcium levels in the blood and hence has potential for interactions with calcium channel blockers (a class of allopathic medications used for high blood pressure and heart problems).

The Chinese system considers the root to possess sweet, pungent and cooling properties.

Adverse effects: Skin eruptions (maculo-papular rash) have been reported with its use. There is also a report of a patient developing bleeding after surgery which has been attributed to kudzu. The patient developed bleeding 1–2 weeks after taking kudzu, approximately one month after surgery. The cause–effect relationship with kudzu intake was not firmly established, but it is considered necessary to be aware of this report. There have been reports of adverse reactions in patients taking kudzu along with verapamil (an allopathic drug classed as a calcium channel blocker) or triptans (used in the treatment of headache).

Precautions: May interact with antiplatelet and antidiabetic medications. Kudzu is not recommended for use during pregnancy in traditional Chinese medicine and also for patients with yin deficiency with heat or aggressive blood problems (usually patients with low blood pressure and a fast heart rate).

LADY'S MANTLE

Alchemilla vulgaris

The genus name *Alchemilla* is derived from the word alchemy because the herb was believed to bring about miraculous cures. The plant has also been associated with Virgin Mary, because the lobes of the leaves resemble the scalloped edges of a mantle. Used in cosmetics.

Approved by Commission E for:
- diarrhoea.

Medicinal part: Herb collected in the flowering season and dried.

Uses: Mild and non-specific diarrhoea and gastrointestinal disorders

Other uses: In folk medicine, the herb is used internally for menopausal complaints, dysmenorrhoea (painful menstruation), gastrointestinal disorders and as a gargle for mouth and throat inflammation. Used externally for skin ulcers, eczema and rashes and as an additive in baths for the treatment of lower abdominal ailments.

Probable mode of action: The effect to contract cells (skin and other) following inflammation (astringent) has been attributed to the presence of tannins. Constituents have been shown to inhibit tumour growth. Herbal extracts have also been shown to inhibit some enzymes (e.g. trypsin).

Adverse effects: The tannin constituents may cause liver dysfunction. Periodic monitoring of liver function is recommended.

Precautions: Avoid during pregnancy and whilst breastfeeding. Herbalists recommend that subjects taking this herb should report fatigue, weakness, darkening of the urine or any yellowish discoloration of the eyes.

LADY'S SLIPPER – AMERICAN VALERIAN

Cypripedium pubescens

Has a reputation for its sedative and relaxing effects on the nervous system. Used by the Native North Americans for sedative and antispasmodic properties to ease menstrual and labour pains, to counter insomnia and nervous tension. Utilized by the early settlers as a substitute for valerian, hence the term American Valerian.

Medicinal part: Roots.

Uses: Insomnia, irritability, hysteria, emotional tension, anxiety states.

Other uses: For relief of discomfort such as mild pain and for inducing sleep. Often used in combination with other herbs.

Probable mode of action: The effects of the constituents appear to be primarily on the nervous system. The constituents include volatile oils, volatile acid, resins, starch, fixed oil and sugar. The precise effects of the constituents are not known with certainty.

Adverse effects: Roots may cause psychedelic reactions and large doses may result in dizziness, restlessness, headache, mental excitement and visual hallucinations. May cause allergy and contact dermatitis due to the quinine constituents.

Precautions: To be avoided by subjects with allergies. The safety in pregnancy has not been established and there is very little toxicological data. Best avoided during pregnancy.

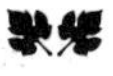

LARCH

Larix decidua

Larix was the name give to pine resin in the time of Dioscorides. The tree, indigenous to the hilly parts of Europe (e.g. the Alps), has been used medicinally and also for ship building and as sleepers for railway tracks. Has been used for making varnishes and in commerce was referred to as 'Venice turpentine'.

Native Americans used the needles and inner bark to make a tea to treat coughs. The resin was used by them as a chewing gum and to relieve indigestion.

Approved by Commission E for:

- fevers and colds
- coughs/bronchitis
- tendency to infections
- blood pressure problems
- inflammation of mouth and pharynx
- common cold.

The FDA has approved the use of the constituent arabinogalactan as a food additive and as a fibre supplement.

Medicinal parts: Outer bark separated from its outermost layer.

Uses: Mainly as an expectorant in chronic bronchitis. Also as a stimulant, diuretic and astringent. Has been used to treat neuralgic discomforts and furuncles (boils).

Other uses: External applications have been used in the treatment of eczema and psoriasis. Has been rarely used internally in haemorrhage and cystitis. Has been considered for use as a disinfectant for gangrene in hospitals. Was also considered for use as an antidote for cyanide and opium poisoning. Used in veterinary medicine.

Probable mode of action: The bark contains tannic acid, larixinic acid and turpentine. When used externally, the herb causes an increase in blood flow and also has antiseptic properties which have been attributed to the essential oil content. The polysaccharide constituent arabinogalactan was

herbs

considered to stimulate the immune system and also to assist in preventing the spread of cancers to the liver. These reports are unconfirmed.

Adverse effects: Inhalation may cause acute inflammation of the airways. Kidney damage is thought to occur following oral intake of the bark or following local application of the oil over large areas of the skin. Allergies (e.g. hives, rashes, contact dermatitis) may also occur.

Precautions: Arabinogalactoside contains galactose and should be used cautiously by those with lactose intolerance.

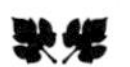

LAVENDER

Lavandula officinalis
Lavandula augustifolia

The name is derived from the Latin word *lavare* which means to wash. The herb was used by the ancient Greeks and Romans and was introduced to Britain by the Romans who used lavender in their bath water.

Medicinal parts: Flowers, leaf.

Uses: To relax muscles, ease anxiety and relieve depression (may be combined with rosemary, kola or scull cap), and to promote sleep.

Other uses: Decongestant, promotes removal of secretions from the lung and upper airways (expectorant) and as an antibacterial agent. Has been used to relieve flatulence and to promote appetite. Was considered to repel fleas which transmitted the plague. Externally, lavender oil has been used to minimize scarring and heal wounds, and to relieve irritation caused by insect bites and stings.

Probable mode of action: Constituents include a volatile oil (which contains camphor), coumarins and flavonoids. Considered a versatile herb but the exact effects of the constituents are not known with certainty. Constituents have been studied in the laboratory for effects on breast tumours and also for effects on methicillin-resistant *Staphylococcus aureus* (MRSA).

Adverse effects: The oil should not be taken by mouth. Local applications are best used in dilution as toxic skin reactions may occur.

Precautions: Infusions may be taken orally but the oil should not be taken orally and should only be rubbed on the skin or used in baths. Lavender oil should be considered as poisonous. No other precautions are available in the literature. Some herbalists do not advise the use of lavender during pregnancy and breastfeeding. Be cautious in patients who are taking other sedatives.

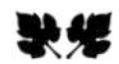

LEMON

Citrus limon

Possibly the first citrus fruit known in the Mediterranean. Has been described in Pliny's *Natural History* as the malum medicum. Recorded in the 10th century Arabic treatise on farming by Qustus al-Rumi. Has been depicted in Roman mosaics in North Africa. Lemons have been identified among the ruins of Pompeii.

Were used by the British Royal Navy to combat scurvy (a disease caused by lack of vitamin C).

Medicinal part: Fruit. Lemon is used internally in the form of oil, tincture or fresh fruit.

Uses: Commonly used as a source of vitamin C in cases of low resistance, scurvy and colds. **In folk medicine**, lemon juice was recommended as a drink for fever, as a remedy for acute rheumatism and as an antidote to intoxicants.

Other uses: Additional traditional uses that are still recommended are for sunburn, as a substitute for quinine in malaria and to reduce temperature in patients with typhus. **In Indian medicine**, it is used as a remedy for shaking and heartburn. Has been used to relieve the pain of bee stings.

Probable mode of action: The juice contains a high amount of citric acid which gives it the sharp flavour. Lemons are a good source of vitamin C and of flavonoids. Has properties which are anti-inflammatory and also believed to stabilize blood vessel walls to prevent leakage.

Adverse effects: Low potential for sensitization through skin contact with volatile oil.

Precautions: None known.

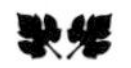

LEMON BALM

Melissa officinalis

Melissa is derived from the Greek word meaning bee as bees are strongly attracted to this plant. Paracelsus (1493–1541) called the plant 'the Elixir of Life'. Has been previously recorded in Roman writings and the Arabs have used the plant for centuries to treat depression and anxiety.

The *London Dispensary* published in 1696 stated 'An essence of balm given in canary wine will renew youth, strengthen the brain, relieve languishing nature and prevent baldness'.

Approved by Commission E for:

- nervousness and insomnia.

Medicinal parts: The oil extracted by distillation, the dried leaves, the fresh leaves and the whole plant.

Uses: Used mainly as a tea to produce mild sedation (to treat agitation and insomnia) and to induce perspiration to bring down the fever of colds and flu.

Other uses: In folk medicine, the drug is utilized as decoctions of the flowering shoots for nervous complaints, abdominal disorders, nervous gastric complaints, hysteria, melancholia, chronic bronchitis, nervous palpitations, vomiting, migraine, headache and high blood pressure. Used externally for rheumatism, nerve pains and stiff neck. The crushed leaves aid in healing wounds and insect bites. An infusion added to a bath is believed to promote the onset of menstruation.

Probable mode of action: The active constituents have been shown to possess mild sedative, carminative, spasmolytic (relieves spasms), effective against bacteria and viruses (antibacterial, antiviral), antioxidative and antihormonal effects. As a sedative, only the very fresh preparations should be used. The polyphenol constituent has been found to have antiviral properties.

Adverse effects: Can cause irritation if used in high concentrations.

Precautions: Avoid during pregnancy and be cautious when applying locally in those with sensitive skin.

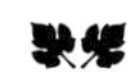

LEMON VERBENA

Aloysia triphylla

Named after the wife of King Carlos IV of Spain. Was brought to Europe by Spanish explorers in the 17th century from Argentina and Chile.

In the USA, lemon verbena is listed as GRAS (Generally Recognized As Safe) for human consumption in alcoholic beverages. Lemon verbena is also used in herbal teas.

Medicinal parts: Fresh twigs and the dried leaves and stems.

Uses: Treatment of asthma, cold, fever. Frequently used as a tea.

Other uses: In France, lemon verbena is used in the symptomatic treatment of digestive disorders, agitation and insomnia (inability to sleep). The herb has also been used in the treatment of fever associated with haemorrhoids, varicose veins and for impure skin. In **Morocco**, it is used for chills and constipation. Also used for flatulence, colic, diarrhoea and indigestion.

Probable mode of action: The leaves are considered to be antispasmodic, sedative and to bring down fevers (febrifuge). The active constituents include flavonoids (including apigenin) and iridioids.

Adverse effects: The oil may be irritant and may sensitize the skin to sunlight. Large doses of the tea can cause gastric irritation.

Precautions: The lack of pharmacological and toxicological data makes its use during pregnancy unsafe at present.

LIQUORICE – LICORICE

Glycyrrhiza glabra

Ayurveda term: Yashtimadhu
Liquorice was one of the principal drugs mentioned by the ancient Indian physician Susruta. Widely used in Ayurveda as a medicine and to disguise the unpleasant flavours of other medications. In ancient Chinese pharmacy it was used for its rejuvenating properties. The Greeks recommended the herb for the treatment of peptic ulcers (gastric and duodenal ulcers).

Approved by Commission E for:
- cough/bronchitis
- gastritis.

Medicinal parts: Dried roots and runners.

Uses: Inflammation of the digestive tract (peptic ulcers, heartburn), eczema and cold sores.

Other uses: Cough and bronchitis, rheumatism and arthritis. **In folk medicine**, the herb is used for appendicitis, constipation and to increase milk production and promote passage of urine. Used to treat epilepsy and inflammation of the gastrointestinal and urogenital tracts. Externally the herb is used for skin disorders.

Probable mode of action: Found to have antiviral, anti-inflammatory and antiallergic properties. The active constituents exert anti-inflammatory effects. Liquorice has protective effects against gastric ulcers that are caused by aspirin. The ability to release carbenoxolone, a compound which protects against gastric ulcers, is considered to be a major effect. The roots contain glycyrrhizin (a saponin) which is much sweeter than cane sugar.

Adverse effects: Excessive quantities can cause headache, sluggishness and dangerously low levels of potassium in the body.

Precautions: Not recommended for those suffering from high blood pressure. Not to be used in women during premenstrual syndrome as it causes water retention and possible bloating. Use with caution in those with cirrhosis of the liver and during pregnancy. Avoid using liquorice for longer periods than six weeks. Maintain a potassium-rich diet when using liquorice.

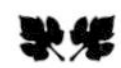

LIFE ROOT – GOLDEN RAGWORT

Senecio aureus

Senecio has had a reputation as a general tonic for use in debilitating diseases such as tuberculosis.

Life root is not used as a food, although many *Senecio* species are used as a form of spinach in South Africa.

Medicinal parts: Aerial (above ground) parts.

Uses: Treatment of menstrual disorders (amenorrhoea, dysmenorrhoea, menorrhagia) and also for whitish discharge from the vagina (leucorrhoea).

Other uses: For menopausal symptoms, male impotence and has been used in the treatment of gonorrhoea.

Probable mode of action: The exact effects of the constituents are not known with certainty. Constituents include a bitter principle, tannin and mucilage. *Senecio* is a uterine tonic often used for absent or delayed menstruation.

Adverse effects: Contains pyrrolizidine alkaloids which have the potential to cause liver damage. Life root is toxic if taken internally and is legally restricted in some countries.

Precautions: Should not be ingested. Contra-indicated during pregnancy and lactation as it is well known following studies and traditional use that life root is an abortifacient, emmenagogue and uterine tonic. Placental transfer and secretion to breast milk have been documented in animals. Most *Senecio* species contain pyrrolizidine alkaloids, though not always in toxic concentrations.

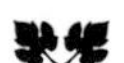

LILY-OF-THE-VALLEY

Convallaria majalis

The leaves and flowers have been used for centuries to treat heart disease as they contain substances (glycosides) that act on the heart muscle.

The crude drug is known as ling lan in Chinese traditional medicine.

The plant was traditionally used as an antidote to poison gas. Russian herbalists have used it as an anti-epileptic.

Approved by Commission E for:

- arrhythmia
- cardiac insufficiency
- nervous heart complaints.

Medicinal parts: Dried flower tips, herb, dried root rhizome with roots, the flowering aerial parts and the whole fresh flowering plant.

Uses: The herb is used for mild cardiac insufficiency, heart insufficiency of old age and chronic cor pulmonale (severe lung disease usually as a result of a heart disorder).

Other uses: In folk medicine, uses were for weak contractions during labour, epilepsy, dropsy (swelling, usually of ankles), strokes and resulting paralysis, conjunctivitis, leprosy. Flowers have been used as fomentations to remove the red spots that have resulted from bruises.

Probable mode of action: The constituents are very similar to digitoxin and strophanthin, which are referred to as cardiac glycosides and act on heart muscle. Hence considered to increase the power and speed of heart muscle contraction (inotropic and chronotropic effects). The heart beat frequency is reduced. Animal tests have shown a diuretic effect and a constrictor effect on the veins.

Adverse effects: Nausea, vomiting, stupor, disorders of colour perception and cardiac arrhythmias can occur. These are particularly seen with overdose.

Precautions: Dangers of poisoning are low with oral use due to the poor absorption of the glycosides. Preparations for internal use are no longer considered safe.

LOBELIA – INDIAN TOBACCO – PUKEWEED

Lobelia inflata

Has a long history as an herbal remedy for chest diseases such as asthma, bronchitis, pneumonia and cough.

Native Americans smoked the herb to treat asthma. In the 19th century, American physicians prescribed the herb to cause vomiting, hence the term pukeweed.

Medicinal parts: Fresh and dried herbs and seeds.

Uses: As an effective expectorant in bronchitis and asthma.

Other uses: Topically for muscle inflammation (myositis) and rheumatic nodules.

Probable mode of action: Pharmacological properties are attributed to the alkaloid constituents, principally lobeline which has peripheral and central effects similar to those of nicotine but is less potent. Lobeline also promotes removal of secretions from the lung and upper airways (expectorant), hence the use in respiratory disease. Lobeline has been used as a substitute for nicotine in many antismoking products.

Adverse effects: Nausea, vomiting, diarrhoea, coughing, tremors and dizziness. Overdose causes profuse sweating (diaphoresis), tachycardia (increase in heart rate), convulsions, fall in body temperature (hypothermia), fall in blood pressure (hypotension), coma and death.

Precautions: Should not be used during pregnancy and lactation. Excessive use even for cessation of cigarette smoking or nicotine addiction is not recommended. Best avoided by subjects with high blood pressure, tendency to fits (epileptics) and heart disease.

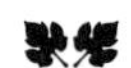

LOVAGE

Levisticum officinale

A traditional spice in Southern Europe and was popular in Roman cooking. Not a popular herbal remedy at present. Used as a fragrance in cosmetics, soaps and lotions.

Approved by Commission E for:
- infection of the urinary tract
- kidney and bladder stones.

Medicinal parts: Roots, leaves, fruits.

Uses: To 'flush' out inflammations of the kidney and urinary tract. Also used to prevent the formation of debris or gravel in the kidney and consequently of kidney stones.

Other uses: In folk medicine, the herb has been used for common gastric complaints such as indigestion, heartburn, flatulence, for menstrual complaints and for catarrh of the respiratory tract. Used externally for aphthous ulcers (ulcers in the mouth usually caused by stress) and for sore throats.

Probable mode of action: One of the active constituents prevents or decreases spasm of smooth muscles. It also contains an essential oil which has a similar antispasmodic effect on smooth muscle. It also has a bitter taste which increases salivary and gastric secretions and hence the use for gastrointestinal complaints.

Adverse effects: The volatile oil is an irritant. Has a low potential for sensitization. May increase photosensitivity in susceptible individuals.

Precautions: Contraindicated in the presence of inflammation of the kidneys or urinary passages. Not to be used during pregnancy.

LYCOPODIUM – CLUB MOSS

Lycopodium clavatum

Found in almost all parts of the earth, the spores have been used for centuries as a dusting powder for wounds and skin lesions. Pharmacists have used the spores to prevent tablets from adhering to each other when stored in boxes or bottles.

Medicinal parts: Spores and fresh plant.

Uses: Orally, club moss is used for bladder and kidney disorders, and as a diuretic. Spores prevent itching.

Other uses: In folk medicine, it is used internally for bladder and kidney complaints, for pharyngeal catarrh and tonsillitis, menstrual complaints, rheumatism and impotence. It is used externally for wounds, itching and suppurating eczema of the skin.

Probable mode of action: Club moss has a diuretic action. Active constituents include alkaloids such as traces of nicotine, triterpenes, steroids and flavonoids. Plant contains the toxic compound lycopodine which is known to paralyse the nerves to muscles (motor nerves).

Adverse effects: Possibly unsafe because of toxic alkaloids (no poisonings known). Irritation could be expected with extended use.

Precautions: May cause central nervous system stimulation. Should be taken under supervision of a physician.

MADDER

Rubia tinctorum

This herb is connected to the Magus card in the Tarot. The Druids incorporated it into girls' coming-of-age ceremonies, probably because of its blood colour. This root has been used for dyeing for at least 3000 years. The earliest example found so far was madder-dyed linen in the tomb of King Tutankhamen from 1350 BC.

In India, it has been used to redden lips and cheeks. It also has a 2000-year history as a medicinal herb in China, India and ancient Greece for breaking kidney stones, to promote the flow of menses, cure jaundice and for intestinal problems. Madder was also used to colour the trousers of French soldiers and the Turkish fezzes.

Rarely used as a herbal medicine at present.

Medicinal part: Root.

Uses: Although not as a general rule employed medicinally, Madder has been reputed as effective in amenorrhoea (absence of periods), dropsy (swelling, usually of the ankles) and jaundice.

Other uses: Treatment of rickets (bone deformities usually due to lack of calcium).

Probable mode of action: The root contains many active constituents including tannins, sugar and a substance called alizarin which is an important colouring substance. The constituents are considered to possess antibiotic and anti-inflammatory effects.

Adverse effects: When taken by mouth, the root colours the urine and milk. One of the main reasons for the herb not being used in medicine is the probable potential to cause cancers, particularly of the liver and kidney.

Precautions: Best not taken as herbal medicine with the information available at present.

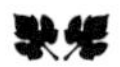

MANDRAKE

Mandragora officinarum

One of the oldest of the medicinal plants. The name mandragora is derived from two Greek words which mean 'hurtful to cattle'. The Arabs called it 'Satan's apple'. During the days of Pliny, mandrake was used as an anaesthetic for operations – a piece of mandrake root been given to the patient to chew before the operation. Anglo-Saxons believed mandrake protected them from being possessed by demons.

Medicinal parts: Dried underground part, fresh herb and the root.

Uses: In folk medicine, a tincture of Mandragora radix was used for stomach ulcers, colic, asthma, hay fever and whooping cough. Today mandrake is used only in homeopathy.

Probable mode of action: The constituent alkaloids include hyoscyamine which changes under storage conditions to some extent to atropine and scopolamine. The activity is mainly due to the antagonism of the effects of the chemical messenger or neurotransmitter acetylcholine (anticholinergic effect) by the main alkaloids (atropine, hyoscyamine and scopolamine). These substances are used in allopathic medication to produce drying of secretions, increase of heart rate and dilatation of pupils.

Adverse effects: Skin reddening, dryness of the mouth, increased heart rate (tachycardia), heart beat irregularities (arrhythmias) and dilatation of the pupils (mydriasis) are early warning signs of toxicity. Decrease in secretion of sweat, disorders in the passing of urine and constipation often follow.

Precaution: Not to be used as a herbal medicine.

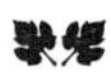

MARJORAM

Origanum hortensis
Origanum vulgare

The Greeks used it extensively, both internally and externally as fomentations. It was a remedy for narcotic poisons, convulsions and dropsy. Among both Greeks and Romans, it was a custom to crown young couples with marjoram.

The ancient Greeks believed that if marjoram grew on one's grave, the deceased would enjoy eternal peace and happiness.

Goat and sheep eat this herb, but horses are not fond of it and cattle reject it.

Used in Italian, French, North African, Middle Eastern and American cuisines and spice blends such as bouquet garni.

Medicinal parts: Herb, oil.

Uses: It is so acrid that it has been employed as a rubifacient (a substance which when applied to skin causes redness due to its effect on blood vessels causing an increase in blood flow to the skin), and often as a liniment and as a caustic. A few drops put on cotton wool and placed in the hollow of an aching tooth may relieve pain.

Other uses: Early treatment of measles to produce a gentle perspiration and bring about the eruption (appearance of the rash). Used as an infusion to treat spasms, colic and relief from stomach ailments (dyspeptic complaints) and relieve nervous headache. Externally the dried leaves and tops are applied in bags as a hot fomentation to painful swellings and rheumatism as well as for colic.

Probable mode of action: The oil from marjoram is considered to be a stimulant and carminative, to induce perspiration (diaphoretic) and be a mild tonic and useful regulator of menstruation (emmenagogue). The active constituents (camphoraceous components) are considered to relieve headaches.

Adverse effects: Cross-allergy may occur with other plants of the same family. Ingestion of large amounts causes gastrointestinal upset. May cause systemic allergic reactions particularly in those allergic to basil, hyssop, lavender, marjoram, sage and mint.

Precautions: Avoid use in those allergic to herbs such as marjoram, basil, sage, mint and related herbs. Women who experience heavy menstruation should avoid marjoram. The herb is not recommended for infants and small children.

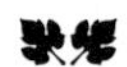

MARSHMALLOW

Althaea officinalis

Althaea is derived from the Greek word meaning 'to heal'. Marshmallow candy dates back to ancient Egypt where it was a honey-based candy flavoured and thickened by the sap of the root of *Althaea*. Hippocrates described the value of *Althaea* in the treatment of wounds. The peeled root was given to teething children to chew and the candy was used during the 19th century to soothe sore throats of children.

Marshmallow is listed by the Council of Europe as a natural source of food flavouring.

Approved by Commission E for:

- Roots and leaf – irritation of mouth and throat lining and associated dry cough/bronchitis.
- Root – for mild inflammation of stomach lining.

Medicinal parts: Flowers, leaves and roots.

Uses: For most diseases of the gastrointestinal tract including mouth ulcers, hiatus hernia, peptic ulcers, enteritis and colitis, constipation and diarrhoea. Also for respiratory diseases, e.g. catarrh, cough. Treatment of peptic (stomach and duodenal) ulcers, ulceration and inflammation of the mouth and pharynx.

Other uses: Cystitis, urethritis, urinary calculus, enteritis. Topically for abscesses, boils, varicose veins, insect bites and thrombotic ulcers (ulcers caused by clots blocking blood flow to the part), constipation, diarrhoea.

Probable mode of action: Marshmallow root is documented to stimulate destruction of foreign particles or bacteria by white blood cells by a process called phagocytosis, and to release oxygen radicals and leukotrienes from human white blood cells called neutrophils. Thus these properties provide a basis for its marked anti-inflammatory and immunomodulatory properties. The polysaccharide extract inhibited coughing. The relatively large amounts of mucilage make the herb an excellent demulcent which coats the mucosa of the mouth and pharynx and decreases the acidity in the stomach.

Adverse effects: No documented adverse effects. However, anecdotally, there are reports of allergic reactions and of a tendency to lower blood sugar.

Precautions: To be used with caution by diabetics who are on allopathic treatment. The absorption of other drugs concurrently administered may be affected and separation of doses are recommended.

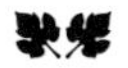

MATE – YERBA MATE – CUP-HERB

Ilex paraguariensis

Native to Argentina, Paraguay, Uruguay and Brazil. The infusion called mate is made from dry leaves and twigs that have been steeped in hot (not boiling) water. Drinking mate with friends from a shared hollow gourd is a very common social practice in Argentina, Uruguay, Paraguay, Chile, Bolivia and Brazil. Also a popular social drink in Syria.

Has been used by the ancient Indians of Brazil and Paraguay. A Spanish explorer reported that the Guarani Indians of Paraguay brewed a leaf tea that 'produced exhilaration and relief from fatigue'. The Jesuits developed plantations in Paraguay and mate became known as 'Jesuit's tea'.

Mate is listed by the Council of Europe as a natural source of food flavouring. Mate is commonly consumed as a beverage. In the US, mate is listed as Generally Recognized As Safe (GRAS). In China, the herb is used parenterally for the treatment of cardiovascular disease (to produce a decrease in blood pressure). Has been used as an appetite suppressant and for weight loss in Germany, France and China.

Approved by Commission E for:
- lack of stamina.

Medicinal parts: Dried or roasted leaves.

Uses: Headache (psychogenic), mental and physical fatigue, nervous depression.

Other uses: Rheumatic pains. **In folk medicine**, Mate is used internally for ulcers, rheumatism, anaemia, neurasthenia, depression, as a diuretic for decreased passing of urine (oliguria) and as a prophylaxis against fever and infections. Mate is used as a poultice for ulcers and inflammation. Used for weakness and fatigue (asthenia) in France and for mental fatigue and depression in Germany and other European countries.

Probable mode of action: The xanthine principles, in particular caffeine, are the active constituents in mate. In rats, a fall in blood pressure has been observed following the use of an aqueous extract of *Ilex pubescens*. Studies suggest that mate differs from other brews containing caffeine in that it causes relaxation of smooth muscles and also strengthens the heart muscle. Has also been found to be an inhibitor of monoamine oxidase (an enzyme involved in the breakdown of substances like adrenaline). Monoamine oxidase inhibitors are a group of drugs used as antidepressants.

Adverse effects: Sleeplessness, anxiety, tremor, palpitations and withdrawal headaches as for other xanthines – a group of drugs in allopathic medicine which include theophylline or aminophylline. Long-term consumption was considered to be the cause of veno-occlusive disease of the liver in a young woman. In **Uruguay**, there was a link between the use of mate and oesophageal cancer.

Precautions: Should be avoided by subjects with heart disease or high blood pressure. Excessive consumption should be avoided during pregnancy and lactation as xanthine derivatives are excreted in the breast milk.

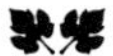

MEADOWSWEET

Filipendula ulmaria

Regarded as sacred by the Druids and has been for centuries a traditional remedy for an acidic stomach. The fresh root continues to be used in homeopathy.

In 1897, Felix Hoffmann synthesized a new drug salicin from the pure salicylic acid found in meadowsweet species, which was less irritant to the stomach. This new drug, acetylsalicylic acid, was named aspirin by Bayer AG who employed Hoffmann. The old botanical name for the plant was *Spiraea ulmaria*.

Meadowsweet is listed by the Council of Europe as a natural source of food flavouring. In the US meadowsweet is listed by the FDA as a Herb of Undefined Safety.

Approved by Commission E for:

- cough
- bronchitis
- fever and cold

Medicinal parts: Aerial parts of the flowering plant.

Uses: Taken by mouth to relieve the symptoms of the common cold. Gastric complaints known as dyspepsia including heartburn and hyperacidity. Also used in the prophylaxis and treatment of peptic ulcer.

Other uses: Cystitis (bladder infections), rheumatic muscle and joint pain, diarrhoea in children.

Probable mode of action: The extracts from the flower have been shown to prevent the development of stomach ulcers in rats and mice. The flavonoid fraction was shown to have a positive effect on the healing of stomach ulcers. However, meadowsweet has been shown to potentiate the ulcers caused by the agent histamine in the guinea pig. The tannins have an effect of contracting cells (skin and other) following inflammation (astringent). Salicylates are a major constituent, which is possibly the basis for its use in rheumatic, muscle and joint pain.

The herb's antimicrobial, antipyretic and diuretic effects have been attributed to salicylate and related constituents. Some experimental work has suggested the presence of constituents with heparin (an anticoagulant) like activity in the flowers and seed.

Adverse effects: The salicylate constituents may contribute to adverse effects such as nausea. Has been known to cause narrowing of the small airways of the lung – bronchioles – to cause bronchospasm and asthma-like symptoms. Handling of the fresh or dried parts of the plant may give rise to skin rashes. Consider allergy to salicylates. Specific adverse effects for meadowsweet have not been documented.

Precautions: To be avoided by asthmatics as meadowsweet may cause bronchospasm. Due to the salicylate content the use in children for diarrhoea is not advocated. The high tannin content is a factor to be borne in mind and excessive consumption should be avoided. Constituents have been shown to increase uterine tone in rabbits. Use in pregnancy and lactation is not recommended. Due to the salicylate content, it would be advisable not to use meadowsweet in children under the age of 12 years (risk of Reye's syndrome). Reye's syndrome is a rare but dangerous condition caused by aspirin in children. The first signs are intense vomiting and drowsiness, behavioural changes, confusion and seizures which may lead to coma.

Because of its heparin-like constituents and the salicylates, meadowsweet should be used cautiously with the following allopathic medications and herbal medicines that could possibly cause delays in blood clotting: warfarin, heparin, ticlopidine, devil's claw, garlic, ginger, ginkgo, saw palmetto.

MILK THISTLE

Silybum marianum

Origin is from Kashmir (India–Pakistan border). Was considered to help nursing mothers to produce milk. Later became known for its protective effects on the liver. Pliny the Elder (23–79 AD) referred to the plant as being excellent for 'carrying off bile'. In 1949, German researchers found milk thistle to protect the liver of animals exposed to high doses of the potent liver toxin carbon tetrachloride. The active constituents, collectively called silymarin, are currently used in Europe to treat many types of liver disorders. Considered to be useful in acute mushroom poisoning. In 1968, it was found that the active principle of milk thistle is in the seed.

Approved by Commission E for:
dyspeptic complaints
liver and gallbladder complaints.

Medicinal part: Ripe seeds.

Uses: To protect the liver against infections such as hepatitis and also against cirrhosis. Also used as an antioxidant, to mop up or prevent the formation of toxic radicals within the body.

Other uses: Antihyperglycaemic (to lower blood sugar), in premenstrual tension, candidiasis (a fungal infection) and psoriasis. Has been used as an antidote to death cap mushroom poisoning.

Probable mode of action: The active constituent called silymarin has been shown experimentally to protect the liver against a wide range of toxic compounds. Silymarin undergoes a process called enterohepatic circulation where it enters the liver circulation and concentrates in the liver cells. Its two main mechanisms of liver protection are an ability to alter the outer liver cell membrane structure and hence block toxin damage, and to stimulate protein synthesis which aids liver regeneration. In animal studies, silymarin protects liver cells against a variety of hepatotoxins, including drugs (acetaminophen, amitriptyline and erythromycin), toxins (alpha amanitin from death cap mushrooms, alcohol and carbon tetrachloride), haemosiderin, viruses and radiation. Silymarin scavenges free radicals, blocks entry of toxic products into cells by competing for receptor sites, inhibits inflammation and stimulates liver regeneration. As a result, it lowers serum transaminase levels (liver enzymes), maintains coagulation factor production and limits necrosis. It also prevents kidney toxicity of the allopathic drug cisplatin.

Adverse effects: May cause headache, nausea, irritability and minor gastrointestinal upset, even though the herb is claimed to have very few or no adverse effects. Rarely a laxative effect may occur. The long-term side-effects of milk thistle are not known as yet.

Precautions: Diabetic patients taking silymarin should carefully monitor their blood glucose and may require reduction in standard antihyperglycemic agents to avoid hypoglycemia. Should not be used in patients with decompensated liver cirrhosis.

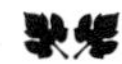

MISTLETOE

Viscum album

Mistletoe is a true parasite for at no period does it derive its nourishment from the soil or decaying bark. Found throughout Europe but considered to be scarce in Scotland.

Held in great reverence by the Druids who considered the possessor of the mistletoe to be protected from all evil. In Brittany, where mistletoe grows abundantly, it is called Herbe de la Croix because according to an old legend, the Cross was made from its wood and thereafter it was destined to become a parasite.

Approved by Commission E for:
- rheumatism
- tremor therapy (adjuvant, i.e. enhances effect of other drugs).

Medicinal parts: The leaves and twigs collected before the berries form.

Uses: Treatment of high blood pressure, arteriosclerosis, nervous tachycardia, headaches due to high blood pressure (hypertension). European mistletoe tea has been used for treatment of high blood pressure, epilepsy, whooping cough, asthma.

In Chinese medicine, mistletoe has been used for joint pain, tendon and muscle pain, lumbago, back pain, vaginal bleeding during pregnancy, agalactia.

Other uses: Chorea (a nervous disease disorder characterized by involuntary movements), hysteria. A proprietary product Iscador, which is produced from naturally fermented mistletoe plant juice, has been investigated for the treatment of cancer. Has also been used to treat degenerative diseases of joints (e.g. osteoarthritis) and as palliative therapy for cancers.

Probable mode of action: The mode of action of cytotoxic activity (activity against cancer cells) has been linked to the ability of the basic amino acids present in mistletoe to maintain the integrity of cells, or the same structure of the cells, during cell division. Sensitivity to mistletoe extracts has been documented for acute lymphoblastic leukaemia cells resistant to methotrexate and cytabarine – two allopathic medications used in the treatment of leukaemias. The constituents, some of which are very similar to the chemical messengers or neurotransmitters in the human body, are considered responsible for the blood pressure lowering effects, which is possibly due to the effects of the constituents on the blood pressure controlling centre (vasomotor centre) in the brain stem.

Adverse effects: Hepatitis may occur following its use. Lowering of blood pressure (hypotension), coma, seizures, dilatation of pupils and death may follow ingestion of toxic doses. Large doses of the plant or its berries may aggravate convulsive disorders and young children have suffered convulsions after eating excessive amounts of berries.

Precautions: Mistletoe berries are highly poisonous. The herb should only be prescribed by a qualified or trained practitioner. Mistletoe therapy has the potential to interfere with the allopathic drug management of high blood pressure, heart disease, antidepressant and anticoagulant treatment. Use of mistletoe during pregnancy is contraindicated. Tyramine and a cardioactive constituent of mistletoe have been shown to have a uterine stimulant effect. The herb should not be used for progressive disorders such as tuberculosis. The use of mistletoe in the treatment of cancers and leukaemias is under review at present.

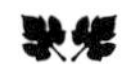

MOTHERWORT

Leonurus cardiaca

An important herb since Roman times, the name *Leonurus* is derived from a Greek word meaning lion's tail, describing the shaggy shape of the leaves. The ancient Greeks used motherwort to relieve anxiety in mothers after childbirth.

Chinese herbalists use the related species *Leonurus heterophyllus* mainly for menstrual disorders, raised blood pressure, heart disease and conjunctivitis. The aerial (above ground) parts (yi mu cao) are also used for eczema and sores, while the seeds (chong wei zi) are used for menstrual irregularities, and as a stimulant of the circulation. They are also believed to act specifically on the liver. Considered especially effective on the eyes to 'brighten the vision'. A weak decoction of the seeds may be used in conjunctivitis, or sore and tired eyes.

Approved by Commission E for:

- nervous heart complaints.

Medicinal parts: Aerial parts collected during the flowering period, between June and September.

Uses: Disability due to cardiac disease, increased heart rate disorders (tachycardia), amenorrhoea.

Specifically indicated in heart (cardiac) symptoms associated with neurosis. It is a specific remedy for tachycardia caused by anxiety, and may be used in all heart conditions associated with anxiety and tension.

Other uses: *Leonurus* is valuable in the stimulation of suppressed or delayed menstruation, and to ease dysmenorrhoea (painful menstruation). Used to ease false labour pains, and the infusion, taken after childbirth is used to restore the uterus and reduce the risk of postpartum haemorrhage (bleeding after child birth). Relieves menopausal symptoms.

In **Germany**, the plant is used as an adjuvant in treatment of an overactive thyroid gland. **In folk medicine**, it is used for bronchial asthma, climacteric symptoms and amenorrhoea.

Probable mode of action: Constituents include alkaloids, glycosides and flavonoids, volatile oil, tannins and vitamin A which have sedative and antispasmodic, and emmenagogue, properties. It is also mildly hypotensive, a cardiac tonic, a gentle uterine stimulant, a relaxant and a carminative and it induces perspiration (diaphoretic). The constituent alkaloid is considered to produce central nervous depression and hypotensive effects in animals. The glycosides have a short-term ability to lower blood pressure.

Adverse effects: No adverse effects or hazards are known following the proper administration of recommended therapeutic doses.

Precautions: *Leonurus* is a uterine stimulant and so should be avoided in pregnancy, although it has been used during labour. Also has the effect of hastening childbirth.

MUSTARD

Brassica/Sinapis spp.

White mustard (*Brassica alba* syn. *Brassica hirta*, *Sinapis alba*); Black mustard (*Brassica nigra* syn. *Sinapis nigra*, *Brassica sinapioides*); Brown mustard (*Brassica juncea* syn. *Brassica integrifolia*).

The Chinese have used it for thousands of years, and the ancient Greeks used it routinely, as well as holding it in very high esteem as a medicine. For the Romans, it was a condiment and pickling spice, and it got its modern English name when they brought it north in mixtures with new wine (mustum, which was combined with the word *ardere*, 'to burn').

Although the volatile oil of mustard is a powerful irritant, in dilution as a liniment or poultice it soothes, creating warmth and drawing blood to the surface. Over the years mustard has been prescribed for a variety of ailments, from scorpion stings and snake bites to constipation and respiratory troubles.

Medicinal part: Seeds.

Uses: Common cold and rheumatism.

Probable mode of action: Active constituents include isocyanates. The exact mechanism of effects of the constituents is not known with certainty.

Adverse effects: Allergic reactions to mustard start very early in life, usually below three years of age. Mustard allergy may result in irritating and uncomfortable skin reactions including angioedema and urticaria. Children and adolescents appear to also be especially affected

A skin burn from culinary mustard has been recorded. Irritant contact dermatitis has been induced by a mustard compress. Pancreatitis as a complication of mustard-induced anaphylaxis has been reported.

Precautions: The internal use of the seeds can be problematic because of the possibility of retention in the intestines. The volatile active ingredients that can be released from mustard require caution in applications of all forms.

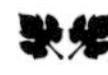

MYRRH

Commiphora molmol (African myrrh)
Commiphora abyssinica (Arabian myrrh)

Was used by the Egyptians in embalming mixtures. Has also been used as an aromatic for perfumes and insect repellents. Ancient Greek and Roman physicians used the herb to treat wounds and prescribed it internally as a digestive aid and to promote menstruation. Mentioned in an Egyptian papyrus dated 2000 BC.

Myrrh is listed by the Council of Europe as a natural source of food flavouring. In the US, myrrh is permitted for use in alcoholic beverages. A popular ingredient of toothpaste in Europe to fight bacteria that cause tooth decay.

Approved by Commission E for:

- Topical use – for mild inflammation of the oral and pharyngeal mucosa.

Medicinal parts: The resin which has exuded from the bark and dried in the air. Myrrh is the pale yellow granular secretion that is discharged into cavities in the bark when it is wounded. The exudate hardens to a red brown mass about the size of a walnut.

Uses: Myrrh is used for the topical treatment of mild inflammations of the mouth and pharynx mucosa. **In folk medicine**, myrrh is used occasionally internally for non-specific intestinal infections and also to promote removal of secretions from the lung and upper airways (as an expectorant) and for coughs. **Folk medicine** uses have also included stimulating the appetite and the flow of digestive juices, aphthous ulcers (ulcers on the mouth and tongue often caused by stress) pharyngitis, catarrh, common cold.

Other uses: The Indian plant *Commiphora mukul*, commonly known as guggulipid, has been used by **Indian physicians** for lowering blood cholesterol levels. Among uses in **Indian medicine** are menstrual disorders, stomach complaints, wounds, ulcers and inflammation of the mouth and skin. **In Chinese medicine**, it has been used for carbuncles, furuncles, wounds, amenorrhoea and abdominal tumours.

Probable mode of action: A ketosteroid has been identified as the active constituent lowering blood cholesterol in the Indian plant (guggulipid). This is believed to occur as a result of stimulation of the thyroid gland. Myrrh is documented to contract cells (skin and other) following inflammation (astringent) and to show antimicrobial activity in laboratory experiments. Other effects attributed to constituents (essential oils) include disinfectant properties and the promotion of formation of granulation tissue. Other properties attributed to the constituents include pain relief (analgesia) and inducing of menstruation (emmenagogue).

Adverse effects: No reported adverse effects for *Commiphora molmol* and *Commiphora abyssinica*. Hiccup, diarrhoea, restlessness and apprehension were documented as side-effects for guggulipid when administered to 20 patients. However, there are records of large amounts causing diarrhoea, nausea, vomiting and an increase in heart rate.

Precautions: May interfere with allopathic treatment of diabetes mellitus. As myrrh is known to affect the menstrual cycle, avoid use during pregnancy. Found to be addictive herb in Somalia. If bleeding of the gums or pain in gums persists for more than two weeks after the use of this herb, a dental surgeon should be consulted.

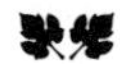

NASTURTIUM – INDIAN CRESS

Tropaeolum majus

Native habitat is Peru. The origin of its use followed the Spanish conquests of Peru and Mexico in the 16th century. Derived its name because of the pungent and peppery odour: *nasus* (nose), *tortus* (twisted).

Approved by Commission E for:

- infections of the urinary tract

- cough
- bronchitis.

Medicinal parts: Fresh herb, leaves, flowers, seeds.

Uses: Unproven uses include infections of the urinary tract and catarrh of the upper respiratory tract. Also used internally for mild muscular pain, skin diseases, scurvy, tuberculosis and menstrual disorders.

Other uses: The herb is used externally for hair loss and for infected and poorly healing wounds.

Probable mode of action: Active constituents include viatmin C, oxalates, flavonoids and carotinoids. The fresh unbruised plant has a constituent that yields benzyl isothiocyanate after cell destruction. The oil extracted from nasturtium is bacteriostatic (prevents multiplication of bacteria), virostatic (prevents multiplication of viruses) and antimycotic (effective against fungi) in laboratory tests. Constituents have been found to lower blood sugar and also to possess stimulant properties.

Adverse effects: Irritation of the mucous membrane of the gastrointestinal tract. Long-term intensive contact with the fresh plant can lead to skin irritation. Low potential for sensitization.

Precautions: Do not use in infants or small children. Do not administer to patients with gastrointestinal ulcers or with kidney disease.

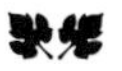

NEEM – MARGOSA

Antelaea azadirachta

The margosa tree has been closely associated with Ayurvedic medical practice and agriculture for centuries, particularly in India and other South Asian countries where millions of trees line the roads. It is cultivated all over India and is commonly grown in Indonesia, Sri Lanka, Myanmar, Pakistan, Japan and in the tropical regions of Australia and Africa. The neem or margosa tree is considered to be an air purifier and to prevent malaria and cholera.

Medicinal parts: All parts of the tree are considered to have medicinal properties. The parts frequently used are the leaves, the bark, the roots and the gum discharged by the stem.

Uses: Leprosy, eye disorders, epistaxis, intestinal worms, anorexia, skin ulcers, contraception (when used intravaginally) and to induce abortion.

Other uses: Also used in diabetes, fever, hepatic disease, malaria, asthma (twigs), haemorrhoids and as an insecticide.

Probable mode of action: More than 130 active ingredients have been isolated from neem. Nimibidin, a constituent of neem seed oil, is suggested to have anti-inflammatory, antiarthritic, antipyretic, hypoglycaemic, diuretic, antifungal and anti-ulcer effects. Nimbidin and nimbin have spermicidal (kills sperm) activity. Preliminary clinical research suggests usefulness as a long-term vaginal contraceptive. The bark contains tannins and polysaccharides that may have anti-inflammatory activity. Sulphur-containing neem leaf extracts appear to have antifungal activity. Neem leaf extracts have been attributed to affect sperm mobility and viability.

Adverse effects: Neem oil is toxic to infants and children. Orally severe poisoning in this age group causes vomiting, loose stools, drowsiness, metabolic acidosis, anaemia, seizures, loss of consciousness, coma and cerebral oedema and Reye's syndrome-like symptoms. Death has been reported to occur within hours of ingestion of neem oil.

Theoretically neem might have additive effects with herbs that decrease blood sugar levels. Herbs with hypoglycaemic potential include devil's claw, fenugreek, garlic, guar gum, horse chestnut, *Panax gingseng*, psyllium and Siberian ginseng.

Precautions: To be avoided if subjects suffer from autoimmune diseases, e.g. multiple sclerosis, lupus. To be avoided by patients awaiting organ transplants and by diabetics. Can interfere with conception and is thus to be avoided in infertility. May decrease the effectiveness of allopathic immunosuppressant drugs such as Imuran, Zenapax and Prednisone (azathioprine, daclizumab, prednisolone).

NETTLE

Urtica dioica

Nettle is a common name for any of between 30 and 45 species of flowering plants of the genus *Urtica*. The most prominent member is the stinging nettle (*Urtica dioica*). The sting of *Urtica ferox*, the onga onga or tree nettle of New Zealand, has been known to kill horses, dogs and at least one human.

The herbs and leaves are listed by the Council of Europe as a natural source of food flavouring. Nettle is used in herbal teas and soups. In the USA, nettle is listed by the FDA as a Herb of Undefined Safety.

Approved by Commission E for:

- internal use of leaf, as supportive therapy for rheumatic ailments
- irrigation therapy, for inflammatory disease of the lower urinary tract and prevention of the formation of 'gravel' in the kidney
- difficulty in urination from benign prostatic hyperplasia (root approved).

Medicinal parts: Root, leaf.

Uses: Uterine haemorrhage, cutaneous eruptions, eczema, epistaxis (bleeding from the nose), malaena (blackish stools due to blood).

Other uses: Urinary tract disorders, rheumatic ailments. Nettle is used in shampoos to control dandruff and is said to make the hair 'more glossy'. Nettle root has been extensively studied in human clinical trials as a treatment for benign prostatic hyperplasia. It has also been used by body builders in an effort to increase the circulating levels of the male hormone testosterone.

Probable mode of action: A constituent has been shown in the laboratory to inhibit some chemical substances that cause inflammation. In similar experiments nettle extracts have been shown to suppress the expression of inflammatory agents, which possibly forms the basis for its use in rheumatic ailments. In clinical studies, nettle has been shown to enhance the effectiveness of the allopathic anti-inflammatory drug diclofenac (a non-steroidal anti-inflammatory drug). An aqueous extract of nettle root inhibited the proliferation of cells in the prostate gland, hence its use in benign prostatic hyperplasia. The extracts were shown to interfere with the binding activity of the sex hormone binding globulin. One of the constituents has been found to occupy sex hormone binding sites and consequently increase the circulating levels of sex hormones such as testosterone. Some constituents have an effect on the uterus. The high potassium content in nettle is believed to be responsible for the diuretic action.

Adverse effects: Consumption of nettle tea has caused gastric irritation, a burning sensation of the skin, oedema and a decrease in the output of urine (oliguria). The leaves are extremely irritant in view of their acetylcholine- and histamine-containing glandular hairs.

Precautions: Likely to interfere with the allopathic drug control of diabetes mellitus, high blood pressure (hypertension). May also interact with drugs that cause depression of the central nervous system (e.g. pain relieving drugs such as morphine, alcohol). Reported to be an abortifacient and avoid use during pregnancy. Excessive use during lactation is best avoided.

NIAULI – CAGE OIL

Melaleuca viridiflora

Native to Australia and Tasmania. Native Australians have used tea tree oil for centuries. Introduced to Europe after the expeditions of

Captain James Cook. A botanist who accompanied Captain Cook observed how the aborigines used the herb to heal infected wounds. Captain Cook's crew brewed a lemon flavoured tea from the leaves, hence the name tea tree. In the 1920s scientists (A.R. Penfold et al.) studied tea tree oil and found it to be a potent antiseptic – 12 times as potent as phenol. Later, bushmen and adventurers would not enter the wilderness without tea tree oil.

This plant is a variant of the tea tree discussed on page 228 and is referred to as the 'broad leaved tea tree'. The oil, Niauli oil, is marketed as tea tree oil and the properties and uses are nearly identical.

Approved by Commission E for:

- cough/bronchitis.

Medicinal parts: Young or shrubby plants and oil which is distilled from the fresh leaves and twigs.

Uses: Used for catarrh of the upper respiratory tract, rheumatism, neuralgia and cystitis.

Probable mode of action: Constituents are considered to be antibacterial and to stimulate the circulation.

Adverse effects: Internal administration of the oil can lead to nausea, vomiting and diarrhoea.

Precautions: Contraindicated for internal use in inflammatory diseases of the gastrointestinal tract or of bile ducts and in severe liver disease. Preparation containing the oil should not be applied to the face of infants or small children as spasm of the glottis (situated at the opening of the windpipe) may lead to symptoms similar to that of bronchial asthma and could also lead to respiratory failure and death.

Considered to increase the metabolism of drugs by the liver. Hence be cautious about lack of efficacy or potency during co-administration with some allopathic medications.

Doses greater than two teaspoonfuls have been considered to be life-threatening.

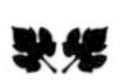

NOTOGINSENG ROOT – SAN QI

Panax notoginseng
Panax pseudoginseng

A traditional Chinese remedy for internal and external bleeding. By Chinese standards it is a relatively new remedy being first recorded for use in 1578 by Li Shizen who pronounced the root as 'more valuable than gold'. The Chinese refer to it as 'three-seven root' because the plant has three leaves on one side and four leaves on the other.

Medicinal part: Roots.

Uses: Taken internally for nosebleeds and for blood in the stools, urine or lungs. Applied externally, it is used to relieve pain and swelling from fractures, sprains, bruises, cuts and wounds.

Other uses: Occasionally for treatment of Crohn's disease, angina and high blood pressure. Also used as an alternative to hormone replacement therapy.

Probable mode of action: Active constituents include saponins and flavonoids. The exact mechanisms of actions of the constituents are not known as yet.

Adverse effects: No reported effects with recommended doses and routes of administration. Known to have caused abortions.

Precautions: Avoid during pregnancy (as it can cause miscarriage) and breastfeeding. Should not be taken by patients on anticoagulants or ticlodipine (a drug given to prevent the formation of blood clots).

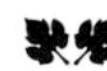

NUTMEG

Myristica fragrans

Hindi name: Jaiphal
Sri Lankan name: Saadikka
Nutmeg ingestion has been reported among prisoners, college students and adolescents attempting to achieve euphoria, although intoxications have occurred with the unintentional misuse of the

herbs

herbal preparation. In **Cambodia**, the nut is used as a remedy for loose stools.

Medicinal parts: Nutmeg seeds through various processes yield several therapeutic components. They include the essential oil of the seed, the compressed, dried aril, the mixture of fat and oil from the pressed seeds, the dried seed kernel freed from the aril and shell of nut, calcified seed kernels and the dried seed kernels.

Uses: Used in flatulence, dyspepsias, musculoskeletal and arthritic disorders, and psychiatric disorders.

Other uses: Used as an emmenagogue and an abortifacient. May also cause euphoria. **In folk medicine**, uses of nutmeg include diarrhoea and dysentery, inflammation of the stomach membranes, cramps, flatulence and vomiting. Externally the oil has been used for rheumatism, sciatica, neuralgia and disorders of the upper respiratory tract.

Probable mode of action: In animal experiments, eugenol in the essential oil inhibits in a dose-dependent manner, medicinally induced diarrhoea. Myristicin, one of the active constituents of the oil, has weak monoamine-oxidase inhibitor properties that are responsible for some of the cardiovascular symptoms. It is metabolized in the body to an amphetamine-like compound (amphetamine is a stimulant of the brain). An effect on prostaglandin synthesis and an antimicrobial effect has also been demonstrated.

Adverse effects: Poisoning may cause nausea, vomiting and central nervous system effects.

These symptoms occur within several hours of ingesting 5–15 mg of nutmeg. Within 24 hours, following an acute delirium and subsequent deep sleep, the patient often recovers uneventfully.

Hypothermia (lowering of the body temperature) may occur following large ingestions. Nutmeg can trigger allergic reactions and contact dermatitis.

Precautions: Not to be used during pregnancy. Be aware of the potential for abuse.

OAK

Quercus robur

The oak was sacred to the Greeks, while the Romans dedicated it to Jupiter. It was venerated by the Druids. Galen applied the bruised leaves to wounds. Its botanical name is believed to derive from the Celtic *quer*, meaning fine, and *cuez*, tree. It was much prized in the past for shipbuilding and the construction of railway carriages. The bark is still used to tan leather and the Scottish Highlanders used it to dye yarn.

Acorns are sometimes used as a coffee substitute.

Approved by Commission E for:

- cough/bronchitis
- diarrhoea
- inflammation of the mouth and pharynx
- inflammation of the skin.

Medicinal parts: Dried bark of the young branches and the lateral shoots, the dried bark of the trunk and branches, the dried leaves of various oak species and the seed kernels without the seed coats.

Uses: Oak is used internally for non-specific diarrhoea and in smaller doses as a stomach tonic. Used externally for inflammatory skin diseases, inflammation of the mouth and throat as well as in the genital and anal area, suppurating eczema, increased sweating, bruises and ulcers, intertrigo (inflammatory condition affecting skin folds) and as an adjuvant in the treatment of chilblains.

Other uses: Used as a gargle for bleeding of the mouth and throat. As a footbath for sweaty feet. The powdered bark used as a snuff for nosebleeds. Used **in folk medicine** internally for haemorrhagic stools, non-menstrual uterine bleeding, haemoptysis (coughing of blood) and chronic inflammation of the gastrointestinal tract. Used externally for bleeding haemorrhoids, varicose veins, uterine bleeding, vaginal discharge, rashes, chronic itching and scaly skin disorders.

Probable mode of action: Constituents include tannin, gallic acid and ellagitannin which are considered to contract cells (skin and other) following inflammation (astringent), and have haemostatic (stop bleeding), antiseptic, anti-inflammatory and tonic properties. The oak is considered to have antiviral and antihelminthic properties.

Adverse effects: Internal administration could lead to digestive complaints because of the secretion inhibiting the effect of the tannins.

Precautions: Oak may delay the absorption of alkaloids and other alkaline drugs. These drugs should be administered at least two hours apart.

ONION

Allium cepa

Onion has been used as a herbal remedy from time immemorial. The physicians of ancient **Egypt** prescribed onions for a wide range of medical disorders. Dioscorides in the first century AD attributed the effects of many herbal remedies to the onion content. In 1835 an onion and milk diet was advocated for dropsy. **In folk medicine**, onion has been used to treat cough (including whooping cough), bronchitis, asthma and angina, stimulate the gallbladder and be an aid to menstruation.

Approved by Commission E for:

- loss of appetite
- arteriosclerosis
- dyspeptic complaints
- fevers and colds
- cough/bronchitis
- hypertension
- tendency to infection
- inflammation of mouth and pharynx
- common cold.

Medicinal part: The bulb.

Uses: Used to improve loss of appetite, prevent atherosclerosis and treat stomach ailments (dyspepsia), fever and colds.

Other uses: Hypertension (high blood pressure), inflammation of mouth and pharynx. **In folk medicine**, onion is administered internally for cough, whooping cough, bronchitis, asthma and angina. Onion has been used to stimulate gallbladder function, for digestive disorders with bloating and colic. Onion has also been used in worm infestations (ascariasis). Externally onion was used for insect bites, wounds, light burns, furuncles, warts and in the after care of bruises. **In Indian medicine**, onion is used for dyspeptic conditions, respiratory conditions, wounds, pain and malarial fever. **In Chinese medicine**, onions were used for worm infestations, fungal and bacterial infections.

Probable mode of action: Active constituents include essential oils, diphenylamine and sulphur compounds. Active constituents are responsible for the odour and tearing (lachrymation). Onions are rich in vitamin C. The thiosulphinate constituents have shown an antibacterial effect against *Bacillus subtilis*, *Salmonella typhi*, *Pseudomonas aeroginosa* and *Escherichia coli*. Some constituents are considered similar to those found in garlic and thus considered to be helpful in lowering high blood pressure. Other constituents are considered to have an effect on blood coagulation and cause 'thinning' of the blood. Administration of an alcoholic onion extract was found to reduce allergy-induced bronchial asthma.

Adverse effects: Large quantities taken orally can cause stomach upset. Hand eczema may also occur with frequent handling.

Precautions: Concomitant use of herbs with coumarin constituents or antiplatelet effects could theoretically increase risk of bleeding. May interfere with drug control of blood sugar. A maximum of 35 mg of diphenylamine is recommended per day if used over several months.

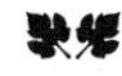

OREGON GRAPE

Mahonia aquifolium

In traditional North American Medicine, *Mahonia aquifolium* has been used to treat loss of appetite and debility.

Current use is mainly in the treatment of skin disorders, particularly psoriasis.

Medicinal part: Bark.

Uses: Internally to treat psoariasis and some other skin disorders. As a tonic for liver and gallbladder disease and to reduce nausea and vomiting and similar stomach ailments.

Other uses: Eczema. Has been used internally to treat syphilis. Externally as a gargle for sore throat and as a wash for tired or bloodshot eyes.

Probable mode of action: Active constituents include the alkaloids berberine and hydrastine, which are also found in goldenseal. Highly bactericidal (prevents multiplication of bacteria), amoebicidal (kills amoebae) and trypanocidal (kills the parasitic worm trypanosome). In one clinical trial, oregon grape was found to be mildly effective for reducing skin irritation, inflammation and itching in people with mild to moderate psoariasis. The constituents have been shown experimentally to reduce flakiness and scaling of skin.

Adverse effects: High doses can cause vomiting, lowered blood pressure and reduced heart rate (bradycardia). Other symptoms of excessive intake may include lethargy, nose bleed, skin and eye irritation and kidney irritation.

Precautions: Berberine-containing plants including barberry, goldenseal and oregon grape should not be used during pregnancy and breastfeeding. This herb should be avoided by patients with overactivity of the thyroid gland (hyperthyroidism). Should not be used with liquorice as *Glycyrrhiza* species nullifies the effect of berberine.

PAPAYA – PAPAIN

Carica papaya

Carica papaya originated in Central America. Popular as an abortifacient in Sri Lanka, Java, Panama and Turkey. Used as an amoebicide in Japan and as a laxative in Panama and Trinidad. In Chinese medicine, it is used as a digestive aid, and in Mexico it is used to treat dyspepsia.

Air-dried seeds have been used in traditional veterinary medicine in Indonesia and Philippines as a 'dewormer'.

Has also been used in the wine making and brewing and the textile and tanning industries.

In **folk medicine**, papaya leaf is used orally for preventing and treating gastrointestinal tract disorders, intestinal parasite infestations and as a diuretic and sedative.

Medicinal parts: Leaves, fruits and latex.

Uses: Papain is used as a digestive aid, for controlling oedema and inflammation following trauma and surgery (used for cuts, rashes, stings and bruises as a local application), for treating parasitic worms and chronic diarrhoea. Has been used to treat arthritis.

Other uses: Papain is used in hay fever, nasal drainage, inflammation of throat and pharynx. Topically used to treat wounds, sores and ulcers. **In Indian medicine**, papaya leaf is used for worm infestations, damage to the urinary tract and kidney stones, haemorrhoids, coughs and bronchitis.

Probable mode of action: Papain, an active constituent, is a mixture of proteolytic enzymes which would aid digestion. Chymopapain, another constituent, also aids digestion. The effects of the other constituents are not known with certainty. The phytochemicals in papaya may inhibit the female hormone progesterone. Leaves also contain tannins. Papain is the main constituent in the fruit and latex.

Adverse effects: Large amounts taken orally may cause oesophageal perforation. Ingestion of papaya latex can cause severe gastritis. Topical use can cause itching. Allergic reactions including attacks of asthma may occur rarely. Allergic reactions have followed inhalation of papaya powder. Frequent use has been reported to be associated with a yellowish discoloration of the palms and soles, similar to carotinaemia (which follows excessive consumption of carrots). This is a harmless condition.

Precautions: Some proteins in potato may inhibit the proteolytic activity of papain. Cross-sensitivity to papain may occur in those sensitive to figs and kiwi fruit. Papaya is contraindicated in pregnancy. This is because of the experimentally proven embryotoxic and teratogenic (ability to cause abnormalities during the formation of organs) effects, as well as abortifacient effects in humans. Unripe papain fruit should not be used during pregnancy. The leaves and root contain cyanogenic glycosides.

PARSLEY

Petroselinum crispum

Since ancient times, parsley has been used to enhance youth and beauty and to boost libido. The Romans used parsley as a remedy for sore eyes and as a tonic to increase the strength of their gladiators. Other traditional uses have been for gastrointestinal disorders (e.g. constipation, flatulence, indigestion, colic). Also used as an aphrodisiac and for the treatment of asthma and rheumatism and to promote menstrual flow.

Parsley herb and root has been approved by Commission E for:

- infections of the urinary tract
- kidney and bladder stones.

Medicinal parts: The oil extracted from the parsley fruit, the fresh or dried aerial parts, the dried underground parts and the whole fresh plant at the beginning of the flowering season.

Uses: As a breath freshner, for urinary tract infections and for kidney and bladder stones.

Other uses: Topically for cracked skin, bruises, insect bites and to stimulate hair growth. **In folk medicine**, the fruit has been used for menstrual disturbances, disorders of the gastrointestinal tract, the kidneys and lower urinary tract and as an aid for digestion. Has also been used in the treatment of asthma. Popular phytotherapy agent for high blood pressure in some regions of **Morocco**.

Probable mode of action: Active constituents include volatile oil containing apiole, myristicin and psoralens. Also contains vitamin B_1, B_2 and C. Apiole appears to be associated with antispasmodic vasodilator and menstrual flow stimulating effects. Both apiole and myristicin appear to possess uterine stimulating properties. Parsley is considered to cause irritation of the kidney epithelium, and to increase kidney blood flow and urine formation. In animal experiments, the fruit has demonstrated a diuretic effect and the production of a moderate increase in the tone of the uterus. Higher doses of the fruit in such experiments caused an increase in the contractile force of the smooth muscle of the intestine, bladder and especially of the uterus. The latter may explain its use in menstrual complaints and also the danger of its use in pregnancy.

Adverse effects: Can occasionally cause allergic reactions. If more than 10 g of the constituent apiole is used, haemolytic anaemia (anaemia following destruction of red blood cells), thrombocytopenic purpura (bleeding due to reduction in the number of circulating blood platelets) and kidney and liver dysfunction may occur. The constituent myristicin may cause giddiness, deafness, hallucinations, bradycardia and hypotension. The apiole and myristicin constituents have been alleged to cause liver failure. The oil from the seed may cause allergic reactions such as contact dermatitis.

Precautions: Theoretically should not be used in patients with oedema as parsley may cause sodium and water retention which may make hypertension worse. Best avoided by patients with kidney disease. Therapeutic doses of the herb and root are contraindicated in pregnancy. The parsley fruit has been associated with abortions and hence should be avoided during pregnancy. Caution is necessary in patients who are taking allopathic medications that are associated with activity of the chemical messenger, serotonin.

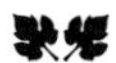

PASSION FLOWER

Passiflora incarnata

The name *Passiflora* is from the Italian *fiore della passione* which is considered to be associated with the resemblance of the flower to the elements surrounding the crucifixion of Christ.

Has been used in Brazilian traditional medicine to cure fevers.

Passion flower is listed by the Council of Europe as a natural source of food flavouring. In the US, the use of passion flower in food is permitted. Passion flower is used in combination with valerian root and lemon balm for conditions of unrest, difficulty in falling asleep due to anxiety. Passion flower is used extensively in homeopathy.

Approved by Commission E for:

- nervousness and insomnia

Medicinal parts: The whole or cut dried herb and fresh aerial parts. The yellow pulp from the berry is edible and has been attributed with medicinal properties.

Uses: Sedation, as a hypnotic in insomnia, as an antispasmodic. Used for treatment of neuralgia, generalized seizures, hysteria, nervous tachycardia.

Other uses: Unproven uses include the use of the passion flower internally for depressive states and also for hysteria, general nervous agitation, insomnia and nervous gastrointestinal disorders. The herb has been used externally for haemorrhoids and as a bath additive for nervous agitation. Also used for asthma. One of the uses has been for the treatment of withdrawal symptoms following long-term use of benzodiazepines (e.g. Valium) because of its sedative and anxiety relieving effects. Has been used topically for burns.

Probable mode of action: The constituents maltol and ethylmatol have been attributed with central nervous system depressant effects, namely sedation and hypnotic actions. These constituents are considered to mask the stimulant effect of the harmful alkaloid constituents. The glycosides in the flower have been shown in animal experiments to cause a lowering of blood pressure and to stimulate respiration. In animal experiments the constituents have been shown to increase the threshold for convulsions (anticonvulsant effect) and it is likely that some of the constituents bind to receptors to which drugs such as Valium bind in the brain.

Adverse effects: Sedation. Hypersensitivity reactions have been noted. Workers making herbal preparations containing passion flower have been diagnosed as suffering from occupational asthma and rhinitis.

Precautions: As toxicological data are lacking excessive use during pregnancy and lactation should be avoided. Likely to potentiate the action of other central nervous system depressants such as alcohol.

PAU D'ARCO

Tabebuia impetiginosa

Few herbal medicines have been used for such long periods for diverse medical disorders as pau d'arco. Initial use is considered to be prior to the Inca civilization. This tree, which is native to the Amazon rain forest, has been used not only in South America, but also in North America and Europe, as a herbal medicine for centuries. Was initially used to make hunting bows. The Guarani and Tupi Indians called the tree tajy, which means to have strength and vigour. The Portuguese who first colonized Brazil named the tree pau d'arco, meaning bow stick.

Has been used in traditional medical systems

for the treatment of malaria, anaemia, syphilis, all types of infections and infestations (bacterial, viral, fungal, parasitic), for rheumatism, dysentery and inflammatory disorders and as an aphrodisiac.

Medicinal part: Bark, wood.

Uses: Has been considered to kill bacteria, viruses, fungi and parasites and also to kill cancer cells (including leukaemic cells) and to relieve pain and reduce inflammation. Thus uses include *Candida*, viral, respiratory tract infections (flu, common cold), diarrhoea and bladder infections.

Other uses: Also used in the treatment of patients with cancer and parasitic infestations. In **folk medicine**, pau d'arco has been used orally for cancer, diabetes, ulcers, gastritis, liver ailments, asthma, bronchitis, gonorrhoea and syphilis.

Probable mode of action: The bark and the wood have the naphthoquinone derivative lapachol which is considered to increase the risk of bleeding by prolonging prothrombin time. These effects can be reversed by vitamin K. Preliminary data suggests lapachol to possess antibacterial, antifungal, antimalarial and antiparasitic actions. The bark and the wood contain about 15 quinone compounds including lapachol, beta lapachone and tabebuin, an anthraquinone. One of the major contributors to the difficulties in obtaining scientific evidence associated with the efficacy of the constituents has been the inconsistencies of the products that have used for analytical work.

Adverse effects: High doses would cause nausea, vomiting, diarrhoea, dizziness, anaemia and increase the risk of bleeding. Has been associated with the passage of pink-coloured urine. It is not known whether this is a manifestation of the increased bleeding tendency.

Precautions: Avoid in those on anticoagulant drugs, namely drugs that increase the time taken for blood to clot. Should not be used in those with bleeding diseases, usually inherited, such as haemophilia and Von Willebrand's disease. Do not use doses providing more than 1.5 g per day of the lapachol constituent. Not to be used during pregnancy and breastfeeding. Some herbalists do not recommend the use of the bark or wood in patients under the age of 18 years.

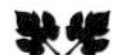

PEANUT – GROUNDNUT

Arachis hypogaea

First grown by the Inca of ancient Peru. Believed to have originated in either Argentina or Bolivia. It is estimated that half a billion of people on earth rely on peanut as their primary source of protein.

Medicinal part: The oil.

Uses: To lower blood cholesterol and prevent heart disease.

Other uses: To lose weight and decrease appetite, prevention of cancer. Topically for arthritis, skin ailments (scalp crusting, dry skin, eczema, ichthyiosis). The peanut oil was applied rectally for constipation. Has been used as a bath additive for subacute and chronic eczema and for atrophic eczema and ichthyiosis (a skin condition with dry scales, sometimes called 'fish-scale' disease). The pharmaceutical industry used the oil as a vehicle for medication in external, internal and parenteral preparations. The cosmetic industry uses the oil in skin, sun and massage oils. **In Indian medicine**, peanut oil is used for constipation, neuralgia and dislocated joints.

Probable mode of action: Peanuts are a rich source of protein (roughly 30 g per cup after roasting), as well as a rich source of monounsaturated fat. Research has identified some antioxidants and other chemicals which are likely to be beneficial to health. Some of the consituents may contribute to cardioprotective and cancer protective effects. The high monounsaturated and low saturated fat content of peanut oil is considered to prevent heart attacks and lower cholesterol. However there is some animal evidence to suggest

herbs

that the oil is atherogenic (promotes the deposition of fat plaques or atheromatous plaques inside arteries). The effect obtained when used as an enema for constipation and in dermatology is achieved primarily from the drug's oiliness. Peanuts are a good source of resveratrol, a chemical studied for potential anti-ageing effects. Peanuts are devoid of omega-3 fats.

Adverse effects: Can cause severe allergic reactions in those allergic to the Fabaceae family (e.g. soy beans). In those allergic to peanuts, eating a single nut or just breathing the dust from peanuts can cause a fatal reaction. Though the allergy is considered to last a lifetime, recent work suggests that approximately 20% of children will outgrow a peanut allergy.

Precautions: To be absolutely avoided if there is suggestion of allergy. Peanuts may be contaminated with mould *Aspergillus flavus*, which produces a carcinogen, aflatoxin.

PEEPAL

Ficus religiosa

Indian name: Peepal

The peepal is one of the best known trees in the Indian subcontinent. It is venerated by Hindus and Buddhists. The rishis in the past meditated under the peepal trees. It was beneath a peepal tree that Gautam Buddha attained enlightenment and that particular tree came to be known as the Bodhi tree – 'the tree of wisdom'.

Medicinal parts: Leaves, bark.

Uses: The leaves are used as a laxative and to prepare tonics. The tonics reduce fever. Used in **Indian medicine** to stop or decrease bleeding and also to reduce secretions. Infusions of the leaves are used to treat heart disease.

Other uses: Peepal leaves have been used in mumps and to treat boils. A popular remedy in India for excessive urine output is to soak a piece of the tender bark in water overnight and allow the water to be taken the following morning.

Probable mode of action: The nature of constituents and their exact mode of action are not known with certainty as yet.

Adverse effects: No information available.

Precautions: No information available.

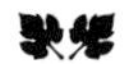

PENNYROYAL

Mentha pulegium
Hedeoma pulegioides

Has a traditional folk medicine use of inducing abortions and as an emmenagogue. Pulegium of the Romans, named by Pliny for its reputed power of driving away fleas. *Pulex* is the Latin name for flea. Has been hung in the rooms of patients recovering from ill-health in the belief that the herb would hasten the process. The oil has a scent similar to that of citronella and has been used in soaps and detergents.

Medicinal parts: The essential oil is extracted from the fresh plant, the herb.

Uses: Used orally as an antispasmodic, antiflatulent and for bowel disorders.

Other uses: As an abortifacient, menstrual regulator, for colds and respiratory ailments and in the treatment of gout. Used externally for skin diseases. The oil has been used to repel fleas in pets and the dried form has been used to repel spiders.

Probable mode of action: The volatile oil and its metabolites may be responsible for hepatotoxicity and neurotoxicity and bronchial cell destruction. The metabolites of one of the active constituents cause depletion of hepatic glutathione making the liver more vulnerable to damage by agents such as paracetamol. The oil is high in pulegone, a highly toxic volatile agent which can stimulate uterine activity.

Adverse effects: Oral intake can cause abdominal cramps and pain, fever, nausea and vomiting. There may be nervous system effects such as confusion, delirium, auditory and visual hallucinations. With severe toxicity, kidney and liver failure occurs which may progress to acidosis, respiratory failure and death. May also cause abortion. Severely acute poisonings have been observed following administration of 5 g of volatile oil. Vomiting, elevation of blood pressure, anaesthesia-like paralysis and death due to respiratory failure has been reported following larger doses.

Precautions: Considered unsafe and to be avoided during pregnancy. Cases of death have been described following misuse of the volatile oil to cause abortions. In 1978, a pregnant woman died after consuming two tablespoonfuls (approximately 30 ml) of pennyroyal oil, and another death occurred in 1994 after consumption of a tea containing pennyroyal extract. Should not be used in subjects who have or are likely to develop fits (seizures) and in those with liver and kidney disease. Contraindicated in children.

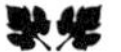

PEPPERMINT – MINT

Mentha piperita

Peppermint oil is one of the world's oldest medicinal herbal preparations with use documented in ancient Egypt, Greece and Rome.

Referred to in the New Testament as *hedyosmon* – 'sweet smelling'.

Possibly used in England since the 17th century.

In folk medicine, peppermint was used to treat nausea, vomiting, morning sickness, respiratory infections and dysmenorrhoea.

Peppermint oil is approved by Commission E for:
common cold
cough/bronchitis
inflammation of the mouth and pharynx
liver and gallbladder complaints
dyspeptic complaints
tendency to infection.

Peppermint leaves have been approved by Commission E for:
- liver and gallbladder complaints
- dyspeptic complaints (indigestion).

Medicinal parts: The medicinal parts are the oil extracted from the aerial parts of the flowering plant, the dried leaves and flowering branch tips, the fresh flowering plant and the whole plant.

Uses: Peppermint leaf is used for loss of appetite, for flatulence, gastritis and enteritis. The oil has been applied to teeth to relieve toothache, and has also been applied topically to relieve itching associated with rashes and insect bites.

Other uses: Also used in the treatment of spasms of the gastrointestinal tract, gallbladder and bile ducts. The oil has been used for catarrh of the respiratory tract and inflammation of mucosa of the mouth and pharynx. Peppermint oil has been used externally (as a massage) for muscle pains (myalgia) and neuralgia. Inhaled to relieve nasal congestion. Has been used as lozenges or suppositories to relieve muscle spasms associated with procedures that involve viewing the intestinal lumen using a telescope (e.g. colonoscopy). **In folk medicine**, the leaves are used for nausea, vomiting, morning sickness, respiratory infections, painful menstruation (dysmenorrhoea) and colds.

Probable mode of action: Mint has a refreshing odour and pungent taste. Active constituents which include menthol and flavonoids are known to relieve spasms of the smooth muscle of the gastrointestinal tract and decreases flatulence. Considered to stimulate production of bile acid. Flavonoids stimulate bile production and another constituent has been attributed with anti-inflammatory and anti-ulcer properties. Documented to be a carminative, antibacterial, insecticide and secretolytic agent. Also has a cooling effect on the skin.

Adverse effects: Can induce biliary colic in patients with existing bile stones. May worsen heartburn and cause a burning sensation in the mouth. Decreases the rate at which the immunosuppressant drug ciclosporin is broken down in the body and may cause ciclosporin toxicity. The application of the oil to the face of infants and children has caused narrowing of the tubes or airways of the lung (bronchospasm), swelling and spasm of the opening to the breathing tract (laryngeal oedema and spasm). These are potentially life-threatening complications.

Precautions: The oil is toxic to infants and can cause cessation of breathing (apnoea). Many herbalists recommend that peppermint be avoided during pregnancy. Avoid in those with gallstones, or use only under medical supervision. Drugs that are used to reduce acidity in the stomach (e.g. H_2-receptor antagonists and proton pump inhibitors such as cimetidine, ranitidine, lanzoprazole, pantoprazole) may cause the release of mint from enteric-coated capsules in the stomach due to decreased acidity, thus decreasing its therapeutic efficacy. Peppermint oil capsules should be taken at least two hours before other medications. Due to relaxation of the oesophageal sphincter, may worsen the symptoms of hiatus hernia.

PHELLODENDRON – HUANG BAI – CORK-TREE

Phellodendron amurense

The name huang bai comes from the bright yellow colour of the plant's inner bark, which is used in herbal preparations in Chinese medicine.

In Russia the tree is referred to as barkhat amurskiy.

Medicinal part: Bark.

Uses: Diarrhoea, dysentery, swollen joints in legs.

Other uses: Treatment of jaundice.

Probable mode of action: The berberine constituent has antibacterial and fungicidal properties. Another constituent may be antimutagenic. May possess vasodilatory properties due to other constituents.

Adverse effects: High doses may cause nausea and vomiting.

Precautions: Should not be taken by patients diagnosed with spleen and/or stomach disorders. Should not be used during pregnancy due to the high berberine content.

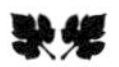

PILEWORT – LESSER CELANDINE

Ranunculus ficaria

An ancient remedy for piles, which gave it its old name, pilewort.

Medicinal parts: Whole herb, flowers collected in March and April.

Uses: Haemorrhoids by topical application or as a suppository.

Other uses: Reported to contract cells (skin and other) following inflammation (astringent).

Probable mode of action: The saponin constituents are possibly responsible for the local antihaemmorhoidal activity. Two other constituents have been shown in laboratory tests to possess antibacterial and antifungal properties.

Adverse effects: The sap of pilewort is irritant to the skin. Topical use may cause irritant skin reactions: 'It was not uncommon for beggars to produce sores about their bodies by the medium of various species of Ranunculus, for the sake of getting alms, afterwards curing these sores by applying fresh Mullein leaves to heal them'. Other reported side-effects include nausea and vomiting.

Precautions: Pilewort should not be used internally. Do not take by mouth. Safety during pregnancy has not been established. Stop taking the herb if breathing problems or tightness in the chest or throat develops. Also stop using the herb if there is pain in the chest and/or skin hives, rash or itchy swollen skin.

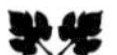

PIMPINELLA – GREATER BURNET

Pimpinella major

An essential oil from the root is used as a flavouring in candy and liqueurs.

Approved by Commission E for:
cough/bronchitis.

Medicinal parts: Flowers, root.

Uses: Leaves are diaphoretic, diuretic and relieve stomach upset. Preparations of the roots are used for colds, chills and catarrh of the upper respiratory tract.

Other uses: Unproven uses in **folk medicine** include internal use for disorders of the urinary organs, inflammation of the bladder and kidney, bladder and kidney stones and oedema. It is also used for flushing out therapy in bacterial infections of the urinary tract. Externally it is used for inflammation of the mucosa of the mouth and pharynx. It is also added to baths for treating poorly healing wounds. When chewed, the fresh root may relieve toothache.

Probable mode of action: The herb contains essential oils. Active constituents include furocoumarins and volatile oils. Exact effects of constituents are not yet known with certainty. The root is attributed with anti-inflammatory, mildly astringent and expectorant properties.

Adverse effects: No reports of adverse effects following recommended therapeutic doses. Photosensitivity may occur in light-skinned individuals.

Precautions: None known. However, pimpinella contains essential oils and saponins.

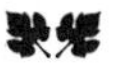

PINE – PYCNOGENOL

Pinus maritama
Pinus pinaster
Pinus strobus

Ancient Mexicans used pine resin to make ointments. The *Aztec Herbal* published in 1552 describes the use of pine needles and flowers in a liquor which was placed under the armpits of the sick in order to remove the 'evil smell'.

Several species of pine that grow in North America have been used by Native Americans to treat cuts and wounds by making a decoction of the tree bark. Teas were made from pine needles to promote removal of secretions from the lungs and upper airways.

In the US, pine bark extract is included in a number of non-prescription face creams that claim to fight ageing or restore wrinkled skin.

Pycnogenol is the patented trade name for a water extract of the French maritime pine (*Pinus pinaster*) or *Pinus maritama.*

Medicinal parts: Bark, resin, needles, seeds.

Uses: Preventing and treating a condition known as chronic venous insufficiency (when blood collects in the veins due to a defect in the valves within the veins or heart), varicose veins, swelling of the legs and ulcers or blood clots in the veins. Known to provide relief of abdominal pain caused by endometriosis (presence of the uterine lining [endometrium] outside the uterus in the abdominal cavity). Has also been used to decrease low density lipoproteins in the blood and is thus useful in the prevention of heart attacks.

Other uses: Pine bark has anti-inflammatory actions. Has been reported to slow the degenerative changes in the eye (retinopathy). Reported to be used to boost sperm quality and sperm movement and for erectile dysfunction. Has been considered for use in attention deficit hyperactivity disorder (ADHD) and in diabetes mellitus. In **China**, a prescription product containing pine bark extract has been approved for treating skin pigmentation conditions.

Probable mode of action: Active constituents prevent leakage of fluid from veins and strengthens the walls of blood vessels. Pine bark is considered to possess antioxidant activity thus limiting the free radicals, which are potentially harmful chemicals that are produced during the breakdown of foods in the body. Probably causes an increase in the production of nitric oxide in the body.

Pycnogenol is a mixture of flavonoid constituents extracted from the bark of pine trees and possesses antioxidant properties.

Adverse effects: Theoretically, the herb can affect blood sugar levels. The astringent taste may cause some stomach discomfort.

Precautions: Not recommended for use by people who have allergies. Not to be taken internally by patients suffering from asthma or bronchitis. The essential oil has to be taken under medical supervision. If on allopathic medication for control of diabetes mellitus, inform your physician of the intake of pine as control of blood sugar may be affected.

PINEAPPLE

Ananas comosus

On the second voyage to the New World in 1493, Columbus and his crew encountered a fruit which they had never seen before. One of them described it as being 'in the shape of a pine cone, twice as big, which fruit is excellent and it can be cut with a knife, like a turnip and it seems to be wholesome'. Its resemblance to a pine cone gave rise to the fruit's English name, while its Latin name *Ananas* came from the word 'nana' which was the local people's name for the plant. People in the Caribbean area at that time valued the fruit highly, placing it outside their homes to welcome visitors. Later, the Europeans adopted this habit with pineapple motif used on gate posts and in carvings.

Approved by Commission E for:
wounds and burns.

Medicinal part: Fruit.

Uses: Unproven uses include internal application for post-traumatic and postoperative swelling to stimulate healing and as an enzyme subsite for digestive symptoms after pancreatic disease. The fruit has also been used for oedema, digestive complaints and for febrile and inflammatory disorders in the **Hawaiian Islands**, **Philippines** and **South America**. Has been used for asthmatic conditions in **Zaire** and as a vermifuge in **Brazil**. Pineapple bran has been used for weight reduction regimens.

Other uses: In Indian medicine, the fruit is used for dyspeptic symptoms, constipation, amenorrhoea and painful menstruation (dysmenorrhoea) as well as for black vomiting (possibly vomiting of old blood in the stomach) and fever.

Probable mode of action: Pineapple contains an enzyme known as bromelain that is best known for its ability to break down proteins. Bromelain also has an anticlotting action that may help prevent heart attacks and strokes. Pineapple has been described as an antiphlogistic (anti-inflammatory), fibrinolytic (breaks down fibrin blood clots) and proteolytic (breaks down proteins). The proteolytic enzymes promote wound healing. In animal experiments, bromelain has also been found to have properties that influence the immune system by increasing the activity of some white blood cells (e.g. monocytes) against cancer cells and also by increasing the production of chemicals associated with the immune response such as tumour necrosis factor and interleukin 1.

Adverse effects: Gastric complaints (nausea, vomiting) and diarrhoea may occur as side-effects of internal administration. Allergic reactions following repeated administration have been observed. Has been known to induce contractions of the uterus.

Precautions: Consumption of pineapple juice in large quantities is contraindicated during pregnancy. In folk medicine, it is considered to induce abortions.

PIPSISSEWA

Chimaphila umbellata

Pipsissewa is a Cree name meaning 'It-breaks-into-small-pieces'. Was listed in the US Pharmacopeia from 1820 to 1916. Used by the Native Americans to induce sweating and to treat fevers such as typhus. Also used for kidney and bladder complaints and to treat smallpox and regulate menstruation.

Medicinal parts: Leaves.

Uses: Diuretic and urinary antiseptic, used in acute and chronic cystitis.

Other uses: Was applied externally for skin diseases. Fresh leaves were applied to rheumatic joints or muscles, as well as blisters, sores and swellings. The **European settlers** used the herb for rheumatism, urinary and kidney problems. Was used as a hypoglycaemic, tonic and an anti-inflammatory agent.

Probable mode of action: The herb contains quinine which is considered to be a urinary antiseptic. Also considered to increase blood flow to the kidney and to increase the function of the kidney tubules. Hydroquinones (including arbutin), flavonoids, triterpenes, methyl salicylate and tannins are among the active constituents. Alcoholic and aqueous extracts of the plant are said to have antimicrobial properties in laboratory tests. Laboratory experiments have also demonstrated a blood sugar lowering effect.

Adverse effects: Weak sensitizing effects (on the skin) due to some of the constituents. May cause diarrhoea, nausea and vomiting.

Precautions: Not suitable for long-term use. Reduces the absorption of minerals from the gut (the tannins may cause complexes with medications that would decrease absorption) and it is best to take Pipsissewa 2 hours before or after any other medication that needs to be taken. Effects on mothers who are breastfeeding are not known. Best avoided in those with iron deficiency and malabsorption syndromes, and in those with gastric disease (e.g. ulcers).

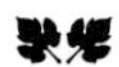

***PISTACIA LENTISCUS* – MASTIC – PISTACHIER LENTISQUE**

Pistacia lentiscus

The resin from the tree is used for chewing gum. The berries have been used for liqueurs and sweets. The tree was the beginning of the world famous Grasse perfume industry.

Medicinal part: Resin.

Uses: Leaf decoction for stomachache, chew leaf for hypertension, eat leaf for fever.

Other uses: Fruit is taken orally for stomach ailments and used externally for rheumatism. Was formerly used in dentistry as a material for fillings. The masticated resin releases substances that 'freshen' the breath and tighten the gums.

Probable mode of action: In animal experiments, a constituent was shown to protect against ulcer formation. Some of the constituents have an effect of contracting cells (skin and other) following inflammation (astringent). Contains essential oils.

Adverse effects: Occasional risk of diarrhoea in small children.

Precautions: Best avoided in small children. Essential oils are not to be taken orally.

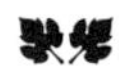

PLANTAIN

Plantago major

This medical and edible plant has a long history of use in traditional herbal medicine and is considered a panacea for diverse medical conditions particularly in Asian countries. Native Americans carried the powdered root as a protection against snake bite or to ward off snakes. These people also called it the 'Englishman's foot' or 'White Man's foot' as it was said to grow wherever their feet touched the ground and this is mentioned in Longfellow's *Hiawatha*. Further, an American Indian native name means 'life medicine'.

A related species (*Plantago lanceolata* L.) is listed by the Council of Europe as a natural source of food flavouring.

Medicinal part: Leaf, fruit.

Uses: Traditional use of the leaves and seeds has been for their antibacterial, astringent, anti-inflammatory, antiseptic and antitussive (stopping cough) properties. Has also been used as an anti-helminthic, expectorant (to facilitate removal of secretions from the chest), laxative and haemostatic, to stop bleeding quickly and to promote healing of tissues.

Other uses: There is some medical evidence for the use of plantain in complementary medicine for respiratory disorders (e.g. asthma, emphysema, bronchitis), to treat fever, high blood pressure and rheumatism and to control blood sugar. Plantain leaves have been used to cool inflamed skin. Hot plantain tea has been used to treat hay fever and asthma. The seeds have been used as a laxative. An extract has been used in the treatment of snake bite. In **folk medicine** it has been used for bladder infections where the patient passes blood cells in the urine. A decoction of the roots has been used for diverse medical disorders ranging from diarrhoea, dysentery and haemorrhoids to catarrh, sinusitis, coughs and hay fever. As stated earlier, the root has been used as an antivenom for rattle snake bites.

Some experimental work suggests that seeds of *Plantago psyillium* may be an effective substitute for patients who cannot tolerate salicylate-based anti-inflammatory drugs for the treatment of ulcerative colitis.

Probable mode of action: The young leaves are rich in vitamin B_1 and riboflavin. The plantain seeds contain up to 30% mucilage which enables the fruit to act effectively as a bulk laxative. The constituent acubin has been demonstrated in experiments to be a powerful antitoxin. The other constituents include apigenin, baicalein and the acids benzoic, citric, salicylic, oleanolic and ursolic. An aqueous extract was shown to possess anti-inflammatory activity in the rat using various models of inflammation, and a strengthening of capillary vessels has also been documented. Both the anti-inflammatory and wound healing activities of plantain have been attributed to some of the constituents which are acidic in nature. Plantain has also been documented to lower concentrations of plasma lipids, cholesterol, beta lipoproteins and triglycerides in rabbits with experimental atherosclerosis.

Adverse effects: Allergic contact dermatitis to plantain has been reported. The green parts of the plant have been found to release an irritant principle (isothiocyanate) upon enzymatic hydrolysis. The seed may also cause sensitization and dermatitis. Abdominal distension and flatulence may occur particularly following excessive consumption of fruit. Experimental work has shown that subjects with a positive skin prick test to weed pollens may also react adversely to plantain pollen extracts. Allergy to *Psyllium* seeds has been reported in people who had no previous allergy and in those with a history of occupational exposure to plantain.

Precautions: Excessive doses may cause diarrhoea and fall in blood pressure. In laboratory work, plantain has been found to exert effects on the uterus. This in combination with its laxative effects may cause adverse effects during pregnancy if used in excessive amounts. Should not be used in patients with abdominal discomfort or pain which may be due to intestinal obstruction. May inhibit the absorption of drugs such as carbamazepine and lithium, which is important as therapeutic blood levels are required in the disorders for which these drugs are used. Some herbalists recommend that plantain should not be taken by patients on digitalis treatment.

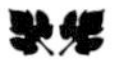

POKE ROOT

Phytolacca decandra
Phytolacca americana

Called pocon by the Native Americans, poke root was used as an emetic and externally for skin diseases. The Delaware people took it as a heart stimulant and in Virginia it was regarded as a strong purgative. The early American settlers used it to treat venereal disease. Even today Appalachian backwoodsmen chew the seeds and berries for arthritis.

Medicinal part: The dried root.

Uses: Chronic rheumatism, chronic respiratory catarrh, tonsillitis, laryngitis, adenitis, mastitis, mumps.

Other uses: Externally as an ointment for scabies, tinea, acne also as a poultice for mastitis (inflammation of the breasts) and mammary (breast) abscess, inflammatory conditions of the upper respiratory tract and lymphatic adenitis, mumps.

Probable mode of action: Constituents include saponins, alkaloids, resins, tannin, formic acid, sugars and proteins which have antirheumatic, stimulant, anticatarrhal and purgative effects and is an emetic in large doses. Also known to have an effect on parasites (parasiticide) and fungi (fungicide). By stimulating the formation and activity of protective white blood cells (leucocytes) it has an anti-inflammatory effect.

Adverse effects: All parts of the plant are poisonous. The saponins cause irritation of the mucous membranes. Symptoms include nausea and vomiting with abdominal pain and diarrhoea, hypotension (low blood pressure), tachycardia (increase in pulse rate).

Precautions: It should be used only as prescribed by a qualified practitioner, and the recommended dosages should never be exceeded. The seeds in the berries are poisonous and have caused fatalities in children. It may produce foetal abnormalities, so should not be used during pregnancy. Emergency poison treatment procedures should be instituted for small children who consume even one berry. Up to 10 berries are considered harmless for an adult.

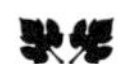

POMEGRANATE

Punica granatum

The fruit has long being a religious and artistic symbol. It is described in the most ancient of Asian literature. In the Old Testament, Solomon sang of an 'orchard of pomegranades'. Because of its role in the Greek legend of Persephone, the pomegranate came to symbolize fertility, death and eternity and was an emblem of the Eleusinian Mysteries. In Christian art it is a symbol of hope. According to authoratitive sources, the weapon grenade derived its name, attested in 1532, from the French name for the fruit which is *la grenade.* Jewish tradition teaches that the pomegranate is a symbol for righteousness because it is said to contain 613 seeds which corresponds with the 613 *mitzvot* or commandments of the Torah.

Medicinal parts: Root, bark, the fruits, the peel of the fruit and the flowers.

Uses: Intestinal infections, reduces some risk factors associated with heart attacks (lowers low density lipoproteins, reduces macrophage oxidative status and foam cell formation).

Other uses: To treat high blood pressure. Has been used to treat diarrhoea, dysentery, worm infestations and eye pain.

Probable mode of action: One pomegranate is considered to deliver 40% of an adult's daily vitamin C requirement. It is also a rich source of folic acid and of antioxidants. Pomegranates are rich in tannins which act as antioxidants and are responsible for free-radical scavenging ability. The plant also contains alkaloids and is antihelminthic (effective against tapeworms, ringworms) and amoebicidal. The tannins in the herb contract cells (skin and other) following inflammation (astringent), and it is useful in treatment for sore throats, diarrhoea and dysentery.

Adverse effects: Gastric irritation. Vomiting (including the vomiting of blood), dizziness, chills, vision disorders, collapse and death may occur due to respiratory failure. Total blindness could occur within a few hours or few days.

Precautions: Take precaution not to exceed recommended doses and watch for early signs of overdose.

POPLAR

Populus tremuloides

The name *populus* is from the Latin word for poplar and *tremuloides* means 'shaking, trembling, quivering'. It is the most widely distributed tree in North America, growing on a wide variety of soils. Most frequent use is in the manufacture of pulp products such as speciality papers, newsprint and books. Also used in the making of tongue depressors and spoons.

Poplar is listed by the Council of Europe as a natural source of food flavouring. In the US, poplar is permitted for use in foods.

Poplar leaf buds are approved by Commission E for:
haemorrhoids
wounds and burns.

Medicinal parts: Bark, leaves and leaf buds.

Uses: Muscular and arthritic 'rheumatism', specifically rheumatoid arthritis. Used mostly as a tonic and to bring down fevers when subjects have intermittent fever.

Other uses: Cystitis (bladder infections), diarrhoea, anorexia with stomach or liver disorders. The buds of *Populus tremula* (European white poplar, aspen) and *Populus nigra* (black poplar) are used reputedly to promote removal of secretions from the lung and upper airways (expectorant) and to stimulate the circulation. Also used for upper respiratory tract infections and rheumatic conditions.

Probable mode of action: One of the main constituents is very similar to salicylates, hence the use in rheumatic disorders and for muscular pains. Salicin is a prodrug that is metabolized to saligenin in the gastrointestinal tract and to salicylic acid following absorption. Poplar buds are considered to have antiphlogistic (anti-inflammatory), antibacterial (kills bacteria) and wound healing effects.

Adverse effects: Toxic effects associated with salicylates (e.g. heartburn, tinnitus) may occur following ingestion.

Precautions: Safety during pregnancy has not been established. Same precautions as for salicylates (not to be used in children under the age of 12 years). Contraindicated in patients hypersensitive to salicylates. It is necessary to consider that propolis and balsam of Peru may be components in commercially available preparations. To be avoided by subjects with ulcers in the stomach or duodenum (peptic ulcers).

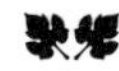

POTENTILLA – SILVERWEED

Potentilla anserina

Potentilla means 'little powerful one'. The ability of the plant to survive trampling along with the soft texture of the leaves led to the leaves being stuffed into shoes to relieve and cool the sore feet of travellers. Called 'traveller's ease' or 'traveller's joy', it was put in shoes to absorb sweat.

The herbal tea from the underground roots was

used to help delivery (childbirth) and as an antispasmodic for diarrhoea.

Approved by Commission E for:

- diarrhoea
- inflammation of the mouth and pharynx
- premenstrual syndrome.

Medicinal parts: Leaves and root.

Uses: Internal application for topical treatment of inflammation of the mouth and pharynx. As an adjuvant in the treatment of non-specific diarrhoeas and for painful menstruation (dysmennorhoea).

Other uses: In folk medicine, *Potentilla* is used externally as a wash for poorly healing wounds.

Probable mode of action: The herb is known to contract cells (skin and other) following inflammation (astringent) because of the tannin concentration. On isolated rat uterus, a paralysing effect was observed attributed to the presence of ammonium salts.

Adverse effects: Possible irritation of the stomach.

Precautions: None known. Best avoided during pregnancy due to possible effects on the uterus.

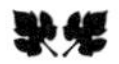

PRICKLY ASH – NORTHERN

Zanthoxylum americanum

Zanthoxylum is from the Greek meaning yellow wood.

Prickly ash is listed by the Council of Europe as a natural source of food flavouring. In the US, prickly ash is listed as a Generally Recognized as Safe (GRAS) herb.

Medicinal part: Resin extracted from the fruit and bark.

Uses: Cramps, intermittent claudication (pain in the calves of the leg when walking short distances, possibly due to poor blood supply), Raynaud's disease (a disease of blood vessels which affects peripheral circulation), peripheral circulatory insufficiency.

Other uses: Chronic rheumatic conditions, as a stimulant for gastrointestinal disorders and for relief of toothache.

Probable mode of action: The active alkaloids are considered to promote the peripheral circulation. It is also considered to stimulate the central nervous system in a rather non-specific manner. Northern prickly ash contains alkaloids and coumarins, resins, tannins and a volatile oil. The constituents differ from those in Southern prickly ash.

Adverse effects: May cause stimulation of the nervous system. Tannins present may reduce the absorption of iron from the gut.

Precautions: Excessive ingestion may interfere with anticoagulant therapy, i.e. drugs affecting the coagulation of the blood such as warfarin. Safety of use during pregnancy has not been established. Ingestion of parts of this plant has been stated to have caused death in sheep and cattle.

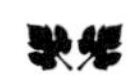

PRICKLY ASH – SOUTHERN

Zanthoxylum clava-herculis

Historically prickly ash bark was chewed to relieve toothache.

Southern prickly ash is listed by the Council of Europe as a natural source of food flavouring.

A related species in Nigeria, *Zanthoxylum zanthoxyloides* is used as a 'chewing stick' which is believed to have antimicrobial properties towards more than 20 organisms.

Medicinal parts: Berries, bark.

Uses: Cramps, intermittent claudication (pain in the calves of the leg when walking short distances, possibly due to poor blood supply), Raynaud's disease (a disease of blood vessels which affects peripheral circulation), peripheral circulatory insufficiency.

Other uses: Rheumatic conditions, to stimulate digestion and relieve flatulence (dyspepsia).

Probable mode of action: Hypotensive (lowering of blood pressure) properties have been documented for the alkaloid constituents. One of these was also shown to antagonize angiotensin (a naturally released hormone which increases blood pressure) induced hypertension. The constituents also have anti-inflammatory activity in rats and potentiate the painkilling effects of morphine. The constituents are predominantly alkaloids, amides, lignans, resins, tannins and a volatile oil. Does not contain coumarins.

Adverse effects: Reduction of the absorption of iron from the gut, sun sensitivity, bruising and bleeding.

Precautions: May interfere with digoxin and other cardiac glycoside therapy. The alkaloid constituents are considered to be potentially toxic. May interact with drugs affecting clotting of the blood such as warfarin. Safety in pregnancy has not been established. Ingestion of parts of this plant has been stated to have caused death in cattle.

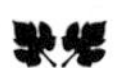

QUINCE

Cydonia oblongata

The modern name derives from the 14th century plural of *quoin*, via old French *cooin* from Latin *cotoneum malum/cydonium malum*, ultimately from Greek *kydonion malon*. Among the ancient Greeks, the quince was a ritual offering at weddings, for it had come from the Levant with Aphrodite and remained sacred to her. Plutarch reports that a Greek bride would nibble a quince to perfume her kiss before entering the bridal chamber 'in order that the first greeting may not be disagreeable or unpleasant'. Quinces are mentioned for the first time in the later 13th century.

Medicinal parts: Fruit and seeds.

Uses: As a demulcent (to prevent inflammation and irritation) in digestive disorders and diarrhoea. As a lotion it is used to soothe the eyes. The seeds are also used treat coughs and gastrointestinal catarrh. Additionally the herb is used as compresses or poultices for injuries, inflammation of joints, injuries of the nipples and gashes or deeply cut fingers.

Other uses: A decoction from the seeds was taken by mouth to treat dysentery, gonorrhoea and thrush.

Probable mode of action: The main active principles are mucilage, some tannins and vitamin C. There is little or no information on the mode of action. The constituents have been reported to possess astringent, demulcent and diuretic effects and also some effects on the heart. A decoction of the plant has been shown to kill the bacterium that causes cholera (*Vibrio cholerae*).

Adverse effects: There is a need to be aware of the potential toxicity of the cyanogenic glycosides present in the seeds.

Precautions: Avoid during pregnancy and whilst breastfeeding. The seeds are potentially toxic because of the amygdalin (laetrile) content. Should not be kept within the reach of children or pets.

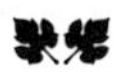

RASPBERRY

Rubus idaeus

An edible and medicinal plant.

Both the leaf and fruit are listed by the Council of Europe as natural sources of food flavouring.

Medicinal part: Leaves, roots.

Uses: Diarrhoea, in pregnancy to facilitate parturition (childbirth – a tonic made from the leaves is used to 'strengthen the uterus'), stomatitis, tonsillitis (as a gargle), conjunctivitis (as an eye lotion). Acts as an astringent on irritated skin.

Other uses: Has been used to stop vomiting (antiemetic). Externally the leaves and roots have been used as a poultice for wounds, sores, conjunctivitis, burns and varicose ulcers. In women who are not pregnant, raspberry is used to regulate menstruation.

Probable mode of action: Raspberries contains polyphenol antioxidants which are reputed to maintain the integrity of the cardiovascular system and also of the lining cells of the blood vessels (endothelial cells). Xylitol, a naturally occurring sweetener chemically referred to as five carbon sugar alcohol, has been extracted from the raspberry. The activity on the uterus has been demonstrated in both the pregnant and non-pregnant rat and on the human uterus.

Adverse effects: None documented as there have been very few studies on the use of raspberry leaf in humans.

Precautions: Excessive consumption is to be avoided because of the tannin constituents. Best avoided during pregnancy, and if to be used during labour, it should be undertaken under the supervision of a medical practitioner. Women with hormone-dependent conditions such as endometriosis, uterine fibroids or cancers of the breast, ovaries or uterus should not take raspberry leaf. Should not be taken by men with cancer of the prostate. Little is known about the effects of raspberry leaf on infants, hence it is best avoided during breastfeeding. As large amounts of raspberry leaf (like blackberry leaf) may lower blood sugar, subjects on allopathic medications for control of blood sugar should be cautious. In theory, tannins in the raspberry leaf can interfere with the absorption of drugs taken at the same time. Some herbalists recommend that raspberry leaf tea should be drunk 2 hours before or after taking other medications.

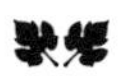

RAUWOLFIA

Rauwolfia serpentina (Indian snake root)
Rauwolfia cafra (South African quinine tree)

Rauwolfia is believed to have been used in India for about 4000 years. It has been mentioned in the work of ancient Indian physicians such as Charaka. Its roots have been valued in India and the Malaysian peninsula from ancient times as an antidote for the bites of poisonous reptiles and insects. Plant is used medicinally in Ayurveda, Unani and allopathic medicine.

Approved by Commission E for:
- hypertension
- nervousness and insomnia.

Medicinal part: Dried roots.

Uses: To reduce blood pressure, depress activity of the nervous system; a hypnotic (to treat insomnia).

Other uses: Flatulence, vomiting, eclampsia, hypertension and liver disease. Used to encourage uterine contractions during birth and has been used locally to treat wounds. **In Indian medicine**, the herb is used as an antidote for snake bites and poisonous bites of other reptiles and for the control of high blood pressure, dysuria, fever, colic and in the treatment of wounds. It is popularly known as *pagal-ka-dawa* as a medicine for insanity.

Probable mode of action: Snake root depletes the amines (catecholamines) that are secreted by the nervous system to cause narrowing of blood vessels thus increasing blood pressure.

Adverse effects: Can cause serious lowering of blood pressure. Known to cause nasal congestion, states of depression, tiredness, erectile dysfunction. The herb may cause drowsiness and caution is necessary if driving motor vehicles or using machinery.

Precautions: Avoid during pregnancy and breastfeeding or if you are planning a pregnancy. Avoid in chronic diseases of the gastrointestinal system (stomach and duodenal ulcers), oesophageal reflux, ulcerative colitis, diverticulosis. Do not use in children under two years of age. Rauwolfia is contraindicated in depressed patients.

RED CLOVER

Trifolium pratense

One of the world's first agricultural crops. In China and Russia, red clover was used to treat chest infections, speed wound healing and relieve water retention. Has been investigated as a mode of treatment for cancers since 1800s. Has been implicated as a cause of infertility in livestock. At present, red clover is included in some herbal supplements which claim to cause enlargement of the breasts.

Medicinal parts: Dried and the fresh flower heads.

Uses: Chronic skin disease, whooping cough.

Other uses: In children with skin problems, childhood eczema, psoriasis. Also used in the treatment of cancers, especially of the breast and ovary.

Used in the treatment of coughs and bronchitis, whooping cough.

The fresh, crushed flowers can be applied to bites and stings; the tincture in water may be used as an eye lotion for conjunctivitis. Has been used as a form of hormone replacement therapy in post-menopausal women due to the possible oestrogen-like activity.

Probable mode of action: Over 125 chemicals have been identified in the red clover plant. Constituents include carbohydrates, phenolic glycosides, flavonoids, saponins, salicylates, coumarins, volatile oil, fats, minerals (aluminium, copper, iron, manganese, potassium), resin, vitamins.

Effects attributed to these active constituents are sedation and to counter spasms (antispasmodic), to promote removal of secretions from the lung and upper airways (expectorant). Also used for skin disorders, as a diuretic and as an anti-inflammatory agent. Considered to possess effects similar to the female hormone, oestrogen. Contains coumarins and coumarin-like compounds. Also contains tocopherol, a form of vitamin E which has been associated with reduced incidence and occurrence of heart attacks and cancer.

Adverse effects: Reported oestrogenic side-effects in grazing animals have been attributed to the isoflavone constituents. May cause breast tenderness or enlargement and weight gain.

Precautions: Avoid use during pregnancy and when breastfeeding. Also to be avoided in subjects with female hormone-dependent or sensitive cancers. Some herbalists recommend avoidance prior to surgery due to the possibility of causing an increase in the tendency to bleed.

REHMANNIA – CHINESE FOXGLOVE – DI HUANG

Rehmannia glutinosa

One of the most popular herbal tonics in Chinese medicine and is a constituent of the 'Four Things Soup', possibly the herbal tonic most widely used by women in China. Considered to be one of the 50 fundamental herbs in Chinese Traditional Medicine.

Used in Chinese medicine in its unprocessed form (sheng di huang) or processed form (shu di huang).

Medicinal part: Root.

Uses: To replenish vitality, strengthen the liver, heart and kidney, to treat anaemia, to treat dizziness and urinary tract infections.

Other uses: Rheumatism, eczema, hypertension, respiratory disorders and other conditions as part of a traditional Chinese herbal formula. Has been used to treat fungal infections (e.g. *Candida*).

Probable mode of action: Rehmannia contains vitamins A, B, C, D, amino acids and other constituents that have an anti-inflammatory action. It helps prevent depletion of glycogen and thus prevent reductions in blood sugar (hypoglycaemia). Is considered to dispel heat from the body. Constituents were also found to help stop bleeding from ulcers and reduce inflammation of the digestive tract. Other constituents were reported to be antibacterial, immunosuppressive and had a protective effect on the liver when exposed to toxins. One of the iridoid constituents is considered to stimulate the adrenal glands to produce anti-inflammatory substances (possibly corticosteroids) and also to stimulate the production of sex hormones in postmenopausal women.

Adverse effects: Considered to be relatively safe and no adverse reactions or drug interactions are known to date. Mild effects may occur when taken for the first time. These include loose stools, abdominal pain, dizziness and palpitations. These resolve with continued use.

Precautions: Not used in isolation, only as part of a herbal formula.

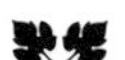

RHATANY – RAIZ PARA

Krameria triandra

Rhatany is a traditional South American plant remedy. The name rhatany is said to describe the creeping character of the plant in the language used by the Peruvian Indians while its Spanish name is derived from its dental properties (root for teeth).

The indigenous people of Baja used the plant as a red dye for wool and leather and for diarrhoea and dental problems. It is still a staple of Mexican traditional medicine for haemorrhoids, sore throat, sore gums and sore nipples.

Approved by Commission E for:

- inflammation of the mouth and pharynx.

Medicinal parts: Air-dried root, bark, flowers, stem.

Uses: As a tonic. Has been found to be useful when taken by mouth for chronic diarrhoea, dysentery, menorrhagia (heavy bleeding during periods), incontinence of urine, haematuria and passive blood loss from the bowel. **In folk medicine**, the herb is used internally as an antidiarrhoeal agent for enteritis and for inflammation of the female genital organs and urinary tract.

Other uses: Used as an infusion locally for anal fissures, prolapsed piles and for whitish discharges from the vagina (leucorrhoea). Used as a gargle for sore throat. Has an effect of contracting cells (skin and other) following inflammation (astringent). Used as solution for mucous membranes of the eyes, nose and gums. The powder is also used in dental practice. When applied externally to wounds, it helps to decrease or stop bleeding. **In folk medicine**, the herb is used externally to strengthen gums and clean teeth (used particularly for infections of the gums and mouth which cause pyorrhoea and a foul smell from the mouth).

Probable mode of action: The essential constituent is a tannic acid which is similar to the amine tyrosine. In laboratory tests, the constituents have been found to be effective against bacteria and fungi. Constituents contract cells (skin and other) following inflammation (astringent) which is considered by many to be the main therapeutic effect.

Adverse effects: The high tannin content may irritate mucous membranes. Likely to cause allergies such as breathing problems or tightness of chest or throat, chest pain and skin rashes.

Precautions: Do not use for periods longer than two weeks without medical supervision. Excessive doses may cause damage to the liver due to excessive absorption of tannic acids. Chronic application on the skin may cause damage.

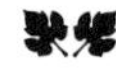

ROSEMARY

Rosmarinus officinalis

Has been used for centuries to promote menstrual flow and as an abortifacient. Widely used in cosmetics and for cooking.

Rosemary is listed by the Council of Europe as a source of natural food flavouring. In the US, rosemary is listed as Generally Recognized As Safe (GRAS).

Approved by Commission E for:

- blood pressure problems
- dyspeptic complaints
- loss of appetite
- rheumatism.

Medicinal parts: Leaves, twigs.

Uses: Used internally for stomach ailments (dyspeptic complaints such as flatulence or stomach spasm) and externally for hypotensive circulatory disorders (disorders of the circulation associated with low blood pressure) and rheumatic conditions.

Other uses: In folk medicine, the uses include treatment of digestive symptoms, headaches, migraine, menstrual disorders (dysmenorrhoea, amenorrhoea and oligomenorrhoea), states of exhaustion, dizziness and poor memory. It is used externally as a poultice for poorly healing wounds, for eczema, as an analgesic for injuries of the mouth and throat, topically for myalgia (muscle pains), intercostal neuralgia and sciatica. Also used to improve mental clarity and concentration. The hot tea has been used to fight infections. A rosemary oil massage is considered to relieve muscular and nerve pain.

Probable mode of action: The constituent rosemarinic acid has been shown to suppress the processes that are involved in the production of harmful substances by toxins which cause lowering of blood pressure and reductions in some of the blood constituents such as platelets. The mode of action of rosemary is different from that of non-steroidal anti-inflammatory drugs as rosemary does not interfere with cyclo-oxygenase activity or prostacyclin synthetase (two enzymes that are important in inflammation and the production of pain). Other constituents are attributed with antimicrobial and antiviral activity. Animal tests have demonstrated a reduction in the spasm of the gallbladder and bile ducts and of the upper intestine. Animal tests have also shown anticonvulsive activity, liver protective activity and tumour-inhibiting effects. As regards the latter, some experiments have suggested that rosemary would decrease the activation or production of chemicals that could cause cancer and also promote the destruction of such chemicals within the body. One of the constituents, carnosic acid, is reported to have antioxidant effects.

Adverse effects: Bath preparations, cosmetics and toiletries containing rosemary oil may cause redness (erythema) of the skin and dermatitis. Photosensitivity has been associated with rosemary oil. Large quantities of the volatile oil in rosemary may cause gastrointestinal irritation.

Precautions: The oil should be used cautiously by individuals with allergies. Rosemary oil contains 20–50% camphor and oral intake of camphor could lead to epileptiform convulsions.

Reportedly, rosemary is an abortifacient and should not be used during pregnancy. Use of very large quantities of rosemary leaves for the purpose of abortion has caused deep coma, spasm and vomiting along with gastroenteritis, uterine bleeding, kidney irritation and death in humans.

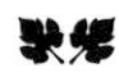

RUE

Ruta graveolens

A popular spice in ancient Rome. Mentioned as peganon in the New Testament. Widely used in Ethiopia as a flavouring agent for coffee and in spice mixtures.

Medicinal parts: Leaves, root, oil extracted from the herb.

Uses: Used as an emmenagogue (to regulate menstruation), antispasmodic and abortifacient.

Other uses: In folk medicine, rue is used for menstrual complaints, as a contraceptive and as an abortive agent. The herb is also used for inflammation of the skin, mouth and pharynx, earache, toothache, for feverish infectious disease, for cramps, as an obstetric remedy, for hepatitis and for stomach ailments (dyspepsia), diarrhoea and intestinal worm infestations. There are also reports of its use to promote production of breast milk. In **Chinese medicine,** it has been used for snake and insect bites.

Probable mode of action: Active ingredients include alkaloids and coumarins. The alkaloids in the plant prevent loss of fluid following inflammation (antiexudative). A constituent inhibits fertility and the coumarin derivatives and alkaloids prevent spasms. In addition, the constituents have been shown to possess antimicrobial activity and the potential to cause photosensitization. Constituents have been found in laboratory experiments to selectively block channels through which ions move in and out in nerve fibres (ion channels which allow passage of sodium and potassium ions).

Adverse effects: Photosensitization due to its constituents.

Photodermatitis has been observed following skin contact with the fresh leaves. Misuse of the herb for abortions have caused vomiting, epigastric pain, liver damage, kidney damage, depression, sleep disturbances, vertigo, delirium, fainting, tremor and spasm. On occasions fatalities have occurred. May cause a fall in blood pressure.

Precautions: All parts of the plant are potentially poisonous. Not to be used during pregnancy. Cautious use in patients who are receiving allopathic medications for control of blood pressure is recommended.

SAFFLOWER

Carthamus tinctorius

Indian name: Koosumbha
Chinese name: Hoang-tchi

One of oldest crops grown by humans. Safflower contains two colouring matters, yellow and red, the latter being more valued. It is chiefly used for dyeing silk. Safflower oil is flavourless and colourless. There are two types of safflower that produce different kinds of oil, one high in monounsaturated fatty acid (oleic) and the other high in polyunsaturated fatty acid (linoleic acid). Though suggested to lower blood cholesterol levels, there is no supporting medical research at present.

Medicinal parts: Seed, flowers, oil extracts.

Uses: Seed for lowering of blood cholesterol, flower extracts for menstrual problems, heart disease and pain and swelling associated with trauma and as a laxative.

Other uses: Male and female sterility, respiratory diseases. In **folk medicine,** flowers are used in children's and infants' complaints such as measles, fevers and eruptive skin disorders. **In Chinese medicine**, safflower flowers are used in the treatment of amenorrhoea and stomach tumours as well as for external and internal wounds. **In Indian medicine**, safflower is used for scabies, arthritis and chest pain. Unproven use is the oil for the prophylaxis of arteriosclerosis.

Probable mode of action: Flowers are reputed to have a laxative effect and to induce perspiration (diaphoretic). Active constituents include flavonoids, linoleic acid and carotinoids. Several chemicals with antioxidant properties have been isolated from the plant. The linoleic acid constituent is possibly converted to prostaglandins, substances involved with immunity.

Adverse effects: No health hazards or side-effects are known following the proper administration of recommended doses. May increase the immunosuppressant activity of some drugs such as ciclosporin, which is not an adverse effect. However, this effect on immunity can interfere with the protective responses expected following vaccinations.

Precautions: Not to be used during pregnancy. Has to be used with great caution in those patients with suppressed or decreased immunity (e.g.

herbs

patients with burns or septic wounds and recipients of transplants).

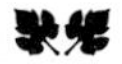

SAGE

Salvia officinalis

Was known as the herb of immortality. Revered for thousands of years, sage has been used as an effective antimicrobial agent to treat colds, flu, catarrh, sore throats and chest infections.

Approved by Commission E for:
- loss of appetite
- inflammation of the mouth
- excessive perspiration.

Medicinal parts: Fresh leaves and the fresh flowering aerial parts, the dried leaves and the oil extracted from the flowers and stems.

Uses: Used to improve appetite and as an antiseptic, hormonal stimulant, carminative and as an abortifacient.

Other uses: Sage is used externally for inflammation of the mucous membranes of the nose and throat and internally for stomach ailments (dyspeptic symptoms) and to induce perspiration (diaphoretic). **In folk medicine**, sage is used internally for gastric disorders such as loss of appetite, bloating, flatulence, diarrhoea, enteritis and also for excessive perspiration. Sage tea has been used as a diuretic and for the treatment of gout and arthritis. Externally as a rinse and gargle for light injuries and skin inflammations, bleeding gums, stomatitis, laryngitis, pharyngitis and for firming of gums.

Probable mode of action: The constituents of sage (including alpha and beta thujone) have been attributed with effects against bacteria, viruses and fungi (antibacterial, fungistatic, virostatic) and to contract cells (skin and other) following inflammation (astringent). Also said to promote secretions (secretolytic) and have perspiration inhibiting effects. Considered to act on the central nervous system and also act as a spasmolytic. In mice experiments, sage was shown to have an inhibitory effect on the nervous system.

Adverse effects: Long-term use may cause restlessness, vomiting, vertigo, tremors and rarely seizures. A sense of heat, tachycardia (increased heart rate), feelings of vertigo and epileptiform convulsions may occur following prolonged use of alcoholic extracts of the herb or volatile oil or following the intake of leaves in excess of 15 g. May also cause local irritation.

Precautions: Contraindicated during pregnancy. To be used cautiously in patients who are likely to have low blood sugar due to allopathic medications. To be avoided in those who have epilepsy or other disorders that may predispose to convulsions.

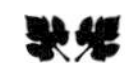

SANDALWOOD

Santalum album

Indian names: Chandan, Srigandha

Sandalwood is believed to be indigenous to India and occupies a very important place in Hindu rituals. The Parsis use it for the fire of their temples. The wood was highly prized in ancient India and China owing to the sweet odour. This tree is mentioned in the earliest of Sanskrit and Chinese literature. Of importance to Buddhists and is used during meditation and at religious ceremonies. Reported to have been used to embalm the bodies of royalty in Sri Lanka since the 9th century. Very popular as an incense in China and Japan during worship and at ceremonies.

Used traditionally in Ayurveda for skin disorders (acne and bacterial skin infections). In Traditional Chinese Medicine, sandalwood is considered to be an excellent hypnotic.

Approved by Commission E for:
infections of the urinary tract.

Medicinal parts: Oil extracted from the trunk wood, the heartwood freed from the sap wood and the bark and the dried wood.

Uses: One of the main uses has been for acne and other disorders of the skin. Used for inflammatory conditions of the urinary tract. Generally used in combination with herbs having diuretic and disinfectant effects. **In Chinese medicine**, sandalwood is used primarily for epigastric pain, chest pain and vomiting. **In Indian medicine**, uses include heat stroke, sunstroke and resulting fever. Used as an infusion mixed with honey in the state of **Kerala** and with water cooked in rice in **Nepal**.

Other uses: Also used in the treatment of gonorrhoea and as an antiaphrodisiac in Ayurveda.

Probable mode of action: The active constituents include alpha and beta santalol which have been found to have antibacterial properties as well as sedative effects. Essential oil from sandalwood has a disinfectant effect on the urinary tract. Effects of other constituents are not known.

Adverse effects: Intake can occasionally lead to skin itching, queasiness, gastrointestinal complaints and haematuria.

Precautions: Avoid in patients with kidney disease. The smoke from sandalwood should not be inhaled. There is little or no information on safety during pregnancy.

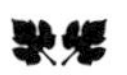

SARSAPARILLA

Smilax aristolochiaefolii
Smilax regelii
Smilax ornate
Smilax febrifuga

From around the 16th century sarsaparilla was considered as an effective treatment for syphilis. This use has not been scientifically substantiated. Reported to have been a favourite drink of the cowboys in North America. Has been publicized as a performance enhancing agent which is essentially unsubstantiated.

Sarsaparilla is listed by the Council of Europe as a natural source of food flavouring. In the US, sarsaparilla is permitted for food use.

Approved by Commission E in 1992 for:

- psoriasis
- rheumatic complaints
- renal disease as a diuretic.

Medicinal parts: Dried roots, the entire underground part and tuberous swellings produced by the runners.

Uses: Preparations of the root are used for skin diseases such as psoriasis and other skin disorders, kidney disease as a diuretic and to induce perspiration (diaphoretic).

Other uses: Chronic rheumatism, rheumatoid arthritis, adjunct in the treatment of leprosy.

Probable mode of action: Anti-inflammatory and liver-protective effects have been shown in animal experiments (rats). The steroid saponins are responsible for the irritating effect on the skin and the strong diuretic diaphoretic effects with high doses. Other active constituents are considered to produce emulsifying effects.

Adverse effects: The saponin constituents if taken in large doses can cause gastrointestinal irritation which may result in diarrhoea and vomiting. Saponins also produce haemolytic effects (destruction of red blood cells) but this occurs only when injected and not when taken orally. Inhalation of the dust from the root has caused asthma. Also reported to have caused a lowering of blood pressure (hypotension).

Precautions: Avoid excessive intake. As effects on pregnancy and breastfeeding are not known with certainty, sarsaparilla should be avoided. It is best to take other drugs orally 2 hours before or after oral intake of sarsaparilla.

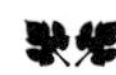

SAVORY

Satureja hortensis

Considered to increase sexual drive by the ancient Romans.

FDA classifies savory as Generally Recognized as Safe (GRAS).

Medicinal parts: Fresh leaves, dried leaves and stems.

Uses: As an appetite stimulant, promote removal of secretions from the lung and upper airways (expectorant) and for treating nausea, diarrhoea and gastrointestinal disturbances (abdominal cramps, flatulence).

Other uses: Traditionally used as a tea for sore throats. Also contracts cells (skin and other) following inflammation (astringent) and as an aphrodisiac.

Probable mode of action: The astringent effect has been attributed to the tannin constituents. Some other constituents have been effective against bacteria and fungi. Also contains a volatile oil.

Adverse effects: Topical use may cause irritation.

Precautions: Avoid during pregnancy as safety during pregnancy has not been established.

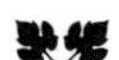

SAW PALMETTO – CABBAGE PALM

Serenoa repens

Staple food of the Native Americans in the south eastern US. The berries were used as a source of food and also for medicinal purposes, e.g. impotence, inflammation, infertility and as an expectorant.

Approved by Commission E for:

- prostatic complaints
- irritable bladder.

Medicinal parts: Berries dried and ground into a powder. Partially dried ripe fruit, ripe fresh fruit.

Uses: Benign prostatic hyperplasia (BPH) and prostatitis. The medication is considered to relieve only the difficulties associated with an enlarged prostate without reducing the enlargement.

Other uses: In folk medicine, saw palmetto is used for inflammation of the urinary tract, bladder, testicles and mammary glands. Has also been used for nocturnal enuresis (increase in the passing of urine at night), persistent cough, eczema and for improvement of libido. In Germany, over 90% of patients presenting with benign hyperplasia of the prostate gland are first treated with this herb which is required to contain 85–95% fatty acids and sterols.

Probable mode of action: A constituent of the herb has been shown to inhibit binding of the male hormone to the receptors in the prostate, thus preventing the accumulation of a steroid which may lead to prostatic hyperplasia (increase in size of the prostate gland). Saw palmetto extracts inhibit an enzyme and the conversion of testosterone (male hormone) to dihydroxytestosterone, an important factor for stimulation of growth in the prostate gland. Saw palmetto extracts also block the uptake of testosterone and dihydroxytestosterone by the prostate without affecting serum testosterone levels. In addition, anti-inflammatory activity is thought to be important in decreasing the swelling of BPH and prostatitis. The lipophilic extract of the powder from the dried ground berries is thought to contain the medicinal properties.

Adverse effects: Rare effects include mild headaches and gastrointestinal (stomach upset and diarrhoea) symptoms. It has been suggested that by interfering with the action of testosterone, saw palmetto may affect sexual drive in males (decreased libido). May cause back pain and there are reports of increased blood pressure (hypertension).

Precautions: Avoid use with other hormonal drugs. Should be taken only following appropriate consultation by patients with cancers that are hormone-dependent because of its antioestrogenic, oestrogenic and antiandrogenic effects. Not to be used during pregnancy and lactation. Best taken with food to minimize gastrointestinal side-effects.

SCOPOLIA

Scopolia carniolica

Was used instead of belladonna by physicians in Padua, Italy in the early 19th century. Was included in the US Pharmacopeia in 1900.

Approved by Commission E for:
liver and gallbladder complaints.

Medicinal part: Dried rhizome.

Uses: For spasms and colic like pain of the gastrointestinal tract, bile ducts and urinary tract for adults and children over six years of age.

Other uses: Not known.

Probable mode of action: The herbal constituents oppose the action of the chemical transmitter acetylcholine by competing for its action and hence relax smooth muscle and eliminate spasms of the gastrointestinal tract and bile ducts. Broadly the effects are considered as parasympatholytic/anticholinergic similar to that of belladonna.

Adverse effects: Visual disturbances, heat build up due to lack of sweating.

Micturition disorders may occur with overdose. These effects are due to its effects on the parasympathetic nervous system.

Precautions: The drug is contraindicated in closed angle glaucoma (increased pressure in the fluid within the eye), prostatic adenoma (a benign growth of the prostate gland) with residual urine, tachycardia (increased heart rate), and obstruction of the gastrointestinal tract. Should be used only under the supervision of a physician. The drug is contraindicated in any state where increased anticholinergic activity is harmful.

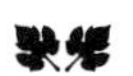

SCULL CAP – AMERICAN SKULLCAP

Scutellaria lateriflora

American skullcap is different from Baikal or Chinese skullcap (*Scutellaria baicalensis*).

In the US, skullcap is listed by the FDA as a herb of Undefined Safety.

Medicinal parts: The leaves and root.

Uses: Has been used mainly as a mild sedative and to treat nervousness and insomnia. Has also been used to treat menstrual disorders such as cramps associated with menstruation.

Other uses: In Chinese medicine, the roots of *Scutellaria baicalensis georgi* have been used traditionally as a remedy for inflammation, suppurative dermatitis, allergic disease, hyperlipidaemia and atherosclerosis. Has been used traditionally to expel the placenta (afterbirth) after childbirth and to promote menstruation. Has also been used as a bitter tonic and febrifuge.

Probable mode of action: *Scutellaria* species contain flavonoids and other constituents, the exact mode of action of these been not known with certainty. Primarily, this is so as American skullcap is rarely used today. The flavonoid constituents in *Scutellania baicalensis* have been shown to possess properties that inhibit the release of histamine from mast cells, comparable to the allopathic medication sodium cromoglicate. Flavonoids have also been shown to lower cholesterol levels in rats. Found to be effective in stroke-like conditions in man after clinical studies. The herb is considered to possess sedative, antispasmodic, anti-inflammatory and lipid peroxidation inhibitor effects.

Adverse effects: Overdose of scull cap tincture caused giddiness, stupor, confusion and seizures. Liver toxicity has also been reported. Some cases of adulteration of scull cap with Teucrium have been considered responsible for liver poisoning that has been attributed to scull cap.

Precautions: Should not be taken during pregnancy. May interfere with the immune response. Be aware.

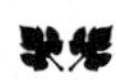

SEA BUCKTHORN

Hippophae rhamnoides

Russian and Chinese scientists consider sea buckthorn oil as the best single source known to man of vitamins E and C, beta carotene and unsaturated fatty acids (omega-3, omega-6 and omega-9 essential fatty acids which are rarely found in fruits). Russian cosmonauts have used the oil to protect themselves from radiation burns in space.

The plant was fed to horses in ancient Greece to improve their health and add gloss to their coats. Hence the Latin name *Hippophae rhamnoides* which means shiny horse.

Berries have been in use for more than 1000 years in Tibetan and Indian medicine. Known as the wonder plant in China, India and Pakistan. In Mongolia and the Middle East, leaves or leaf extracts are used to treat colitis.

Medicinal part: Ripe yellow-red berries.

Uses: Decrease cardiovascular risk, recovery of blood formation (haemopoiesis) after chemotherapy (drugs used in the treatment of cancer).

Other uses: Prevention and treatment of liver disease, colitis, chronic skin diseases – eczema, psoriasis (**in Russia**), keratitis and conjunctivitis (eye diseases). Unproven uses include infection prophylaxis, particularly during the time just before spring and during convalescence. Used externally as a treatment for radiation damage and for sunburn and as a fatty oil for the treatment of wounds. Also used in the treatment of burns and eczema.

Probable mode of action: The berries are documented to contain 120 mg of vitamin C per 100 g weight. The oil is rich in vitamins A, C and E. The phenolic constituents from the berries inhibit the growth of Gram-negative bacteria and another component can inhibit the growth of lactic acid bacteria in the gut. Active constituents include ascorbic acid (vitamin C), flavonoids, carotenoids and fatty oils. Has been used as a vitamin C supplement, the vitamin encouraging healing of wounds, growth of epithelium (covering of the skin after damage – epithelialization), strengthening of sight and inhibiting of sclerosis and the ageing process. Also considered to lower cholesterol and blood sugar. The oil is considered to prevent ulcer formation and to prevent tumour formation. Flavones are considered to improve contractility and pumping of the heart muscle. Some constituents have been studied for the prevention of cancers and also for the treatment of cancers.

Adverse effects: None well documented.

Precautions: Avoid during pregnancy and lactation. Mutagenicity and teratogenicity studies are not available.

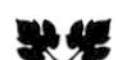

SENEGA – SENECA SNAKEROOT

Polygala senega

The North American Seneca tribe used the herb to treat rattlesnake bites and coughs and colds. Other tribes used the herb for heart complaints and to treat insect bites. Dioscorides used the term polygala as it was considered to promote lactation.

Senega is listed by the Council of Europe as a natural source of food flavouring.

Approved by Commission E for:
cough/bronchitis.

Medicinal part: Dried root.

Uses: Bronchitis, especially chronic bronchitis, asthma and as a gargle for pharyngitis.

Other uses: As a diaphoretic, emetic and to increase salivary secretions (sialogogue). Some uses in **France** have been for the treatment of eczema, graft rejection and psoriasis.

Probable mode of action: The root promotes secretions (secretolytic) and acts to facilitate removal of secretions from the lung and upper airways (expectorant). A clinical study revealed that a fluid extract of senega root reduced the viscosity of sputum in patients with bronchiectasis. This reduction of viscosity of the sputum will promote the removal of secretions in bronchiectasis where the accumulation of secretions is a major disadvantage. One of the constituents was found to increase the blood concentration of the hormones secreted by the adrenal gland (adrenocortocotrophic hormones). Extracts of the herb have been shown to decrease swelling due to congestion of blood (congestive oedema).

Adverse effects: Saponins are generally regarded as irritant to the gastrointestinal tract. Large doses have caused vomiting and diarrhoea. Overdose leads to nausea, diarrhoea, gastric complaints and queasiness. Reported to have caused anxiety, mental dullness and vertigo. May cause disturbances in vision (eyesight).

Precautions: May exacerbate existing gastrointestinal inflammation. Should be avoided by patients with diabetes mellitus on therapy as senega can lower blood sugar. Avoid use during pregnancy and lactation. To be avoided in patients who are hypersensitive to aspirin or salicylates.

SHEPHERD'S PURSE

Capsella bursa-pastoris

Named following the resemblance of the flat seed pouches of the plant to an old-fashioned leather purse. The Irish name clappedepouch is an allusion to the begging lepers who stood at crossroads with bell and clapper receiving their alms in a cup at the end of a long pole.

Found in Greenland where it was introduced by Norsemen 1000 years ago.

Approved by Commission E for:

- nose bleeds
- premenstrual syndrome
- wounds and burns.

Medicinal parts: Leaves and stems.

Uses: Internally for increased bleeding during periods (menorrhagia), vomiting of blood (haematemesis) and passing of blood in the urine (haematuria). Used externally for nose bleeds and superficially bleeding skin injuries.

Other uses: Diarrhoea, cystitis (as a urinary antiseptic). Used in **America** for headaches. In **Spain**, a decoction of the fresh plant is used for bladder inflammation.

Probable mode of action: Constituents have been shown to produce anti-inflammatory effects and to reduce the passage of fluid from small blood vessels caused by agents released during inflammatory reactions (reduce capillary permeability induced by histamine and serotonin). A diuretic effect has been demonstrated in mice following oral and intraperitoneal administration. Laboratory studies have revealed that extracts cause contraction of the smooth muscle of the intestine and of the uterine muscle. Two unidentified alkaloid components of shepherd's purse have been documented to have activity on the uterus. The constituents also yield an irritant (isothiocyantate) which can cause blisters and has been implicated in hypothyroidism.

Constituents that have been identified include saponins, flavonoids, mustard oil, resin, tyramine, acetylcholine, potassium and an essential oil.

Adverse effects: Signs of toxicity are sedation, enlargement of the pupils and difficulty in breathing. Death may occur due to respiratory paralysis. In animals, paralysis of the hind limbs has been observed.

Precautions: To be avoided in patients taking treatment for high blood pressure as the herb can cause either hypertension or hypotension. Should also be avoided by patients with disorders of the thyroid gland and preferably by those with heart disease. May have additive sedative effects with other depressants of the nervous system such as alcohol. Reputed to act as an abortifacient and to be avoided during pregnancy. Some herbalists recommend that preparations of shepherd's purse should not be kept for over one year and the preparation should be avoided by patients with kidney stones. Shepherd's purse has been implicated in some domestic livestock poisonings.

SKUNK CABBAGE

Symplocarpus foetidus

The name is due to the unpleasant odour from the plant particularly when it is bruised.

Medicinal parts: Seeds, the rhizome and the roots.

Uses: Bronchitis, whooping cough, asthma, especially bronchial asthma ('chest tightness').

Other uses: Has been claimed to be useful for nervous disorders and as a diuretic.

Probable mode of action: Constituents include starches, gum sugar, fixed and volatile oils, tannins and several alkaloids, phenolic compounds and glycosides. Considered to act as an antispasmodic, to induce perspiration (diaphoretic) and promote removal of secretions from the lung and upper airways (expectorant) and as a sedative. Some workers have isolated oxalates from the plant.

Adverse effects: Root is bitter and acrid with a disagreeable odour. May cause a burning sensation in the mouth and be an irritant to the lining (mucosa) of the mouth. Nausea and vomiting may follow oral intake. Severe itching and inflammation may occur following contact with the root. There is a theoretical possibility that oxalate crystals may be deposited in the kidney and the tubules.

Precautions: Fresh plant can cause blisters. Always use with caution. Known to affect the menstrual cycle and should be avoided during pregnancy and breastfeeding. Best avoided by patients with kidney stones.

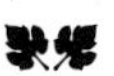

SLIPPERY ELM

Ulmus fulva

The Native North Americans and the settlers valued the inner bark of the tree as a poultice for skin disorders and as a drink to soothe fevers. Has been traditionally passed down generations as a treatment for gastrointestinal disturbances.

It has been recommended by the Food Additives and Contaminants Committee that the use of slippery elm as a flavouring agent in food should be prohibited. However, slippery elm is listed by the Council of Europe as a natural source of food flavouring.

Medicinal part: Dried inner rind separated from the outer bark.

Uses: Internally for inflammation or ulceration of the stomach and duodenum (gastric and duodenal ulcers), colitis, diarrhoea.

Other uses: Locally for abscesses, boils and ulcers, burns, swollen glands, gout and rheumatism.

Probable mode of action: Mucilage is the principal constituent of slippery elm. The mucilage constituents have demulcent (relieve inflammation and irritation) and emollient (soften and smoothen the skin) properties. Tannin constituents contract cells (skin and other) following inflammation (astringent properties). Slippery elm is considered to be a demulcent, emollient and soothing to the stomach and intestines. Some constituents have been attributed with antioxidant properties.

Adverse effects: None documented.

Precautions: The constituents of the outer bark have been known to cause abortions. The preparation is best avoided during pregnancy.

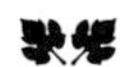

SLOE – BLACKTHORN

Prunus spinosa

Prunus is the Latin name for plum or cherry. It was believed that Christ's crown of thorns was made from blackthorn and that to bring a blackthorn blossom into the house meant certain death.

The wood from the plant is used for making walking sticks and the traditional shillelaghs of Ireland.

Used as flavouring for wine, gin and vodka.

Sloe fruit is approved by Commission E for:

- inflammation of the mouth and pharynx.

Medicinal parts: Flowers, fruit.

Uses: Fruit is used externally (as a gargle) for inflammation of the mouth and pharynx. Preparations of the sloe flower are used for common colds, diseases and ailments of the respiratory tract, as a laxative, for diarrhoea, for prophylaxis and treatment of spasms of the stomach and complaints of flatulence in the stomach and for most disorders of the stomach where the function of the stomach is probably not optimal. Also used for diseases of the intestine.

Other uses: In **folk medicine**, the fruit juice is used as a gargle for mouth, throat and gum inflammation. Syrup and wine are employed as a purgative or diuretic and as a jam for a weak stomach. Considered useful for nosebleeds and a paste has been used to whiten the teeth.

Probable mode of action: Uncertain. The fruit possibly contracts cells (skin and other) following inflammation (astringent). The constituents include tannins. Also present are cyanogenic glycosides. The prunasin produces prussic acid on hydrolysis. The flowers contain flavonoids.

Adverse effects: Acute cyanide poisoning due to accidental or deliberate ingestion of these plants is rare. Acute cyanide toxicity usually results from ingestion of significant amounts of masticated pits of fruits and chronic consumption of non-traditional preparations.

Precautions: Avoid excessive intake and use recommended doses. Safety during pregnancy and breastfeeding is not known.

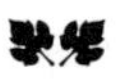

SOAPWORT

Saponaria officinalis

The Latin name of the plant is due to constituent saponins in the root.

A gentle non-irritant soap that can be used on delicate fabrics which may be damaged by synthetic soaps can be made by boiling the root in water. Has been used in complementary medicine since the time of Dioscorides as a stimulant for bile formation and flow, laxative, expectorant, diaphoretic and for scrofulous lesions. In **India**, the rhizome is used to stimulate the formation of breast milk (as a galactogogue). Commonly an ingredient of herbal shampoos.

Approved by Commission E for:

- cough/bronchitis.

Medicinal parts: Rhizome and roots; the aerial parts to a lesser extent. The rhizome is collected and dried in September and October, the aerial parts during the flowering period.

Uses: The herb is used to facilitate removal of secretions from the lung and upper airways (expectorant) in patients with cough and other diseases of the respiratory tract. The root is used for inflammation of the mucous membranes of the upper respiratory tract.

Other uses: In folk medicine, the herb is used internally for constipation, gastrointestinal disorders, liver and kidney disorders, rheumatic gout, neurasthenia. External uses in folk medicine include rashes, eczema and as a gargle for tonsillitis. In **folk medicine**, the root has also been used for diseases of the liver, gallbladder and kidney, constipation, gout and as an emmenagogue. Other external uses include against fungal infections of the tongue and rheumatic complaints.

Probable mode of action: Constituents include saponins, resin, mucilage and a small amount of volatile oil which are considered to promote removal of secretions from the lung and upper airways, act as a laxative and as a cholagogue (increase secretion of bile), detergent and as a purgative. A constituent has aroused interest as a possible therapeutic agent in cancer.

Adverse effects: Localized skin and mucous membrane irritation may occur with large doses. Ingestion is very dangerous and severe adverse effects such as destruction of red blood cells and depression of the brain centre controlling blood pressure may occur.

Precautions: Soapwort is purgative and mildly poisonous in large doses, and should only be used as prescribed by a qualified practitioner. Should not be used for periods longer than two weeks. Should not be taken orally. Avoid during pregnancy and breastfeeding. Long-term use may cause gastric irritation.

SOLOMON'S SEAL – HE SHOU WE

Polygonatum multiflorum

He shou we is considered to be an important Chinese herbal tonic used for diverse medicinal effects. It is considered to be anti-ageing, prevent loss of hair and also increase fertility (sperm counts, ovulation), and in general to restore vitality and virility.

Medicinal parts: Dried rhizome and roots.

Uses: The herb was used in the past for treatment of respiratory disorders and externally for the treatment of bruises, furuncles, ulcers or boils on the fingers, haemorrhoids, redness of the skin, oedema and haematomas.

Other uses: Has been used as a laxative and to lower blood cholesterol. Topically used for skin conditions such as acne and athlete's foot.

Probable mode of action: Constituents include anthraquinones (emodin). Active ingredients are considered to be responsible for the anti-inflammatory effects. Believed to act as a tonic and to relieve an upset stomach. The roots and stems are considered to possess antibacterial activity and to lower blood cholesterol. The exact mode of action of the constituents on reproduction, ageing and other biological systems is not known with any certainty. Also considered to contain oxalic acid which is stated to be inactivated by cooking.

Adverse effects: May cause gastrointestinal irritation with prolonged use. Overdose leads to nausea, diarrhoea, gastric complaints and queasiness. Seven reports of suspected adverse reactions associated with use of *Polygonum multiforum* have been reported to the MHRA in the UK (2006), through the yellow card system. These have all been disorders of liver function ranging from altered liver function tests to jaundice and hepatitis. However, it was suggested that recovery took place on cessation of intake of the herb.

Precautions: As it has laxative properties, it can increase the laxative effects of co-administered herbs such as aloe, rhamnus, senna and yellow dock. This herb needs careful scientific evaluation as regards efficacy and toxicity.

SORREL

Rumex acetosa

The plant is also called 'Cuckoo's meat' from an old belief that the bird cleared its voice by using this herb. In Scotland it is known as 'gowk's meat'. In the time of Henry VIII, this plant was held in great repute in England for table use.

Medicinal parts: Leaves, both dried and fresh, the whole herb.

Uses: As a diuretic and a cooling drink in febrile disorders (fevers). Treatment of scurvy.

Other uses: Both the root and stem were formerly esteemed for their ability to contract cells (skin and other) following inflammation (astringent) and were used to stop bleeding (haemorrhage). Syrup made of the juice of fumitory sorrel had a reputation for curing the itch and sorrel juice with a little vinegar was considered a cure for ringworm and was recommended as a gargle for sore throat. A decoction of the flowers made with wine was said to cure jaundice and ulcerated bowel. It was also used for acute and chronic inflammation of the nasal passages and respiratory tract and as an adjuvant to antibacterial therapy. **Folk medicine** uses include stomach ailments, liver and biliary ailments and purification of the blood.

Probable mode of action: The sour taste of sorrel is due to the oxalate content. Tartaric acid and tannic acids are also constituents.

Adverse effects: Oxalate poisoning may occur following intake of very large quantities of the leaves in salads.

Precautions: None known. Possibly to be avoided in patients with kidney disease.

SOUTHERNWOOD

Artemisia abrotanum

French call it 'garde robe' because when it is laid among clothes it repels moths. Women used to carry sprigs of the herb for its pungent odour, which they hoped might keep them awake during church services.

Medicinal parts: Aerial parts best collected in August and September during the flowering period (it rarely flowers in Britain), and dried carefully to preserve the volatile oil.

Uses: For delayed menstruation, amenorrhoea associated with neurosis, threadworm infestations in children and supporting digestive function.

Other uses: Topically, it may be used as an insect repellent.

Probable mode of action: Constituents include a volatile oil with bitter lactones to which are attributed effectiveness as a digestive tonic, emmenagogue, anthelmintic, antiseptic and uterine stimulant.

Adverse effects: None reported.

Precautions: Safety during pregnancy is not known.

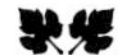

SOY

Glycine soja

The soy plant was possibly used initially as a 'nitrogen fixer' for the soil in agriculture. During the Chou Dynasty (1134–246 BC) the soya bean was designated one of the five sacred grains along with barley, wheat, millet and rice, when it was used as a food. Among the earliest fermented soy foods was shoyu (soy or tamari sauce). Fermentation changed the use of soya to food as the soya bean contained potentially harmful substances (e.g. inhibitors of the enzyme trypsin and similar enzymes needed for digestion of proteins and also haemaglutinins which promote clot formation) which were either destroyed or inactivated by fermentation. Also, like other seeds, the bran or hull of soybean contains phytic acid or phytates – organic acids which inhibit the uptake of essential minerals like calcium, magnesium, iron and zinc from the intestine.

Around 2nd century BC, tofu or soya bean curd was prepared and soya became an accepted source of protein globally, around 700 AD.

In 1999, FDA approved labelling soy products for cholesterol reduction when used in combination with a diet low in saturated fat and cholesterol. The health claim that may be used on labels is 'Diets low in saturated fat products and cholesterol that include 25 g of soy protein a day may reduce the risk of heart disease'. In order to carry the health claim, one serving of a product must contain at least 6.25 g of soy protein and must also be low in total and unsaturated fat, cholesterol and sodium.

Approved by Commission E for:

- raised blood levels of cholesterol.

Medicinal parts: The soya lecithin extracted from the soya bean, the soya oil and soya seed.

herbs

Uses: Soya bean is used for less severe forms of elevated cholesterol levels in the blood (hypercholestrolaemia) when dietary measures are recommended. Also used for liver and gallbladder disorders, anaemia, poor concentration, cerebral and nerve conditions and general debility. Relieving postmenopausal symptoms (particularly vasomotor, e.g. flushes). Also used to prevent osteoporosis (thinning of bones) and cardiovascular disease in postmenopausal females.

Other uses: In **Chinese** medicine, soya bean is used for increased sweating (hyperhidrosis), night sweats, confusion and joint pain.

Probable mode of action: The constituents include isoflavones, genistein, saponins, beta sitosterol and daidzein. Rich in calcium, iron, amino acids and fibre. Also contains linoleic acid, stearic and palmitic acids. The isoflavones are structurally related to plant-derived female hormone – oestrogens (phyto-oestrogens) that are converted to weak oestrogenic ingredients in the body to which are attributed the beneficial effects of the herb on the heart, blood vessels, bone and bladder and in lipid metabolism (reducing cholesterol levels). Soya bean has been documented to decrease low density lipoproteins and triglycerides (fat components in the blood which increase the risk of heart attacks). This has been attributed as stated earlier to the isoflavones which are also considered to relieve menopausal symptoms. Other effects attributed to these constituents are a reduction in breast and prostatic cancers as they inhibit an enzyme, tyrosine kinase, which plays an important role in cell division and tumour growth. The saponins on the other hand are considered to produce antithrombotic and liver protecting effects. As soya contains nearly 35% of protein and eight essential amino acids, it is a good source of protein, particularly in developing countries.

Adverse effects: Constipation, nausea, bloating, allergic reactions such as rash and itching. Inhaled soya dust was claimed to have caused an epidemic of asthma in **Spain**. May inhibit production of the thyroid hormone. Children who are severely allergic to cow's milk are frequently sensitive to soy as well.

Precautions: Avoid prolonged treatment and do not use in patients with asthma and allergic rhinitis (increased risk of soya hull allergy). Use with caution in patients with breast cancer. Children with cystic fibrosis may develop hypoproteinaemia when fed with soya milk. Women with oestrogen receptor positive tumours should exercise caution in the use of soya protein supplements and should only use them if they are recommended and monitored by their physician. There is a concern that more scientific information is required about the absolute safety of soya during pregnancy.

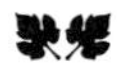

SPINACH

Spinacia oleracea

Spinach was cultivated over 2000 years ago in Iran. Cultivation of spinach began during the Greek and Roman civilizations. The name spinach is derived from the Persian word *ispanai* which means green hand. This later became *spanachia*, the Latin name for spinach. The Arabs named it the 'prince of vegetables' and it was introduced to China around the 8th century.

Medicinal parts: Leaves.

Uses: Used to stimulate appetite and in gastrointestinal complaints and fatigue.

Probable mode of action: Spinach contains a large amount of minerals and vitamins, especially Vitamin A, calcium, phosphorus, iron and potassium. Spinach also has high levels of protein. Also contains vitamins C, E and K.

Adverse effects: May cause renal stones (oxalate content) and may interfere (theoretically) with blood glucose control.

Precautions: When used in children under the age of four months, the nitrate content can cause methaemoglobinaemia. As spinach contains vitamin K, excessive intake should be avoided by those on anticoagulant therapy.

STEVIA – HONEY LEAF

Stevia rebaudiana

For centuries Guarani Native Americans of Paraguay and Brazil used species of *Stevia* (called ka'a he'ê) as a sweetener in yerba mate and medicinal teas for treating heartburn and other ailments. Millions of Japanese people have been using stevia for over 30 years with no reported or known harmful effects. Similarly, stevia has been used for centuries in South America.

In 1985, a study reported that steviol, a breakdown product from two of the sweet compounds in the stevia leaf, is a mutagen. This study was contested but government agencies have expressed concerns over toxicity citing a lack of sufficient conclusive research.

Effects on carcinogenicity remain rather contentious. Beneficial effects in patients with high blood pressure and type 2 diabetes mellitus seem more acceptable.

Japan permits stevia to be used as a food additive as do countries in South America.

Medicinal part: Leaves.

Uses: Sweetener.

Probable mode of action: Sweetening agents are the diterpene glycosides such as stevioside.

Adverse effects: May cause dizziness, headache, flatulence, nausea and muscle pain.

Precautions: Needs to be used with caution in diabetic patients. May increase the blood pressure lowering effect of allopathic medications.

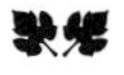

ST JOHN'S WORT – HYPERICUM

Hypericum perforatum

The ancient Greeks believed that the fragrance of St John's wort would drive evil spirits away. Christians considered it a symbol of St John the Baptist because it blooms on June 24th, St John's day. St John's wort is by far the most common antidepressant used in Germany, where physicians prescribe it four times more often than fluoxetine hydrochloride. Used historically for anti-inflammatory and anti-infective properties.

Medicinal part: Herb.

Uses: Antidepressant, for menopausal changes causing irritability and anxiety.

Other uses: Anticancer, antiviral (including human immunodeficiency virus), premenstrual symptoms, seasonal affective disorders, obsessive compulsive disorder, neuralgia, fibrositis and sciatica. Lotion is considered to speed healing of wounds and bruises.

Proposed mode of action: The effects of St John's wort are believed to be due to the combined effects of a number of active constituents; the principal compounds are hypericin and hyperforin but other compounds are also thought to contribute. Extracts of St John's wort have been shown to have high affinity for gamma amino butyric acid (GABA), monoamine oxidase and adenosine receptors in laboratory experiments (*in vitro*). Hyperforin has been shown to be an uptake inhibitor of several chemical messengers including serotonin, dopamine, noradrenaline, GABA and L-glutamate at synapses and inhibits serotonin uptake in the rat peritoneal cells.

Adverse effects: Side-effects of St John's wort are generally mild and it is well tolerated, though there may be interactions with prescribed medications (see below). The most common side-effects are gastrointestinal disturbances, allergic reactions and fatigue. Photosensitivity occurs rarely. Symptoms characteristic of serotonin syndrome (mental confusion, hallucinations, agitation, headache, coma, shivering, sweating, fever, hypertension (high blood pressure), tachycardia (increased pulse rate), nausea, diarrheoa, tremors, muscle twitching, insomnia) may occur if used with drugs classed as serotonin reuptake inhibitors (e.g. fluoxetine [Prozac] and paroxetine [Paxil]). Others include insomnia, vivid dreams, restlessness, anxiety, irritability, agitation, headache, paraesthesias, emotional vulnerability, pruritus and weight gain.

Precautions: Can cause light sensitivity, so susceptible individuals should avoid long exposure to sun. The interaction of St John's wort with a number of prescribed medicines reduces their effectiveness and it should not be taken with the contraceptive pill, antidepressants, immune suppressants, HIV medications, warfarin, digoxin and a number of other medications. If you are taking any medication, consult your doctor before starting St John's wort. Medical advice should also be sought if you are taking St John's wort and a prescribed medicine and intend to stop using St John's wort.

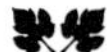

STONE ROOT – HORSE BALM

Collinsonia canadensis

Called stone root as the root is very heavy and very hard and cannot be powdered by usual appliances. The bruised leaves have a tradition of use for bruises and wounds. Listed in the 1st edition of *King's Dispensatory* (1854).

Medicinal parts: Root, whole plant.

Uses: Applied topically for wounds and bruises. Used for gastrointestinal complaints such as haemorrhoids and indigestion.

Other uses: As a diuretic. Also used as treatment for headaches and indigestion.

Probable mode of action: Alcoholic extracts have shown antifungal activity. Other constituents include alkaloids, mucilage, resins, saponins and tannins. The exact effects of these constituents are not known with certainty as yet.

Adverse effects: May cause an elevation of blood pressure.

Precautions: Safety during pregnancy has not been established. Avoid during pregnancy and lactation.

SUTHERLANDIA

Sutherlandia frutescens

(Insiswa, Unwele, Mukakana, Phetola, Lerumo-lamadi, cancer bush, kankerbos, kankerbossie)

Considered to be the most profound multipurpose medicinal plant in Southern Africa which has enjoyed a long history of use by all cultures because of its efficacy as a safe tonic for several medical disorders.

As Sutherlandia assists the body to mobilize its own resources to cope with physical and mental stresses, it is referred to as an adaptogen.

The traditional Tswana name Phetola means 'it changes' the course of an illness towards a favourable outcome. The North Sotho name Lerumo-lamida, means 'spear for the blood' – a powerful blood purifier. The name cancer bush, kankerbos, comes from its reputation as a cure for cancer. The original inhabitants of the Cape, the Khoi San and Nama people, used the plant as a decoction for washing wounds and internally to bring down fevers.

The list of folk, traditional and current uses is enormous.

Medicinal parts: Fresh and dried above ground parts of the plant.

Uses: Improvement of quality of life in the treatment of HIV, tuberculosis and cancer.

Other uses: Also used in diabetes, chronic fatigue syndrome, influenza, rheumatoid arthritis, osteoarthritis, peptic ulcers, gastritis, reflux oesophagitis, menopausal symptoms, anxiety and depression.

Used topically for treatment of eye infections and wounds.

Probable mode of action: The plant is rich in amino acids and pinitol, and contains small amounts of saponins and L-canavarine (non-protein amino acid) which is attributed with anticancer properties. There are also some constituents similar to some of the chemical messengers (neurotransmitters) in the body. Is a potent inhibitor of the metabolizing enzyme system CYP3A4 and of the drug transport system P-gp. A recent study suggested that the plant should be developed as an effective immunomodulator for treatment of diseases associated with overproduction of reactive oxidants by human phagocytes. Is approved by the **African** health authorities for the treatment of HIV.

Adverse effects: Mild diarrhoea, dry mouth, mild diuresis, dizziness, only in very high doses.

Precautions: Needs to be used under guidance because of the potential to cause drug–herb interactions. This is due to the ability of the herb to alter function of drug metabolizing enzymes in the liver. Avoid in pregnancy.

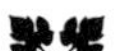

SWEET VIOLET – ENGLISH VIOLET

Viola odorata

Has been cultivated for cosmetics and medicines since antiquity in Europe. Has a long and proven history of use in folk medicine especially for the treatment of whooping cough and cancers.

Leaf and flower extracts have been used in the production of perfumes.

Medicinal parts: Roots, seeds, leaves and flowers.

Uses: As a cough remedy and as a sedative. Its use for headaches, migraine and insomnia is possibly related to its salicylic acid content. The whole plant has been used as a diaphoretic, diuretic, emollient and expectorant.

Other uses: Has been applied topically as an anti-inflammatory agent. The dried root is used for constipation and also to induce vomiting (as an emetic). The flowers have been used for biliary disorders. The petals made into a syrup were used to treat disorders in infants.

Probable mode of action: Extracts from the leaf were found to act like salicylates and aspirin in reducing fever in experimental animals. Contains saponins and also an 'emetine-like' alkaloid. More than 100 volatile oils have been isolated from the leaves.

Adverse effects: May cause vomiting. May have an additive effect with laxatives.

Precautions: Contraindicated during pregnancy and lactation.

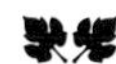

SWERTIA CHIRETTA – SWERTIA CHIRAYITA – CHIRAYATA – KIRATA-TIKTA – INDIAN GENTIAN

Gentiana chirayita

Has a long tradition of use in the Ayurveda, Siddha and Unani systems of traditional medicine in the Indian subcontinent. Grows at altitudes between 4000 and 10,000 feet in the Himalayas from Kashmir to Bhutan.

In India, chirayata has been used as an antimalarial agent, combined with cloves and cinnamon.

Medicinal parts: Leaves, whole plant.

Uses: As a bitter tonic (appetizer), for stomach complaints, to reduce fevers and as an antihelminthic.

Other uses: Laxative and also for diarrhoea. To bring down fevers (as a febrifuge) and to treat asthma.

Probable mode of action: Plant contains two bitter principles which probably produce its effect as an appetizer. Other constituents are resins, gum,

herbs

carbonates and phosphates of potash, lime and magnesium.

Adverse effects: Not considered a toxic hazard in the quantities used.

Precautions: Do not exceed recommended doses. It has been shown in animal experiments that the herb can lower blood sugar. Be aware.

TANGERINE PEEL – MANDARIN ORANGE PEEL – CHEN PI

Citrus reticulata

Has a long history of use in Traditional Chinese Medicine where it is considered to settle, regulate and normalize the flow of qi (life force), break up congestion and enhance the flow of liquids through the body. Chinese herbalists used tangerine peel to relieve indigestion, gas, bloating, nausea, vomiting and loose stools.

Medicinal parts: Red or orange or green coloured peel of fruit.

Uses: Vomiting, belching. Young green peel is used for hernia and for pain in the breast.

Other uses: Combined with pinella root, it is used to loosen phlegm and relieve chest congestion. Has also been used to treat nausea, and muscle pains.

Probable mode of action: The effects of the constituents are not known with certainty. The constituents have been attributed with effects against bacteria (possibly the naringin constituent) and to lower blood fat (lipid) levels (attributed to the bioflavonoids).

Adverse effects: None reported with the usual recommended doses.

Precautions: Do not take tangerine peel if you have a dry cough or an excessively red tongue or if spitting blood.

TEA TREE OIL

Melaleuca alternifolia

Indigenous Australians (Aboriginals) have used oil extracted from the tree's needles for hundreds and possibly thousands of years for burns, cuts and insect bites. Has been recognized anecdotally as a potent antiseptic in Australia. (See also Niauli-Cape oil on page 190.)

Medicinal parts: Oil from the leaves.

Uses: Antifungal agent (antidandruff agent as a shampoo with 5% oil, topically against *Candida*); acne. Commonly used as a local antiseptic.

Other uses: Bug bites, boils, minor wounds. Suggested uses include eczema, lice infestations and wound infections and acne.

Probable mode of action: One of the constituents was shown in laboratory experiments to possess activity against bacteria and fungi. The organisms against which activity was shown included *Staphyloccocus aureus*, *Pseudomonas aeruginosa*, streptococci and *Candida*. Considered to act by disrupting cell walls and causing the loss of intracellular ions and proteins in the organisms. In the treatment of burns, the oil has been observed to bring about cooling – reducing the temperature of the skin – and then to promote healing.

Adverse effects: Possibility of causing central nervous system depression along with disturbances in gait (ataxia) and drowsiness. May cause stomatitis (inflammation of the mouth), vomiting, diarrhoea and gastrointestinal irritation when taken by mouth. May cause dermatitis in sensitive people. Severe skin reaction similar to the skin condition erythema multiforme has been reported.

Precautions: Not to be taken internally. Avoid during pregnancy and lactation.

THUJA

Thuja occidentalis

An ornamental tree in North America used for screens and hedges. Thuja was a Native American remedy for delayed menstruation, headache and heart pain, and was also used to reduce swelling.

Medicinal parts: Young twigs and leaves. The twigs are at their best in summer.

Uses: To treat bronchial catarrh, enuresis, cystitis, psoriasis, amenorrhoea (absence of menstruation), rheumatism and cystitis (bladder infections).

Other uses: Externally it may be used to treat warts, including genital and anal warts. To treat ringworm and thrush, cancers of the chest and breast.

Probable mode of action: Constituents are volatile oil, flavonoid glycosides, mucilage and tannin. The effects are as a nerve stimulant and to promote removal of secretions from the lung and upper airways, and stimulant to smooth muscles, particularly the bronchial muscle and the muscles of the genitourinary system. Also believed to act on the smooth muscle of blood vessels and on the uterus (emmenagogue). Some constituents are attributed with antiseptic, anti-inflammatory, diuretic, contracting cells (skin and other) following inflammation (astringent), counter-irritant and vermifuge effects. Best known effect is possibly its antiviral effect which makes it a remedy for warts, particularly genital and anal warts.

Adverse effects: Nausea, vomiting, flatulence and indigestion have been reported. Considered to have the ability to cause asthma and seizures. The oil is very toxic and should be used very cautiously internally. Stated to counteract the effects of smallpox vaccination.

Precautions: It should not be taken during pregnancy due to its stimulant effect on the uterus. The oil should be used internally only in very small quantities and only under the supervision of a physician. Deaths and convulsions have been associated with improper use of the oil internally.

THYME

Thymus vulgaris

The plant is native to Spain and Italy. Thyme preparations have been used for centuries in folk medicine as an appetite stimulant, for dyspepsia, chronic gastritis and diarrhoea in children. The volatile oil of *Thymus vulgaris* has been suggested as an economical and viable alternative to pesticides in agriculture.

Medicinal parts: Leaves, flowers.

Uses: Bronchitis, sore throat and intestinal colic.

Other uses: As an antihelminthic, antifungal and antiflatulent. Has been popular as a digestive aid. Has also been used as an expectorant.

Probable mode of action: Thyme contains constituents which act to reduce spasms of smooth muscle and to prevent cough (antitussive) and also remove secretions from the chest (promote removal of secretions from the lung and upper airways). Antibacterial and antifungal effects are attributed to the thymol and carvacrol constituents. Thyme is considered to be effective against fungal infections taken internally and also applied locally.

Adverse effects: Thyme oil should not be taken internally. Should be diluted in carrier oil before topical use. Thyme oil can lead to irritation and there is a low potential for sensitization. The oil in particular can cause headache and dizziness and slowing of the heart rate (bradycardia). Also known to cause nausea, vomiting and diarrhoea.

Precautions: Thyme is not be used in patients with inflammatory disease of the gastrointestinal tract. Internal use is contraindicated especially in pregnancy. Be cautious when using thyme in subjects who are sensitive to some grasses.

TORMENTIL ROOT

Potentilla tormentosa or Tormentilla erecta

Hippocrates used *Tormentilla erecta* to treat malaria.

The Lapps use the thickened red juice of the root to stain leather. The Americans use the name tormentil for *Geranium maculatum*, which has similar properties.

Medicinal parts: Dried rhizome and root.

Uses: Diarrhoea (acute or nervous diarrhoea, diarrhoeas due to irritation of the small intestine).

To relieve symptoms of ulcerative colitis and mucus colitis. Useful in conditions where there is alternating diarrhoea and constipation.

Other uses: As a gargle for throat and mouth inflammations and as a lotion for haemorrhoids.

To prevent gastric irritation due to food and also to relieve symptoms or prevent peptic ulcer.

Has been used to treat fever. A douche has been used for vaginal infections. As an ointment, lotion, compress or poultice it will speed the healing of wounds, cuts and discharging sores. A weak decoction is used for conjunctivitis.

Probable mode of action: The tannic acid constituents are attributed with the effect of contracting cells (skin and other) following inflammation (astringent). Other constituents have been shown to possess antiallergic, antihypertensive and antiviral effects. Has also been shown to be a stimulant of the immune system in experiments.

Adverse effects: If ingested in doses in excess of 1 g, the tannins in particular would cause gastrointestinal symptoms such as abdominal pain, constipation, nausea and vomiting. There has also been report of hepatic cirrhosis after intake. Interferes with the absorption of iron and other minerals when taken internally.

Precautions: The herb should not be used in patients with gastrointestinal disorders such as diverticulitis, gastric or duodenal ulcers (peptic ulcers) and ulcerative colitis. Best avoided in inflammatory or ulcerative bowel disease. Should not be used during pregnancy and lactation.

TURMERIC

Curcuma longa

Originally cultivated in India as a dye at least from 600 BC. Is mentioned in the ancient Sanskrit medical script, *Sasuruta's Ayurvedic Compendium* (250 BC) as being useful 'to relieve the effects of poisoned foods'. Was used by Indonesians to paint their bodies for wedding rituals. Was described by Marco Polo during the 13th century as a 'spice very similar to saffron'.

Turmeric is a sterile plant that does not produce seed. Said to have reached China around 700 AD and Africa between 800 AD and 1200 AD.

According to the American Institute for Cancer Research, the constituent curcumin is considered to be beneficial in the prevention of cancers of the breast, colon, oesophagus and skin.

Medicinal part: Root.

Uses: Topically for skin infections, analgesia, leech bites, bruising and infected wounds.

Orally for flatulence, dyspepsia, fever and diarrhoea and other dyspeptic symptoms. Has been used to treat irritable bowel syndrome and also parasitic infestations of the bowel.

Other uses: Chest infections, jaundice, headaches and amenorrhoea. Was used for toothaches and for the treatment of rheumatic disorders.

Ayurvedic medicine: Stomachic and tonic.

Probable mode of action: Rich in potassium and iron. Also contains volatile oils. The oil from the root has shown anti-inflammatory effects. One of the constituents, curcumin, has the ability to stimulate the secretion of bile and to protect the liver. Also known as an anticancer agent. Curcuminoid constituents are responsible for the yellow colour of turmeric. Has been investigated as a medicinal agent for management of cystic fibrosis.

Adverse effects: Overdose or long-term use may cause gastrointestinal disturbances. Theoretically, turmeric may increase the effects and adverse effects of antiplatelet drugs.

Precautions: Should not be used by patients with gallstones or bile duct obstruction and is contraindicated in individuals with stomach ulcers or hyperacidity. Avoid in pregnancy as high doses may stimulate menstrual flow and uterine contractions.

UNICORN ROOT

FALSE UNICORN ROOT – DEVIL'S BIT

Chamaelirium luteum

The Native Americans used false unicorn root for disorders of the female reproductive organs. This plant was used by the Eclectic medical movement of the late 19th and 20th century mainly for female complaints. Now considered an endangered species. This plant is sometimes confused with *Aletris farinose*, or *true* unicorn root which also contains constituents attributed with activity similar to that of the female hormone-oestrogen.

Medicinal Parts: Dried rhizome and roots

Common uses: Used in the management of amenorrhoea (absent menstrual periods) and for pain during menstruation (dysmenorrhoea). Used to treat white discharge from the vagina (leucorrhoea) and vomiting during pregnancy and for menopausal symptoms.

Other uses: Has been used to treat inflammation of the tubes of the uterus (fallopian tubes – salpingitis).To prevent vomiting (as an anti-emetic), to increase the passage of urine (as a diuretic). Also considered to be effective in worm infestations (anti-helminthic). Has a reputation to be useful for impotence in males and to aid digestion and increase appetite. Has been used in combination with Echinacea for inflammatory disease of the pelvis.

Probable mode of action: Active constituents include steroidal saponins (including chamaelirin, a glycoside of diosgenin), helonin (a glycoside), free diosgenin, starch, calcium oxalate. The constituents are reported to act as an emmenagogue (promotes menstruation) and as a uterine tonic. Reported to increase the secretory and cyclical activity of the ovary and thus increase fertility, as the saponin components are considered to possess activity similar to that of the female hormone oestrogen. Also recorded are diuretic effects and prevention of vomiting (anti-emetic).

Adverse effects: Very large doses may cause nausea and vomiting

Precautions: Cattle have died following eating this plant. Though it has been recommended for use in the treatment of vomiting during pregnancy, there is a considerable risk of the plant causing miscarriage as it is an emmenagogue (promotes menstruation). Best avoided during pregnancy.

TRUE UNICORN ROOT – COLIC ROOT

Aletris farinose

Has been used by the Native Americans to relieve digestive complaints and to prevent miscarriages. The Catawbas used the leaves to make a tea to stop diarrhoea. Used in Appalachia for the management of rheumatism and as a tonic. In Argentina it is considered as a remedy for bronchitis.

Medicinal parts: Dried root. The fresh root tends to cause vomiting. The root is bitter, diuretic, narcotic and tonic.

Uses: For poor digestion, loss of appetite, 'nervous stomach' and 'gas' in stomach. Has been used in the treatment of painful menstruation (dysmenorrhoea) and to promote fertility.

Other uses: A tea of the leaves has been used in the treatment of colic, stomach disorders, dysentery and bloody dysentery.

Probable mode of action: The constituents are considered to possess activity similar to that of the female hormone oestrogen. The root contains diosgenin, which has both anti-inflammatory and oestrogenic properties.

Adverse effects: In large doses, the herb can cause drowsiness and sleepiness (narcosis). In large doses the fresh root is somewhat narcotic, emetic and cathartic. The fresh root can cause colic. Has been known to cause vertigo and stupefaction.

Precautions: Known to prevent or decrease the action of oxytocics (drugs used to stimulate contraction of the uterus). Cautious use during pregnancy.

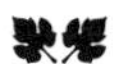

VALERIAN

Valeriana officinalis
Valeriana edulis
Valeriana wallichii
'Valium of the 19th century'

Despite its odour, valerian was considered a perfume in the 16th century Europe.

German health officials have approved valerian for use as a mild sedative and sleep aid, based on several European clinical trials that demonstrated these effects. Approximately 50 tons of valerian are sold each year in France.

Valerian has been classified as GRAS (Generally Recognized as Safe) in the US for food use.

Medicinal parts: Rhizomes, roots.

Uses: To promote sleep, as an anxiolytic, an antispasmodic and for muscle tension.

Commonly combined with sedative agents such as hops, passion flower or St John's wort.

Other uses: To calm hyperactivity in children.

Probable mode of action: Three distinct classes of active ingredients have been associated with the sedative properties. The aqueous extract of valerian has been found to contain substantial quantities of the chemical messenger in the brain, namely, the neurotransmitter gamma-aminobutyric acid (GABA) which binds to the same receptors as benzodiazepines (e.g. Valium), but with less affinity and milder clinical effects. Another substance isolated is glutamine which can be metabolized to the chemical messenger GABA. These constituents are primarily concerned with the effects valerian produces in the central nervous system.

Adverse effects: Headaches (rare), giddiness, nausea, excitability and agitation in some subjects, heart palpitations (rare), insomnia (rare). Habituation or addiction has not been reported.

Precautions: Some constituents have shown cytotoxic and mutagenic activity *in vitro*. Although these effects have not been reproduced *in vivo* even at high doses (1350 mg/kg), valerian probably should not be used by pregnant women. Valerian should not be taken with other sedatives (e.g. alcohol) or before driving or in other situations when alertness is required.

It may be advisable to stop intake of valerian prior to surgery.

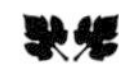

VERVAIN – HOLY HERB – ENCHANTER'S HERB

Verbena officinalis

Vervain was one of the sacred herbs of the Druids. Romans called it the sacred plant (Herba sancta). It was hung around the necks of children to prevent infection. In China it is referred to as ma bian cao and is used to treat the fever of malaria and influenza. The Chinese also used the herb to treat headaches allegedly caused by fluctuations of female hormone secretion.

Indigenous to England and central and southern Europe.

Vervain is listed by the Council of Europe as a natural source of food flavouring. In the US, vervain is listed by the Food and Drugs Administration as a 'Herb of Undefined Safety'.

Medicinal part: Herb.

Uses: Depression, low mood, hysteria, melancholia, to treat generalized seizures or fits and as a sedative. As a poultice for insect bites and bruises and sprains and as an ointment for eczema, sores and painful neuralgia.

Other uses: Management of jaundice, early stages of fever, influenza, painful menstruation (dysmenorrhoea) for which extracts of the fruit are used. Fairly well known as a stimulant of breast milk production (galactogogue).

Probable mode of action: The constituents include iridoid glycosides (e.g. verbenin, verbanalin), bitter principle, saponins, tannins, volatile oil, mucilage and unknown alkaloids. The stimulation of breast milk production is attributed to glycoside aucubin. Verbenelin has been found in experiments to cause a lowering of blood pressure (antihypertensive). Some work has shown that the herb acts like the drug levodopa which is used to treat Parkinsonism. Verbenelin has been reported to exhibit some uterine stimulant activity and possibly is responsible for the emmenagogue effects. The constituents are also reported to have an effect on the secretion of the gonadotrophic hormones (hormones which are associated with reproductive activity) from the pituitary gland. As to the effects attributed to the other constituents- analgesia (pain relief) and aphrodisiac are not clearly defined at present.

Adverse effects: High doses of verbenalin can cause paralysis of the nervous system resulting in stupor and convulsions. May cause contact dermatitis.

Precautions: Vervain can interfere with allopathic drug therapy of high blood pressure (hypertension). Avoid during pregnancy as it may stimulate the uterus. Avoid when breastfeeding. To be used with great caution in patients with allergies and in those with a tendency to have fits (e.g. epileptics).

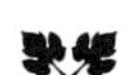

WAHOO – INDIAN ARROW-WOOD – BURNING BUSH

Euonymus atropurpureus

Native to Missouri, US. The thin stems were used as hunting arrows by the Native North Americans who also used the plant as herbal medicine for eye ailments, sores on the face and for gynaecological disorders.

Atropurpureus is derived from the Latin word for dark purple which is likely to be a reference to the colour of the fruits and foliage.

Medicinal parts: Root and bark from stems.

Uses: Specifically indicated in constipation with liver and gallbladder dysfunction. Also used to treat jaundice, gallbladder infections (cholecystitis), skin eruptions and treatment of head lice.

Other uses: As a diuretic, for chest and lung congestion, indigestion and fever.

Considered to stimulate the appetite in small doses. Has been used as a tea to treat malaria and liver congestion (allowing the free flow of bile and so helping the digestive process) and constipation.

Probable mode of action: Constituents include glycosides, small amounts of digitaloids, alkaloids, sugars, fatty acids, tannin and volatile oil. The attributed effects are as a stimulant for secretion of bile, as a laxative and also as a diuretic. Shown to have an effect on the heart and to stimulate the circulation. The constituents are considered to act directly as a bile stimulant. As to how the constituents bring down fever is not known.

Adverse effects: Diarrhoea, vomiting, chills, seizures, syncope and weakness.

Precautions: *Euonymus* is toxic in excessive doses and should not be used during pregnancy and lactation. The leaves and fruit are poisonous. The bark is toxic.

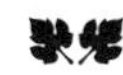

WATERCRESS – SCURVY GRASS

Nasturtium officinale

Used during Greek and Roman times. The Greek general and the Persian King Xerxes ordered their soldiers to eat watercress to keep them healthy. The Greeks also believed that 'eating cress makes one witty'. As watercress is a good source of vitamin C, it was used in the treatment of vitamin C deficiency (scurvy).

Garden nasturtium or Indian cress belongs to a different family, Tropaeolum.

Medicinal parts: All parts of the plant.

Uses: Most popular as a salad green. Has been used medicinally as an anti-inflammatory agent and as an antimicrobial. The juice of the plant has been used to treat acne, eczema, rashes and infections of the skin.

Other uses: Has a long reputation as a stimulant of hair growth on the head and as a hair tonic. Has been used as a poultice for glandular tumours and for swellings involving lymph glands and lymph vessels.

Probable mode of action: Contains vitamins A, C, iron and phosphates and an oil. Also contains gluconasturtiin which is a precursor of isothiocyanates, a metabolite of which has been found to inhibit the carcinogen found in tobacco (nitrosamine). There is some evidence to suggest that the constituents of watercress inhibit the release of histamine.

Adverse effects: None reported.

Precautions: Avoid during pregnancy and breastfeeding as safety is not established. May inhibit the metabolism of paracetamol (acetaminophen).

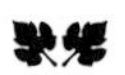

WILD CHERRY

Prunus serotina

The Native Americans had many uses for wild cherry bark, including a tea made from the inner bark to ease labour pains, diarrhoea and lung problems. Chinese physicians prescribe *Prunus yedoensis* for cough.

Medicinal parts: Dried bark from young plants in the autumn when it has its highest prussic acid content. The outer bark is stripped off and the inner bark dried in the shade. It should be protected from light.

Uses: For the irritable and persistent cough of bronchitis, whooping cough (pertussis), and cough due to increased irritability of respiratory mucosa. Treatment of stomach complaints of nervous origin (nervous dyspepsia).

Other uses: As a wash in eye inflammation and to contract cells (skin and other) following inflammation (astringent). Treatment of diarrhoea.

Probable mode of action: Constituents are attributed with effects that reduce coughing and facilitate the removal of secretions from the lung (antitussive, promote removal of secretions from the lung and upper airways). Also considered to have mild sedative effects. Considered to be a bitter and thus useful in digestive disorders. The bark, seeds and leaves of wild cherry trees contain amygdalin which is a cyanogenic glycoside.

Adverse effects: Nausea, vomiting, gastrointestinal irritation, muscle spasms, weakness and coma may occur due to cyanide poisoning.

Precautions: Prunus cause drowsiness. Cyanogenic glycosides are moderately toxic, producing cyanic acid on hydrolysis, and should not be taken in excess. The seeds must be discarded. Death has occurred in children who ate seeds, drank tea made from the plant or chewed on leaves. The plants should be kept beyond the reach of children. The leaves have poisoned cattle. Contraindicated during pregnancy and breastfeeding.

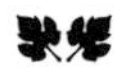

WILD YAM

Dioscorea villosa

In the past, pharmacists used wild yam in the preparation of a contraceptive pill as it mimicked the action of the female hormone progesterone and prevented ovulation. Wild yam was historically the sole source of raw materials for manufacturing contraceptive hormones, cortisone (a hormone from the adrenal gland) and anabolic hormones (hormones which promote growth).

Medicinal part: Roots (rhizomes).

Uses: Painful menstruation (dysmenorrhoea), ovarian pain and muscle cramps after childbirth, intestinal colitis and diverticulitis. Popularly considered to correct hormonal imbalances in the female and used for postmenopausal symptoms.

Other uses: Inflammation of joints due to arthritis (rheumatism) and gout. Also used to treat abdominal cramps and bile stones (gallbladder stones).

Probable mode of action: One of the active constituents, diosgenin, is a precursor of the female hormones oestrogen and progesterone and also has anti-inflammatory activity. A constituent of wild yam is DHEA which is a steroid hormone produced by the adrenal gland.

Adverse effects: May cause vomiting in large ingestions. Known to cause headache, menstrual irregularities and acne. May cause hair loss and an oily skin.

Precautions: Avoid during pregnancy because of the possibility of masculinization of the foetus (a female foetus may develop male features such as body hair). To be avoided by patients with cancers of the breast, ovaries, prostate and uterus.

WILLOW – WHITE WILLOW

Salix alba
Salix fragilis
Salix pentandra
Salix purpurea

The composer Ludwig von Beethoven is believed to been a long-term user of powdered willow bark. Used in ancient Egypt to treat inflammation.

The German Commission E approved internal use of willow for:
diseases accompanied by fever
rheumatic ailments
headaches.

Medicinal part: Bark.

Uses: Muscular disorders and rheumatoid arthritis, inflammatory pain, influenza, catarrh, gouty arthritis, ankylosing spondylitis.

Other uses: To facilitate removal of secretions from the lungs and upper airways (expectorant) and as an astringent.

Probable mode of action: Salicin, possibly the most active metabolite in willow, is metabolized to salicylic acid which is known to possess anti-inflammatory, antipyretic and uricosuric activities. In a randomized double blind study, willow bark extract was proven to have a moderate analgesic effect in osteoarthritis and was well tolerated. It is thought that salicin is converted to salicylic acid *after* absorption so it should not be irritant to the gastrointestinal tract.

Adverse effects: Can cause gastrointestinal bleeding and kidney damage. May cause dermatitis and an 'asthma' like disorder.

Precautions: Drug interactions associated with salicylates are applicable to willow. Concurrent administration with other aspirin-like drugs should be avoided. Avoid use during pregnancy. Salicylates excreted in breast milk have been known to cause rashes in babies. It is necessary to remember that some patients may be allergic to salicylates.

WINTERGREEN

Gaultheria procumbens

In folk medicine, wintergreen leaf has been used orally for headache, stomachache, flatulence, fever and asthma. Children who developed chest infections were made to wear a paper jacket that was coated with camphor and oil of wintergreen.

Medicinal parts: Leaves, bark.

Uses: Contracts cells (skin and other) following inflammation (astringent). Also as a stimulant.

Topically wintergreen oil has been used for rheumatism, sore muscles, lumbago and as an antiseptic.

Other uses: To treat inflamed and swollen muscles, ligaments and joints. Also to relieve the pain in sciatica and trigeminal neuralgia.

Probable mode of action: Active ingredients include methyl salicylate (98%).

When freshly harvested, the plant contains gaultherin that changes to methyl salicylate as the plant is dried. Wintergreen contains less than 1% of wintergreen oil and it is the oil that contains the methyl salicylate.

Adverse effects: Topical use can cause contact dermatitis. Overuse on the skin could also cause salicylate poisoning. Heat and physical activity increases the absorption of salicylates through the skin. Symptoms of toxicity due to salicylates cause tinnitus, nausea, vomiting, stomach pain, confusion.

Precautions: May aggravate stomach ulcers if used orally. The high content of salicylate in the oil necessitates caution as salicylate toxicity could follow even topical applications. Should not be used by those allergic to aspirin. Best avoided by those under the age of 12 years.

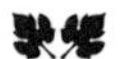

WITCH HAZEL

Hamamelis virginiana

Traditionally, witch hazel is used orally for tumours and cancer and topically for insect bites, minor burns and skin irritations.

Medicinal parts: Bark, leaf.

Uses: Used in diarrhoea, mucous colitis, colds and fevers. Topically for itching, skin inflammation, eye inflammation and haemorrhoids.

Other uses: Has been used to relieve the discomfort after surgical incisions made to aid childbirth (episiotomies) and for operations on haemorrhoids. Also for bruises and varicose veins. Used as a gargle to soothe sore throat and infections of the mouth and gums.

Probable mode of action: Tannin component of the bark and leaf contract cells (skin and other) following inflammation (astringent) and also has anti-inflammatory properties. Tannins applied locally to broken skin or mucous membranes induce the precipitation of proteins, tighten up the superficial layers of the skin and shrink capillaries and promote healing.

Adverse effects: Plants with at least 10% tannins (witch hazel bark contains 12% tannins) can cause gastrointestinal disturbances, kidney damage and necrotic conditions of the liver. Regular consumption of herbs with high tannin content may cause oesophageal or nasal cancers. Ingestion of 1 g of witch hazel may cause nausea, vomiting and impaction. Topical use may cause dermatitis.

Precautions: Avoid long-term use due to risk of cancer. Avoid during pregnancy and breastfeeding.

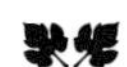

WOOD ANEMONE – WIND CROW FOOT

Anemone nemorosa

Greek legends held that Anemos, god of winds, sent anemones to herald his coming in early spring. Has been used for centuries in traditional medicine. Dioscorides used the flower to treat eye conditions. In Russian folk medicine, the aerial parts of wood anemone are used orally for stomach pains, delayed menstruation, gout, whooping cough and asthma.

Medicinal parts: Dried leaves, stems, flowers.

Uses: Has been used to treat eye disorders.

Other uses: Has been used traditionally for relief of pain (as an analgesic), for earache, as a diuretic and for diseases of the circulation and for gynaecological disorders. In **France**, pulsatilla is used in the symptomatic treatment of nervous disorders, especially minor sleep disorders. In **Germany**, potential uses include disorders of the gastrointestinal tract, disorders of the genital tract and infectious diseases of the skin and mucosal membranes.

Probable mode of action: Constituents include glucosides, tannins, volatile oils and succinic acid. Some constituents undergo change when the fresh plant is crushed and a toxic compound protoanemonin is formed. This and other constituents have caused central nervous system stimulation followed by paralysis in animals.

Adverse effects: Ingestion of freshly harvested wood anemone can cause colic, diarrhoea and severe irritation of the gastrointestinal tract. This is attributed to the glycoside ranunculin which is enzymatically changed to a very toxic compound – protoanemonin. Direct contact may cause severe skin irritation.

Precautions: Safety during pregnancy is not known with certainty. Pulsatilla can be a dangerous and powerful depressant of the central nervous system and heart. The protoanemonin constituent would cause abortion. Avoid during pregnancy.

WORMWOOD

Artemisia absinthium

Has been used for centuries as a moth repellent. Vincent van Gogh was believed to be addicted to absinthe, a green liqueur which was banned in early 20th century. He craved for other substances that contained terpenes. There is a belief that the predominance of yellow in his paintings and the hallucinations he experienced were related to his consumption of absinthe.

Chinese wormwood (*Artemisia annua*) has been used for fevers for over 2000 years.

A thujone-free extract of wormwood is used for flavouring vermouth. Roman wormwood is considered to be less toxic and is also used for flavouring vermouth and Campari.

Medicinal parts: Leaves, herbs.

Uses: Appetite stimulant, liver complaints, antihelminthic.

Other uses: For wound healing (topical application), anaemia, irregular menstruation, worm infestations (antihelminthic). Also used as an insect repellent. Has been used to treat fevers.

Probable mode of action: Constituents include glucosides (absinthin and others) and a sweet smelling volatile oil which has terpenes, primarily thujone. Thujone acts like a narcotic and provides relief from pain and is believed to cause absinthism. Constituents are considered to stimulate the appetite.

Adverse effects: Contains thujone, this may lower the threshold for fits. Renal failure and damage to muscles (rhabdomyolysis) has been reported. Absinthism is characterized by hallucinations, insomnia, loss of intellect, psychosis, tremor and seizures.

Precautions: Avoid in patients with predisposition to seizures. Avoid in pregnancy and during breastfeeding. Long-term use is not recommended by many herbalists.

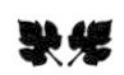

WOUNDWORT – ALL HEAL

Stachys palustris

Name derived from the traditional use of the plant to treat wounds.

The crest of the coat of arms of the Royal Society of Medicine has a hand holding a bunch of herbs – woundwort.

Medicinal parts: Leaves and stem.

Uses: Wound healing, a disinfectant and antispasmodic.

Other uses: Abdominal pain, fever, menstrual disorders. Used externally to stop bleeding and promote healing of wounds.

Probable mode of action: The exact effects of the constituents are not known as yet. Contains flavonoids and iridoids.

Adverse effects: No reported adverse effects at therapeutic doses.

Precautions: Avoid during pregnancy and breastfeeding.

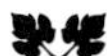

YARROW

Achillea millefolium

Medicinal part: Flowers.

Uses: Used in fever, common cold, amenorrhoea, dysentery, diarrhoea, loss of appetite, coronary and cerebral thrombosis. Fresh leaves are chewed for toothache.

Other uses: Gastrointestinal discomfort and to induce sweating. Used as a solution for eczema. Taken internally, the herb is stated to reduce phlegm (secretions in the chest). Has been used to treat female reproductive disorders.

Probable mode of action: Constituents include ascorbic acid (vitamin C), amino acids, salicylic acid alkaloids and flavonoids. An alkaloid constituent may decrease clotting time and have antipyretic and hypotensive actions. Volatile oil of yarrow may have central nervous system depressant effects.

Adverse effects: Ingesting large amounts may cause sedative and diuretic effects. Topical use can cause dermatitis.

Precautions: Theoretically yarrow can enhance the sedative effect of other herbs (e.g. valerian, kava, German chamomile, hops) and sedative drugs. Avoid in pregnancy as it is reported to be a uterine stimulant. May cause allergic reactions in individuals with a sensitivity to flowers in the Asteraceae or Compositae families.

YELLOW DOCK

Rumex crispus

Has a long history of use on both sides of the Atlantic Ocean as a blood purifier that is associated with skin diseases. The Native North Americans used yellow dock in a mashed form for cuts and applied crushed leaves to boils.

Medicinal part: Root.

Uses: Constipation, obstructive jaundice, upper respiratory tract disorders.

Other uses: Psoriasis, eczema, skin wounds.

Probable mode of action: The constituent anthraquinone glycosides have a laxative effect. The tannins are responsible for the effect of contracting cells (skin and other) following inflammation (astringent). The main use, though not scientifically proven, is as a blood purifier. It is believed that chronic skin disorders also cause blood to be impure. The constituents are reported to promote the flow of bile and have a beneficial effect on the functioning of the liver, kidney and spleen.

Adverse effects: Excessive use can cause abdominal cramps. Prolonged diarrhoea can cause loss of potassium and electrolyte imbalance. Oxalate may interact with calcium resulting in kidney stones. Accidental ingestion of leaf has caused death. Toxic symptoms appear 2–6 hours after ingestion and consist of nausea, vomiting, diarrhoea, mouth irritations, liver and kidney damage.

Precautions: Should be avoided by patients with kidney disease. Potassium loss can increase the toxicity of cardiac drugs such as digoxin. Avoid in any patient likely to have intestinal obstruction. Avoid during pregnancy. Avoid during breastfeeding as anthraquinones can be secreted in breast milk.

YERBA SANTA – MOUNTAIN BALM – SACRED HERB

Eriodictyon californicum

Used by Native American healers for many centuries for bruises and inflammatory disorders. They smoked or chewed the leaves for asthma. Taken up by Spanish settlers who gave it its current name, meaning 'Holy Herb' or 'Holy Weed'.

Was listed in the US Pharmacopeia in 1894.

The US FDA has recognized yerba santa as a flavouring agent for beverages, food and pharmaceuticals.

Medicinal parts: Leaves, roots.

Uses: Treatment of respiratory conditions to promote removal of secretions from the lung and upper airways (expectorant). Used to relieve cough in chronic bronchitis and colds.

Other uses: A poultice made from fresh leaves is applied topically to relieve the soreness of bruises and sprains. Historically a sticky coating of yerba santa leaves was used to seal skin wounds before sterile bandages were widely available.

Probable mode of action: Constituents include five phenolic compounds, free formic and other acids, glycerides of fatty acids. The exact mode of action of the constituents is not known with certainty. One of the other constituents stimulates the flow of saliva. Some constituents have been studied as anticancer agents.

Adverse effects: No side-effects have been reported so far as the studies have been few. However, any unexpected effects should be reported to a physician.

Precautions: Not recommended during pregnancy or breastfeeding. Known to interfere with the absorption of co-administered iron and other minerals.

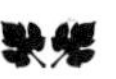

YEW – PACIFIC OR WESTERN YEW

Taxus baccata
Taxus brevifolia

Used by the Native Americans for arthritis, fever and rheumatism. Pacific yew bark is the source of the drug paclitaxel which is approved in allopathic medicine for the treatment of ovarian and breast carcinoma. Paclitaxel inhibits cell division by interfering with the formation of an essential intracellular component called microtubules.

Native Americans used extracts of yew for arthritis, fever and rheumatism.

Medicinal parts: Bough tips and bark.

Uses: In folk medicine, yew has been used to promote menstruation, induce abortion and treat diphtheria, tapeworm infestation, tonsillitis, epilepsy and rheumatism.

Probable mode of action: One of the constituents has been found to inhibit transport of calcium and sodium in heart muscle cells. Pacific yew bark contains 0.01% of paclitaxel, a drug used in allopathic medicine. It belongs to a group of constituents called taxols. Other constituents are lignans, tannins and resins.

Adverse effects: Ingestion of 50–100 g of yew needles can cause death. When taken orally it causes gastrointestinal irritation and slowing of the heart rate. Symptoms of poisoning are dry mouth, vomiting, vertigo, severe abdominal pain, weakness, trembling, shortness of breath (dyspnoea), arrhythmias, hypotension and unconsciousness.

Precautions: All parts of the plant are poisonous except the succulent covering of the seeds. The plant is considered toxic and is not suitable for self-prescription.

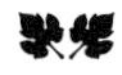

YOHIMBE

Pausinystalia yohimbe

Has been used as an aphrodisiac in Africa for centuries. Derived from the inner bark of the West

herbs

African coryanthe tree. Yohimbe bark is smoked or 'snuffed' for its hallucinogenic effects.

Medicinal parts: Bark.

Uses: Sexual dysfunction, male impotence and to increase libido.

Other uses: Angina, hypertension and diabetic neuropathy. Has been used to treat overdose of the allopathic medication clonidine.

Probable mode of action: Yohimbe bark contains 6% yohimbine. This constituent acts on receptors in the blood vessels to increase blood flow and is used to increase the blood flow to the penis while at the same time preventing blood from flowing out producing erectile stimulation.

Adverse effects: Oral intake of yohimbe causes excitation, tremor, insomnia, anxiety, tachycardia, nausea and vomiting. Yohimbine causes salivation, irritability and fluid retention. Has been documented to cause acute renal failure.

Precautions: Yohimbe can affect blood pressure, heart rate and raise anxiety levels. May prevent the effectiveness of antihypertensive (drugs used in the treatment of high blood pressure) agents like clonidine. May trigger psychosis (psychiatric disorders) in susceptible individuals. Theoretically the concomitant intake of caffeine-containing herbs (coffee, cola, guarana, mate, tea) can increase cardiovascular side-effects. Avoid if using St John's wort, ephedra and ginkgo. Avoid intake of cheese, fermented meats and red wine with yohimbine as the combination can raise blood pressure. Contraindicated in children and during pregnancy and breastfeeding.

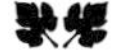

ZOAPATLE

Montana tormentosa
Montanoa frutescens

Zoapatle is a decoction made from *Montanoa tomentosa* which has been used as an oral contraceptive in traditional Mexican medicine for centuries. Records of the use go back to Spanish reports of 1529. It is also documented that for at least five centuries, the aqueous crude extract (ZACE) was used to induce labour, treat excess bleeding after childbirth (postpartum haemorrhage), and induce menstruation in Mexico. Today it is sold in street markets. *Montana tormentosa* differs from *Montana frutescens* in its effect on sperm motility.

Medicinal part: Leaves.

Uses: Used for induction of labour and treatment of bleeding after childbirth (postpartum haemorrhage).

Probable mode of action: Extensive studies have been carried out in laboratories and humans. The extracts of zoapatle caused significant dilatation of the cervix in human studies in Sweden. The antifertility effect apparently depends on the timing of administration in relation to menstruation and ovulation. Though laboratory experiments showed that *Montana tormentosa* did not influence sperm motility or viability, *Montana frutescens* was likely to do so. There are several constituents to which these effects have been attributed. In addition the herb has been found to contain potassium, calcium, magnesium and iron as inorganic constituents and chlorophyll, gum and pectin among the organic constituents.

Adverse effects: Rat studies have shown that the aqueous extract of zoapatle is devoid of acute and sub acute toxicity. In human studies, the extract was found to cause a 'menstrual-like cramp' and bleeding. No gastrointestinal symptoms were reported in this study.

Precautions: Should not be used during pregnancy. In 1998 there was report of cardiorespiratory depression in eight newborn infants whose mothers took yucuyahui (zoaptale) during labour. Hence should not be used in the induction of labour.

FURTHER READING

Bisset N, *Herbal Drugs and Phytopharmaceuticals.* Stuttgart, Germany: CRC Press, 1994:83–87.

Hardin JW, Arena JM. *Human Poisoning from Native and Cultivated Plants.* Durham, NC: Duke University Press, 1974.

3

Potentially Harmful Constituents of Some Herbal Medicines

Whether you are a user or a prescriber, it is important to be aware that herbal medicines can have toxic effects[1]. You should also be aware that though very occasionally there are cases of acute poisoning, toxic effects usually become apparent only after prolonged use of herbal medicines, and because of this the association between the toxic effects and the use of the medicine may not be immediately obvious. Ill-health may be protracted when a diagnosis is delayed, and this is particularly likely to happen when clinicians are unaware that the herbal medicine being used could contain toxic constituents.

Diagnosis and management of ill-health resulting from the use of herbal medicines containing contaminants or adulterants has been very challenging for physicians working in communities that frequently use traditional herbal medicines. For example, a Poison Control Centre in Taiwan reported experiencing difficulties in managing poisonings associated with Chinese traditional medicines, as 47% of the potential toxic effects of Chinese Traditional Medicines were either unknown or could not be found in the scientific literature. They concluded that 'there existed indefinable uncertainty in attributing the clinical effects to the exposures to Chinese traditional medicines'[2].

Children are particularly vulnerable to poisoning from traditional medicines. In Harare, Zimbabwe, of 2873 cases of poisoning in children reported between 1980 and 1989, 23% were associated with traditional medicines. In a second survey of 1456 cases of poisoning reportedly due to traditional medicines, by the same workers, over half (53%) involved patients who were under five years old. The overall mortality rate was

6%[3,4]. In Malawi, traditional medicines were implicated in six out of a total of 11 children who died from poisoning[5].

Harmful constituents may be introduced into herbal medicines unintentionally as contaminants or intentionally as adulterants. In many countries where herbal medicines are manufactured, quality control of manufacturing processes is inadequate and there is often considerable variation in the composition of products marketed at different times or by different manufacturers. The precise amount of adulterant may not be indicated on the label, package or package insert, and in some cases the presence of an adulterant may not be stated at all.

Contamination with toxic metals, such as lead, mercury and arsenic, may occur during the manufacture of herbal medicines. On the other hand, constituent herbs may be contaminated because they have accumulated toxic metals while growing on contaminated soil. The herbs may also have been exposed to polluted air or sprayed with pesticides or herbicides before harvesting. Medicines or their constituents may also become contaminated if stored in unfavourable or wrong conditions or treated with chemicals during storage[6,7].

A survey of imported Asian patent medicines collected from Californian retail herbal stores in 1998 gives some indication of the nature of the problem. Of the 260 products investigated, the Department of Health Services Food and Drug Branch found at least 83 (32%) contained undeclared pharmaceuticals or heavy metals, and 23 had more than one adulterant[8]. Although the remaining products contained no detectable adulterants, they could not be assumed to be free of toxic ingredients, because of the limitations of the analytical methods used, and because of the batch-to-batch inconsistency.

This chapter brings together information from the scientific literature and from our own practice in order to alert you to the potentially toxic constituents of herbal medicines. We wish to emphasize that there should be a greater element of suspicion, particularly with herbal products for slimming and fertility/sexual performance.

We have organized the chapter as follows.

1. A classification of the harmful constituents that have been frequently identified and reported.
2. A profile of the toxicity of each of these groups of constituents.
3. Plants/plant constituents that cause toxicity to the heart and blood vessels.
4. Plants/plant constituents that cause toxicity to the kidney.
5. Plants/plant constituents that cause toxicity to the liver.

If you wish to find further information about a herbal product that concerns you or a particular symptom, there is a list at the end of the chapter that should facilitate quick or easy reference. We list some herbal products which have been found to contain harmful constituents and the symptoms and signs that are commonly associated with toxicity from each of these harmful constituents.

CLASSIFICATION OF IMPORTANT HARMFUL CONSTITUENTS THAT HAVE BEEN FREQUENTLY DETECTED

- Heavy metals (i.e. lead, mercury, cadmium, arsenic, silver).
- Allopathic medications – prescription only and over-the-counter medications.
- Toxic plant constituents, e.g. alkaloids and the whole or parts of toxic plants.
- Animal and human body parts.
- Pesticides.

HEAVY METALS

Introduction

Heavy metals are used intentionally in traditional medicine systems in China, Asia (India), Mexico, Brazil and Africa. For example, the Indian system of medicine known as Ayurveda uses medicines containing lead, copper, iron, gold, silver, mercury, tin and zinc. Ayurvedic herbal preparations known as Bhamsas[9] may contain copper or iron. Kushtas, one of the traditional medicines used in Pakistan, has been reported to contain heavy metals such as lead, silver and mercury[10].

Mercury compounds, cinnabaris (mercuric sulphide), calomel (mercurous chloride) and hydragyri oxydum rubrum (mercuric oxide) are used in Chinese herbal medicines prescribed for tranquillizing, anticonvulsant or hypnotic effects and for ulcers. Chinese traditional physicians may include lead, chromium or cadmium, singly or in combination, in the herbal medicines prescribed for the treatment of heart diseases and disorders of the brain such as strokes[11].

Practitioners of traditional medicine from the ancient systems seem to have been aware of the possibility of toxicity from heavy metals. Some Indian and Chinese medical scriptures include information on adverse effects and also guidelines to minimize or eliminate toxicity during the preparation or formulation of medicines containing these heavy metals.

Prevalence

A number of studies have sought to estimate the prevalence of heavy metal contamination of traditional medicines.

Published evidence from Asia and America reveals that a considerable number of herbal products contain significant concentrations of heavy metals. An Indian survey revealed that 64% of the herbal products tested contained potentially toxic amounts of lead[12]. Further, some Ayurvedic medicines (30 of 31 products analysed) produced in India seem to contain mercury levels that exceed the legal limit of 1 ppm (part per million)[13]. The same survey revealed variability of mercury concentrations between the identical remedies produced by different companies, thus highlighting the lack of standards in their manufacture.

The situation in some parts of Asia is slightly better, possibly due to stringent efforts to maintain quality and safety. For example in Malaysia, where phase 3 registration for traditional medicines has been necessary since 1 January 1992 under the Control of Drugs and Cosmetics Regulation 1984, a survey found that 8% of herbal preparations contained lead levels that exceeded safe limits[15]. Likewise, only 2% of the 2080 Chinese proprietary medicines analysed in Singapore contained metals in amounts that exceeded safe levels[16]. Data from other parts of Asia are not available, but the problem should be a reflection of the rules of the respective regulatory authorities on these products.

Similarly, the issue of heavy metal toxicity from herbal medicines seems to be a significant problem in the West as well. A survey of 260 imported Asian herbal medicines in California[8] found unacceptably high concentrations of lead, arsenic and mercury in 95 products (36%).

In Boston, it was estimated that one in five (20%) Ayurvedic herbal remedies imported from South Asia and available at grocery stores contained potentially harmful levels of lead, mercury and/or arsenic[14].

Herbal products detected to contain heavy metals

Asia and the Middle East

Work done in China using atomic absorption spectrophotometry have revealed the presence of copper, zinc, nickel, cobalt, manganese, chromium, molybdenum, iron, calcium, magnesium, cadmium and lead in nine different kinds of traditional Chinese medicines used for diabetes. All except cadmium and lead were present in high concentrations[17]. Further, some Chinese medicines are known to contain extremely high levels of arsenic and mercury[18].

Of the heavy metals found in herbal remedies, lead is a common constituent of many Asian and Middle Eastern herbal remedies, while mercury too has been found in some preparations[19–24].

Lead has been found in the following folk remedies of this region: paylooah, a Vietnamese folk remedy used in China and South East Asia for childhood fever and rash; ghasard, an Asian Indian folk remedy (usually in the form of a brown powder) used as a tonic to aid digestion; Bint al dahab (daughter of gold), used in Oman and the United Arab Emirates for neonates and children with stomach ailments; santrinj, an amorphous red powder containing lead that is used in Saudi Arabia, principally as a primer for paint for metallic surfaces, but also applied as a home remedy for gum boils and teething; and an orange powder prescribed by traditional medicine practitioners in Saudi Arabia for teething and diarrhoea.

A brick red powder used in the treatment of vitiligo in Oman was found to contain a mixture of cinnabar (HgS) and calomel (Hg_2Cl_2).

US and Mexico

Empacho, a term used to identify a group of Mexican folk remedies for gastrointestinal disorders, has been responsible for lead toxicity. Three products in this group, namely azarcon (also known as alarcon, coral, luiga, Maria Luisa and rueda), greta and albayalde, have been tested in laboratories and found to have lead contents as high as 80–90%[25,26].

Some herbal balls, which are mixtures of medicinal herbs and honey that are added to warm wine or water to make herbal tea, are often contaminated with arsenic and mercury[27].

UK

Cases of lead poisoning from traditional Indian herbal medicines continue to be reported to the poisons units of the UK. Some of these herbal preparations are bought outside the UK while some are bought from dealers within the country. These products are used mainly by patients of Asian ethnic origin for the treatment of chronic disorders such as diabetes mellitus.

There are also reports of Chinese medicines containing mercury (in the form of cinnabar), arsenic and lead being available in the UK. If these products were to be consumed as prescribed for a long period, consumers could develop severe mercury intoxication[28]. The MHRA, based on the analysis of two traditional Chinese medicines containing 11% and 3% of mercury, concluded that the mercuric salts present in these products could have caused unpleasant symptoms such as nausea, abdominal pain, vomiting, diarrhoea, headache and more importantly serious damage to the kidneys and nervous system. Furthermore, any pregnant woman taking these products would have been at risk of miscarriage and possible damage to the foetus[29]. Reports of Ayurvedic medicines containing significant levels of arsenic in isolation (57 ppm of arsenic reported by the MRHA in an Ayurvedic liquid blood purifier seized from a London retail store in 2005[30]) and in combination with lead and mercury continue to appear in the literature[31].

Africa

Lead was detected in traditional medicines in Nigeria in 1984 by Healy et al.[32], and more recently, manganese (as potassium permanganate), chromium (as potassium dichromate) and arsenic[33] were also detected. However contamination of African traditional remedies such as muti with toxic metals has been infrequently reported.

Eye paints[34–36]

Eye paints have been nearly universal since the Bronze Age and were used across North Africa, the Middle East and South Asia from very early times. Egyptians used galena (lead sulphide) and powdered malachite (a green blue mineral which occurs naturally as a surface mineral in the Sinai) to outline their eyes. Ancient Egyptian men and women wore eye paints from childhood throughout their lives and were adorned even in death. Even the statues of Egyptian gods had their eye paints applied daily.

The black paint provided relief from the glaring sun and reflection from the sand before sunglasses were invented. Lamp-black (soot) was the most common source of pigment, though galena (lead sulphide) and stibnite (an antimony compound) were also used for black, and copper compounds for blues and greens. These metals were toxic to bacteria carried by flies and were considered to provide some relief from conjunctivitis and other bacterial infections of the eye. In the 6th century, Alexander of Tralle described kohls made of burnt cadmium, copper, acacia gum, aloes, spikenard, opium, myrrh, lead, burnt ebony, copper, roses and rain water. In the 17th century, Celsus described 26 formulae for kohl and collyria. Five used burnt copper and others used lead, ash from fragrant woods and copper compounds.

Most women applied kohl every week or for any social occasion except during Ramadan and believed that blackening their eyelids and eye brows would protect them from the glance of the 'Evil Eye' and also prevent them from transmitting the 'Evil Eye' to another person. Mothers applied kohl to their infants soon after birth. They blackened the baby's eyes, dabbed kohl on their umbilical cord and darkened their eyebrows. Mothers applied kohl to their children, both male and female, until they were old enough to apply it themselves.

In Afghanistan, women made surma by pounding antimony with almond oil to make a paste and applied it with a small wood stylus. Felix Howland wrote from Kabul in 1936 that students often came to school with blackened eyes as a claim that they had studied so hard that they had strained their eyes.

These eye paint preparations containing lead and antimony were toxic and particularly dangerous when used in children and women. Present day commercial kohl and surma preparations often contain dangerously high levels of lead.

In 2002, Steenkamp et al.[37] described a severe case of multiple metal poisoning in a child treated with a traditional medicine. Analysis of the traditional remedy, a black powder, revealed very high concentrations of iron and manganese.

In the context of traditional medicine toxicity in Africa, the vulnerability and prevalence in children in countries such as Zimbabwe and Malawi were indicated earlier in this chapter[3–5].

The metals most commonly reported in African traditional remedies (muti) are manganese (as potassium permanganate), chromium (as potassium dichromate) and arsenic[38].

Ill-health due to the presence of heavy metals in herbal medications

One of the earliest published cases of heavy metal poisoning due to the use of a traditional medicine was in 1975[39]. Since then there have been a large number of such poisonings published[40–42].

A survey of 5536 exposures to traditional

medicines and food supplements reported to the National Poisons Unit in London from January 1983 to March 1989 and in 1991 included 657 (12%) reports of symptomatic cases and five confirmed cases of heavy metal poisoning resulting from the use of contaminated traditional remedies. The same unit reported 12 cases of poisoning with lead, arsenic or mercury between 1991 and 1995, nine of which were associated with herbal remedies from India, and three with use of Indian cosmetics[43].

In 1988, Venter and Joubert[44] found traditional medicines to account for nearly 16% of all acute poisoning in Pretoria, South Africa, and the associated mortality was 15%.

In 2005, a review by Lynch and Braithwaite[38] found 31 published cases of poisoning by lead, arsenic, mercury and magnesium resulting from the use of Indian traditional medicines. The reports came from the UK, US, Canada, Australia, India, Israel, Germany, The Netherlands, and Qatar. A total of 71% of these patients were of an Indian ethnic origin and 10% were of white ethnic origin. The patients' ages ranged from nine months to 70 years.

Reports of lead poisoning

There have been numerous reports of lead poisoning due to herbal remedies from many parts of the world. Between 1 December 1991 and 31 December 1992, the Californian Department of Health Services received reports of 40 cases of blood lead levels (≥20 μg/dl), exceeding the CDC level of concern in children who had received traditional ethnic remedies[45]. Twelve cases of adult lead poisoning due to Ayurvedic medicines were reported from the US during 2002 and 2003[46].

In Oman, in 1990, 25 infants, ranging in age from one to eight months, were admitted with acute lead encepahalopathy[47]. The source of poisoning in 20 infants proved to be bint al dahab. In a further three infants, there was a strong recent history of administration of this local medication, but the agent could not be identified with certainty. The lead encephalopathy had serious consequences: only 44% of infants were thought to be neurologically normal at the time of discharge. Bint al dahab analysed by Worthing et al. in 1995[24] using X-ray diffraction and X-ray microanalyser studies found that it contained two polymorphs of lead monoxide (PbO). These studies also showed the presence of cadmium and third complex monoxide of lead containing antimony. Bulk analyses showed that the substance contained approximately 91 g of lead monoxide, 600 mg of antimony oxide and 50 mg of cadmium per 100 g of bint al dahab.

A powder prescribed by traditional medicine practitioners for teething and diarrhoea caused lead poisoning in three Saudi Arabian children aged 11, 22 and 44 months[48] and santrinj caused lead poisoning in seven children aged 7 days to 13 months[20].

In 2005, in Rhode Island, two siblings were found to have elevated blood lead levels associated with use of litargirio[49], a remedy traditionally used to treat dysentery in small children, and to calm fright, remove phlegm, relieve convulsions (e.g. epilepsy or convulsions due to fever) and kill intestinal parasites. Litargirio, also known as litharge, is listed by the Illinois Department of Public Health[19] and the Rhode Island Department of Health as a potential source of lead exposure for Hispanic children. Litargirio was a popular traditional remedy, particularly of people from the Dominican Republic, and was sold in 2 inch by 3 inch clear packets by convenience and specialty stores catering to Spanish speaking customers. In 2003, the FDA in the US[50] advised the public to:

- Stop all personal use of litargirio immediately.
- Place unused product in a sealable container or plastic bag and contact the local sanitation/waste department regarding appropriate methods for disposal.
- Thoroughly wash hands and any other body parts that may have come in contact with the powder. Wash affected household surfaces with soap and hot water.

- Ask a healthcare provider to test children or pregnant/nursing women for lead poisoning if they have used litargirio.

Heavy metal poisoning has also been reported from Ayurvedic preparations. In 2006, a report suggested that the heavy metal components of the bhamsas have the potential to cause toxicity[9]. Four adults among 29 who had taken Ayurvedic mineral tonics had established lead poisoning which was successfully treated with chelation therapy[51].

Toxicity due to lead was reported in a five-year-old child after the ingestion of a Tibetan herbal vitamin used to 'strengthen the brain'. Herbal vitamin preparations are commonly used in China, India and Tibet and other South Asian countries[23].

There have been reports of heavy metal poisoning from paylooah and ghasard (an Indian folk remedy used as a tonic to aid digestion)[19]. Lead poisoning has also been caused by bokhoor, a traditional practice of burning wood (Kuwait) and lead sulphide to produce pleasant fumes to calm infants[52].

Products with the highest content of lead were usually being used by male patients for treating fertility disorders[38]. However, it has been shown that high levels of lead exposure in men decreases sperm count and motility, in addition to an increased number of morphologically abnormal sperms. A study had shown that blood lead levels between 40 and 50 µg/dl were associated with low sperm count, decreased sperm motility and abnormal sperm. The effects on fertility are most likely when blood lead levels are >50 µg/dl for prolonged periods[38].

Reports of mercury poisoning

It was recognized in the early 1990s that Chinese patent herbal medicines commonly used in the US, contained cinnabar (red mercuric sulphide) or calomel (mercurous chloride). Medical practitioners were alerted to the need to consider the possibility of mercury poisoning when investigating the cause of ill-health in patients using these medicines, whether or not they were of Asian ethnic background[53].

Wong (2002)[54] reported acute generalized dermatitis, abnormal liver function and elevated blood mercury level (187 nmol/L) associated with Chinese herbal medicine used for rheumatism by an 80-year-old Chinese patient. The elevated blood mercury level returned to normal range upon discontinuation of this Chinese herbal medicine, while his diet remained unchanged.

Daily exposure to 180–252 mg cinnabar in a herbal medicine for four weeks resulted in mercury poisoning[55].

Reports of arsenic poisoning

Tay and Seah (1975)[39] detected arsenic poisoning over a 15-month period in 74 patients. Approximately one-third (64%) of the cases were caused by a local antiasthmatic herbal preparation containing 12,000 ppm of inorganic arsenic sulphide. The other patients were poisoned by six other brands of herbal preparations used for the treatment of asthma and a variety of other illnesses. Subsequent investigations revealed 22 other brands of Chinese herbal preparations, most of which were imported preparations, containing high concentrations of inorganic arsenic ranging from 25 to 107,000 ppm. Nearly 40% of the patients had taken the medicine for less than six months, but the others had a longer history of exposure ranging from one to 15 years. Systemic involvement was confined mainly to the skin (91%), nervous system (51%), gastrointestinal system (23%) and blood (23%). Malignancy of the skin was present in six patients.

Between 1983 and April 1984, physicians at the Saint Paul Ramsay Medical Center in Saint Paul, Minnesota diagnosed arsenic poisoning in three Hmong patients[56]. Hmong were recent immigrants to the US from the highland areas of northern Laos. The source of the arsenic poisoning was suspected to be Hmong folk remedies.

The *Wisconsin Medical Journal* in 2001[57] reported the investigation of two Hmong children aged one and two years for elevated blood lead levels. The investigators were provided with a reddish-brown powder that they had been administered for medicinal purposes. The powder was analysed at the Wisconsin State Laboratory of Hygiene and was found to consist of 36% arsenic, the bulk of the material being arsenic sulphide or realgar. The elevated lead levels were attributed to lead paint in the house. The medicine had been purchased at a store in California and was used to treat chicken pox, flu-like symptoms and nasal congestion.

Other metals

Seven cases of dichromate poisoning in purgative solutions obtained from nyanga (traditional township healers) have been reported[33].

There is also report of kidney damage attributed to Chinese herbal medicines containing cadmium[58].

> Common clinical signs and symptoms of lead, mercury, arsenic, chromium, copper and silver poisoning are presented at the end of the chapter in Appendix I.
>
> Some herbal products in which heavy metals were detected are provided at the end of the chapter in Appendix II.

ALLOPATHIC MEDICATIONS

Introduction

The use of allopathic medicines in herbal preparations may pose considerable problems to both regulators and clinicians[59].

In contrast to heavy metals, synthetic medications are usually added to traditional medicines to increase the speed of response and effectiveness.

Although the addition of allopathic medications to herbal medicines is not permitted in countries with strict regulatory systems, in many of the countries where herbal medicines are manufactured, it is considered acceptable provided that the nature and quantity of the allopathic medication is specified on the label.

Clinicians managing ill-health must be aware of the wide range of allopathic medications that may be included in herbal medications. Products imported, and particularly those regularly used by migrant communities, may include allopathic medications banned in countries such as the UK and US.

Clinicians also need to be aware of the possibility of variations in constituents between batches and between products made by different manufacturers, and the possibility of inaccurate product labelling and product literature, which, as noted at the beginning of this chapter, may not state the presence of adulterants or the precise amounts present. The label will in any case be of no help if written in a language/script which cannot be read by a clinician.

The ever increasing concern about adulterants is highlighted this month in a paper in the *Journal Legal Medicine* where Miller and Stripp record that they analysed 90 samples of randomly purchased tablets, pills, creams and teas from China Town New York and found that 5 samples contained nine different western pharmaceuticals. Two of these samples contained undeclared or mislabelled substances. One sample contained two pharmaceuticals contraindicated in people for whom the product was intended. Drugs identified included promethazine, chlormethiazole, chlorpheniramine, diclofenac, chlordiazepoxide, hydrochlorothiazide, trianterene, diphenhydramine and sildenfil citrate (Viagra).

Another issue of great concern is the use of compounds that are chemically similar derivatives of restricted allopathic medications. This may be a fraudulent attempt to circumvent regulatory restrictions of countries such as the UK or to make detection more difficult. An example of this was reported from Canada, where a compound closely similar to sildenafil was added to a Chinese herbal product, which claimed to restore mental alertness[60].

Similarly N-nitrosofenfluramine has been used instead of fenfluramine in some Asian herbal weight-loss remedies, because fenfluramine is banned in the UK and several other countries. However, N-nitroso compounds have been linked with carcinogenesis in the liver. In 2002, the Japanese authorities received reports of 474 cases of hepatotoxicity associated with the use of herbal weight-loss remedies, many of which were found to contain fenfluramine or N-nitrosofenfluramine. Two patients developed fulminant hepatic failure and in only one was a liver transplant successful[61].

Prevalence

The prevalence of allopathic medicines in herbal preparations has been of particular concern in Asian countries with large Chinese populations.

The Taiwanese FDA (Annual Report of National Laboratories of Foods and Drugs, 1990 and 1991)[62] reported that 30% of the antirheumatic and analgesic herbal products that they sampled contained allopathic drugs including paracetamol, aminopyrine, caffeine, chlormezanone, chloroxazone, diazepam, diclofenac, ethoxybenzamide, hydrochlorothiazide, ibuprofen, indometacin, ketoprofen, mefenamic acid, papaverine, phenylbutazone, piroxicam, prednisolone and salicylamide. Aminopryine and phenylbutazone are no longer prescribed in the UK.

Another study in Taiwan analysed 2609 samples and found that 26% contained at least one adulterant. The most common adulterants included caffeine, acetaminophen, indometacin, hydrochlorothiazide, prednisolone, chloroxazone and ethoxybenzamide. Several of these medications could cause serious adverse side-effects resulting in fatal or debilitating medical disorders[63].

In Hong Kong the Government Laboratory carried out 65,748 tests on Chinese medicines in 2004[64]. Many of the proprietary Chinese medicines on sale for treatment of obesity and impotence caused the most concern. They were found to contain sidenafil, tadalafil, sibutramine and N-nitrosofenfluramine. The problem appears to be increasing: the number of Chinese proprietary samples for the treatment of obesity and impotence submitted to the laboratory for analysis increased six-fold between 2003 and 2004.

In Malaysia in 1991, 83% (25 out of 30) of antiarthritis preparations seized from Chinese medicine shops contained phenylbutazone (an aspirin-like anti-inflammatory drug) in amounts ranging from 0.6 to 198 mg per pill or capsule. Black pills[65] for arthritis known as zhui feng tou gu wan or black pearls have also been reported to contain phenylbutazone.

Adulteration is a widespread practice and has been reported from Australia, Belgium, Canada, The Netherlands, New Zealand, the UK and US[1].

In 1999, eight out of 11 Chinese herbal creams available in London for the treatment of eczema were found to contain dexamethasone at concentrations inappropriate for use on the face or in children[66].

The 1998 Californian survey of imported Asian patent medicines[8] revealed that of the 257 products that were analysed for pharmaceuticals, 17 products contained pharmaceuticals that were not declared on the label (most commonly ephedrine, chlorpheniramine, methyltestosterone and phenacetin).

In India, 38% of 120 samples of alternative medicines that had been dispensed to patients suffering mainly from asthma and arthritis were found to be adulterated with steroids[67].

Dangers

The rather complex combinations of allopathic and traditional herbal medicines could lead to one or more of the following scenarios:

1. The herbal drug been taken in excess of the prescribed dose or for an extended duration leading to the safe dose of the allopathic constituents being unknowingly exceeded.
2. The herbal medicine containing an amount of allopathic medication capable of producing toxic or adverse effects.
3. Exposure to the allopathic constituent within the herbal medicine exacerbating the disease state for which the herbal medicine is taken.
4. Harmful interaction/s occurring between the allopathic constituent in the herbal medicine

and allopathic medicine/s prescribed by a general practitioner or other allopathic medical practitioners.

5. An undeclared allopathic constituent of a herbal medication producing a complication or adverse effect, the diagnosis of which being delayed or completely missed, results in severe ill-health. This is a particularly so in long-term consumers of herbal medicines.

Reports of ill-health

The reports of ill-health associated with most of the herbal medicines documented in this section are not due to the herb but to the allopathic medication which had been introduced to the herbal medicine.

In 1975 a subject who was taking Chinese herbal medicines for the relief of arthritis and back pain developed agranulocytosis (dangerously low levels of neutrophils, cells that protect against infections) and life-threatening infections with bacterial sepsis resulting in death. The herbal medicines were shown to contain substantial amounts of undeclared aminopyrine and phenylbutazone, drugs that are well-known causes of agranulocytosis.

Slimming agents in particular have caused severe liver disease including liver failure due to the allopathic constituent[68,69].

> A list of some herbal medicines which have been found to contain allopathic medicines is provided at the end of the chapter in Appendix III. This list also indicates some of the potential adverse effects of the allopathic medications.

ANIMAL/HUMAN PARTS

Inclusion of animal and human products in traditional herbal medicines can have two possible consequences.

Firstly, they may transmit infections to the user. For example, the ingredients of nu bao include human placenta (placenta hominis), deer antler (*Corna cervi pantotrichum*) and donkey skin (*Colla cori astini*), which are potential sources of bacteria and viruses that could transmit infection.

Secondly, some constituents that are used medicinally are potentially toxic (not a contaminant); the toxin is part of the medicine. For example, venom extracted from skin glands of certain species of toads (*Bufo marinus, Bufo alvarius*) is used in some aphrodisiacs and some other Chinese medications (e.g. chan su). The venom contains bufotoxins, which have similar molecular structure and pharmacological effects to digoxin. These preparations can cause symptoms and clinical findings very similar to digitalis overdose and toxicity (e.g. persistent nausea and vomiting, light-headedness, slowing of the heart rate, palpitations, insomnia, seeing yellow halos around lights) and have led to dangerous alterations in heart rhythm and even death[70].

> A list of some of the herbal medicines known to contain animal and human parts is provided at the end of the chapter in Appendix IV.

TOXINS OF PLANT ORIGIN[71,72]

Some plants have always been known to be toxic to man and even to cause death. These naturally occurring toxins present in plants are commonly referred to as phytotoxins. While most of the information on the toxicity of plants remains anecdotal, studies on toxic components of plants have also resulted as a result of serious 'unexplained' adverse effects in agricultural livestock or when similar disease processes occur in groups of humans who have received a particular form of herbal treatment. For example, the occurrence of kidney disease or liver disease in groups of patients who had received a particular form of herbal treatment has, at least within the past three decades, provoked or 'kick-started' the study of toxic constituents of herbs.

Obviously, concentrations of the toxic constituents in herbal preparations are an important consideration. The presence of a toxic component does not always imply that an adverse effect will follow intake. Thus concentrations of the toxic component, the dosages of the herb taken and the duration of intake are all important factors in the discussion of toxicity of plants.

For example, with herbal teas and honey, the amount or frequency of consumption is important. With herbal teas and honey, the fact that large quantities may be consumed over a long periods is an important factor in the toxicity[73–76].

Toxicological studies on herbal teas have been limited. It is possible for some herbal teas, that during the course of their preparation or formulation may lead to the concentration of some toxic constituents[76]. This would of course be true of water soluble toxic constituents.

Of the known toxic constituents of plants, arguably the best known are the pyrrolizidine alkaloids. Other toxic constituents belong to the chemical classes such as glycosides, glycoalkaloids, saponins and psoralens. An important consideration is that some biologically inactive toxic constituents or phytotoxins may become toxic following metabolism in the human body. Further, some constituents may have the potential to cause changes in genes (mutagenicity) or cause cancers (carcinogenicity).

In addition, some plants such as soya and peanut contain allergens. Also, there is a possibility that some plants may have chemicals that alter the secretion and function of hormones in the body which are then referred to as endocrine disruptors.

According to Chan and Critchley[77], preparations containing aconite, podophyllin or anticholinergics are the cause of nearly all serious poisonings associated with plant constituents of herbal medicines in Hong Kong.

In this section of toxic plant constituents, those that are relatively well-known for causing kidney (renal) and liver (hepatic) toxicity are discussed. Thus there would be some repetition when in the latter part of the chapter there are discussions on plants known to cause renal and hepatic toxicity.

Pyrrolizidine alkaloids (PAs)

Of all plant toxins, the unsaturated pyrrolizidine alkaloids (PAs) have been most frequently associated with disease in humans and animals[78,79].The PAs have been reported to have properties that destroy cells (cytotoxic) including cancer cells and also paradoxically cause cancers (carcinogenic). They are also known to affect genes (genotoxic activity) both under experimental conditions and in the body (*in vitro* and *in vivo*).

They are common constituents of thousands of plant species around the world. More than 350 PAs have been identified in over 6000 plants in the Boraginaceae, Compositae and Leguminosae families. Many of the plants belonging to these families are commonly used in Chinese herbal medicines[80]. However not all pyrrolizidine alkaloids are toxic; it is only the unsaturated form which can be converted to cytotoxic pyrroles that are of health concern.

Comfrey, which has long been one of the most popular herbs in European folk medicine, was found to contain PAs in the 1960s and since then controversy has surrounded its use. Australia banned comfrey for internal use in 1984 and listed it as a dangerous poison available only from pharmacists. Other countries such as Canada and US have also restricted its use[81]. Comfrey and other herbs such as coltsfoot are used topically for injuries or joint pain. They should not be used on broken skin.

Toxicity of PAs

After absorption from the gut, the unsaturated PAs are converted in the liver to toxic metabolites (electrophyllic pyrroles) that damage the liver and may also affect the lungs, kidneys and heart[79].

Comfrey, for example, causes veno-occlusive disease of the small veins in the liver – blocking or occluding the small veins in the liver leading to cirrhosis and eventually to liver failure. Patients may present with clinical signs of portal hypertension (increased pressure in the portal veins which feed the liver). An enlarged liver (hepatomegaly) and abdominal pain are among the main features. These features may be of sudden (acute) origin and may also develop over a longer period of time (chronic).

A further concern is that some PA adducts may be persistent in animal tissues and these metabolites may be re-released and cause damage long after the initial period of ingestion.

Reports of poisoning

There are several historical accounts of toxic exposures involving individual or mass poisonings due to pyrrolizidine alkaloids.

'Bush tea disease', the local name for hepatic veno-occlusive disease, was described in Jamaican children in 1954[82,83]. In 1976, an outbreak of hepatic veno-occlusive disease was reported in Afghanistan. Examination of 7200 inhabitants from the affected villages in Afghanistan showed evidence of liver disease in 22.6%[84].The same year, an epidemic of veno-occlusive disease of liver was reported from Central India, where 42% of the recorded cases died[85,86]. There have been some doubts following further investigation as to causation in this instance.

In 1976, veno-occlusive disease of the liver in a fetus associated with herbal tea consumption by the mother was reported in the UK in a woman addicted to mate tea from Paraguay[87]. The diagnosis was made from liver biopsies and hepatic venography and was confirmed at post mortem. Small amounts of PAs were recovered from a sample of the tea.

More recently a study in two hospitals in South Africa identified 20 children suffering from veno-occlusive disease of the liver thought to be caused by administration of traditional remedies. Most of those who survived progressed to develop cirrhosis and portal hypertension[88].

Also from South Africa is the report of a child given a short course of treatment with a traditional herb remedy who died as a result of hepatic veno-occlusive disease[89].

> Some common sources of PAs, toxic effects and clinical features of PAs are indicated at the end of the chapter in Appendix V.

Kava kava (*Piper methysticum*)[90–92]

Kava, more correctly known as kava kava, is a herbal shrub that has been used for centuries in the South Pacific as a social beverage and in traditional ceremonial rituals as a symbol of welcome and respect to visiting guests and dignitaries.

In the past two decades, kava has been used in the West for treating mild and moderate anxiety, stress, insomnia, restlessness and muscle fatigue and has been one of the 10 top selling herbal preparations. Results from *in vivo* and *in vitro* studies suggest that kava produces most of these effects via a small number of pharmacological mechanisms, namely blockade of voltage-gated sodium and calcium ion channels, reduced transmitter (chemical messenger) release, blockade of receptors for chemical transmitters such as gamma amino butyric acid (GABA) and benzodiazepines (e.g. Valium), and reduction of monoamine (amino acids which produce biological effects) levels.

The kavalactones are thought to be the main active constituents. These will vary depending on the cultivar and other geographic conditions under which they are produced.

The most commonly reported adverse effects include gastrointestinal symptoms, allergic skin reactions and photosensitivity and headache. There is some evidence to suggest that there is a synergistic effect with substances such as alcohol, barbiturates and psychopharmacological agents that act on the central nervous system. There are also concerns about antagonism of dopamine, so it should be used with caution in patients with Parkinson's disease. As it may cause drowsiness it should be avoided by individuals operating machinery. It was not recommended for use in pregnancy, by breastfeeding mothers, by children or in combination with alcohol and other substances which depress the nervous system.

However, in the past few years, severe side-effects including liver damage have been reported in Europe and the US. A total of 110 reports of suspected liver toxicity have been received from around the world – these range from abnormal liver function to acute liver failure requiring liver transplant and death. By January 2003, kava extracts had been banned in the entire European Union and Canada, and were subject to cautions and advisories by the US FDA as a result of 11 cases of hepatic failure leading to liver transplants, including four deaths.

Three possible mechanisms for kavalactone hepatotoxicity need to be considered:

1. Inhibition of cytochrome P450 enzymes which are responsible for the metabolism of a large number of pharmaceutical agents, thus elevating the blood levels of concurrent medications to toxic levels.
2. Direct toxicity of kavalactones or other constituents.
3. Inhibition of cyclo-oxygenase enzyme activity.

The direct toxicity of kava extracts is quite small under any analysis, yet the potential for drug interactions and/or the potentiation of the toxicity of other compounds is large.

There is controversy as regards the mechanism/s and incidence of liver toxicity (hepatotoxicity) and the withdrawal of kava products from sale in many countries. Kava kava and its products are a good example of the difficulties associated with establishing a cause–effect relationship of toxicity with herbal products.

Aristolochic acids93

Aristolochic acid nephropathy

Aristolochia (e.g. *Aristolochia fangchi*) is also known as birthwort, snakeroot, guang fan ji and pelican flower. The various species of *Aristolochia* or other members of the Aristolochiacea family have been used in many herbal traditions for a range of medicinal uses including gastrointestinal colic, as an immune stimulant and as an aphrodisiac. The main species used in Chinese medicine are *Aristolochia manshuriensis, A. debilis* and *A. fangchi.* In India, the main species used, *A. indica*, is reported to be a stimulant, tonic and febrifuge; it is used for snakebites, diarrhoea and intermittent fevers. Other species used in India are *A. longa, A. rotunda, A. roxburghiana*, and *A. serpentaria.*

Although there was some traditional knowledge of possible renal toxicity of the aristolochic acids contained within this genus, this was not investigated fully until the 1990s. This was prompted by the serious incident in Belgium when patients attending a weight loss clinic developed kidney damage and renal failure. Due to confusion over the names and identity of plants, the clinic erroneously used *Aristolochia fangchi* in a combination therapy with other herbs and drugs including acetazolamide, diethylpropion and fenfluramine. This resulted in approximately 112 patients with renal failure requiring dialysis, at least half of whom required kidney transplants.[94,95,96] Approximately a quarter of these patients also developed carcinoma of the urinary tract. Symptoms of kidney damage may be delayed for up to 3 years after stopping use of the herb. Individual patient susceptibility as well as cumulative dose of aristolochic acid are likely to be significant factors in toxicity. In recent years, reports of aristolochic acid-related nephropathy have come from all over the world, including France, the Balkans, Japan, Hong Kong, China and Taiwan. There have been five similar cases reported from the UK.[97–99]

Medicinal use of the herbs has been banned or restricted in most countries, but some products containing *Aristolochia* have been found for sale on the Internet. Products suspected to contain any *Aristolochia* species should not be used for therapeutic purposes.

Ficus insipida[100]

Ficus insipida is a majestic fig tree. Known as ojé in Peru, its latex is still used by indigenous and local people in the Amazonian regions in an antihelminthic (helminths are round-worms) remedy.

A survey of the case files from two hospitals in Peru found 37 patients were admitted with a diagnosis of ojé poisoning in the 12 years from 1992 to 2003. The annual frequency of admission remained fairly steady throughout this period[97].

The time between ingestion and the appearance of adverse or toxic reactions varied between 20 minutes and 2 days in 23 cases where the information was available. The number of days the patients were hospitalized varied between 1 and 12.

Central nervous system and gastrointestinal symptoms dominated in both children and adults. There were slightly more musculoskeletal reactions among children and slightly more cardiovascular and respiratory reactions among the adults. The most common adverse effects were those on the gastrointestinal system. Atypical reactions such as allergic itching and oedema of the lower extremities were also seen. Three patients died.

Atractylis gummifera[101–104]

Atractylis gummifera L is a thistle located in the Mediterranean regions and is especially abundant in Algeria, Morocco, Tunisia, Italy, Greece, Spain and Portugal. Most poisonings occur unintentionally; the plant is easily mistaken for wild artichoke and is popular with small children who enjoy chewing the root as they would chew gum.

Toxicity is attributed to the toxic glycoside atractyloside, which is a powerful inhibitor of oxidative phosphorylation in mitochondria.

In 1954 a report from Algeria described two children, aged four and six years, who arrived at hospital with violent abdominal colic and severe vomiting followed by cyanosis and coma after ingestion of *Atractylis gummifera*. They died the next morning. Histopathology showed congested intestine, peritoneal exudates and haemorrhages in the stomach and kidney. A year later several children in Italy were poisoned, and there were three deaths.

The Tunisian Poison Centre reported that nearly a third of patients (18 out of 56) who were admitted to intensive care units due to plant poisoning between 1983 and 1998 were suffering from *Atractylis gummifera* poisoning[105].

The symptoms usually begin 6–36 hours after ingestion. Typical symptoms are nausea, vomiting, epigastric and abdominal pain, and diarrhoea. There may be accompanying nervous system symptoms such as anxiety, headache, drowsiness, convulsions and coma. There is usually marked elevation of liver enzymes (SGOT, SGPT, bilirubin) and there may be biochemical evidence of renal dysfunction.

No specific pharmacological treatment is currently available to treat *Atractylis gummifera* poisoning: symptoms should be managed supportively.

Aconite[106–109]

Aconites are the dried rootstocks or tubers of *Aconitum* plants. In Hong Kong, they are known as chuan-wu, the main root of *Aconitum carmichaeli*, or cao-wu (the root of *Aconitum kusnezoffi*) and as monkshood or wolf's bane (*Aconitum napellus*) in Europe and the US.

They have been used to treat rheumatism, bruises, fractures, hemiplegia, diarrhoea and abdominal pain. Both chuan-wu and cao-wu have been used in Chinese materia medica, mainly for the treatment of musculoskeletal disorders, and are believed to possess anti-inflammatory, analgesic and cardiotonic effects.

The rootstock is the most toxic part of the plant and is processed to decrease toxicity, usually by soaking or boiling. The principal toxic ingredients are C19-diterpenoid alkaloids (aconitine, mesaaconitine and hypaconitine). Toxicity has occurred after 0.2 mg of aconite or 6 g of processed, prescription rootstocks.

Aconite activates the sodium channels and has widespread effects on excitable membranes of the heart, muscle and nerve tissues. Aconite can produce life-threatening slowing of the heart or increase in heart rate and may stop breathing. Paraesthesia, hypersalivation, dizziness, ataxia, nausea, vomiting, diarrhoea and weakness of the muscles of breathing may begin as soon as a few minutes after ingestion or be delayed for several hours.

In China, 1133 reports of adverse reactions were reported in the Chinese scientific literature during 1993 to 1994. The most common herb-related adverse reactions were associated with Aconite roots followed by *Tripterygium wilfordii*.

Podophyllin[110–113]

The dried roots, rhizomes and resin of *Podophyllum hexandrum* and *Podophyllum peltatum* (American mandrake, devil's apple, mayapple) have been used orally as cathartics and topically for wart removal. Bajiaolian, the root of *Dysoma pleianthum*, also called *Podophyllum pleianthum*, a herb that contains podophyllotoxin, has been used in China for thousands of years in the treatment of weakness, snake bite, tumours and enlargement of lymph nodes.

According to Chan and Critchley[77] podophyllin is one of the phytotoxins most often associated with serious poisonings due to herbal medicines.

Major active components are lignan derivatives including podophyllotoxin. Podophyllin blocks cell division and inhibits the activity of mitochondria.

Toxicity may occur with topical or oral administration and generally occurs within 12 hours. Signs and symptoms of toxicity include abdominal pain, nausea, vomiting, vomiting of blood (haematemesis), kidney failure, bone marrow depression, altered mental state, seizures, paralysis, acidosis and death. Ocular lesions may also follow podophyllin toxicity.

Within one year Kao et al.[112] saw five patients who presented with nausea, vomiting, diarrhoea, abdominal pain, thrombocytopenia, leucopenia, abnormal liver function tests, sensory ataxia, altered consciousness and persistent peripheral tingling or numbness after drinking infusions made with bajiaolian.

The common name of mandrake caused confusion in the case of a 31-year-old man who ingested an unknown amount of podophyllum which he purchased at a local health food store in the mistaken belief that it was the hallucinatory plant *Mandragora officinarum*, also known as mandrake[114]. He presented to the emergency department with nausea and vomiting and recovered uneventfully after a night in hospital. The poisoning was considered to be due to *Podophyllum peltatum* based on chromatographic identification of podophillotoxin in a sample.

Ng et al.[115] reported encephalopathy and neuropathy following ingestion of a Chinese herbal broth (gui jiu) containing podophyllin. Delayed recognition of podophyllum toxicity in a patient receiving epidural morphine has been reported[116].

Camellia sinensis (Chinese green tea)[117]

An association between health supplements containing green tea extract (*Camellia sinensis*) and hepatotoxicity has been recognized since 2002.

It needs to be emphasized that the toxicity is associated with green tea extract and not with green tea.

Eight of the ten cases reported before 2005 involved patients younger than 40 years of age, and seven of the nine were women. All patients improved once they had stopped using the products and had normal liver test results within four months. The approximate cumulative dose ranged from 5.9 g to 120 g, the average being around 30 g. Five patients affected were Caucasian and two were Hispanic. The ethnicity was not recorded in three patients.

A patient who had been using a weight loss supplement called 'The Right Approach Complex' (Pharmanex, Provo, Italy), containing *Camellia sinensis*, for four months, presented to hospital with abdominal pain, nausea and jaundice. All the liver enzymes were elevated and biopsy showed necrosis and inflammation. The temporal pattern of *Camellia sinensis* administration and liver enzyme abnormalities (with a positive re-challenge and exclusion of other possible causes) strongly suggested that the supplement was the inciting agent for two episodes of severe symptomatic drug-induced liver injury.

Black cohosh: *Actea racemosa (Cimicifuga racemosa)*

In North America, the traditional use of black cohosh was to treat snakebite, hence the common name blacksnake root or rattle snake root. It has been used for myalgia, neuralgia and menstrual and rheumatic disorders.

Use of this herb for menopause increased considerably following concerns about the possible risks associated with use of hormone replacement therapy. Side-effects were considered minor and included gastrointestinal irritation, headache, dizziness and vomiting. It is contraindicated in patients with oestrogen-dependent tumours, during pregnancy and with coeliac disease.

There have been reports from Australia and Europe of cases of liver toxicity – including abnormal liver function tests, jaundice, hepatitis and liver failure. The data available suggest that most liver reactions occur within the first three months of starting use of black cohosh. Both Australia and the UK considered that users should be warned of potential risk and have introduced warning labels on products that rare liver reactions may occur. Patients with pre-existing liver disease are advised not to use this herb. Consumers should consult medical professionals for advice if there are health concerns.

Recent publications have cast doubt on the authenticity of some of the herbs used in black cohosh products and it seems likely that there is substitution with some American or Chinese species of *Actea* (or *Cimicifuga*).The relevance of this to safety or efficacy is under review.

CARDIOTOXIC CONSTITUENTS OF PLANTS AND HERBAL MEDICINES[70,118–121]

The first recorded medicinal use of plants containing cardiac glycosides was by the ancient Egyptians and Romans, who used them as emetics and for heart ailments.

The toxicity of herbal cardiac glycosides was well recognized by 1785 when William Withering published his classic work describing the therapeutic uses and toxicity of foxglove, *Digitalis purpurea.*

All parts of the foxglove plants are poisonous, but especially the leaves, the upper leaves being more toxic than lower ones. The toxic properties of these plants do not disappear after drying or cooking.

Exposure to plants containing cardiac glycosides is more common among infants and children under the age of two years than among adults. Poisoning is most likely to occur as a result of drinking teas brewed from plant parts or ingesting leaves, flowers or seeds. Most cases of poisoning have happened when wild-food gatherers have mistaken the plant for comfrey. Accidental poisoning is rare because the plant tastes bitter, as noted in a report of a case of serious poisoning due to accidental intake of foxglove in 2004[68]. Poisoning associated with use of a herbal product was reported recently when a patient developed toxic effects after using a herbal product marketed to cleanse the bowel in which *Digitalis lanata* had been mistakenly substituted for plantain.

Cardiac glycosides predominantly affect the cardiovascular system. They cause alterations in the exchange of ions (e.g. sodium) in heart muscle cells and increase the force with which the heart contracts (increased force of contraction of heart muscle). They also cause slowing of the heart beat (bradycardia) and may lead to excessive slowing or heart block which may be life-threatening. Other toxic effects include effects on the gastrointestinal and nervous systems.

The common symptoms are vomiting, diarrhoea, confusion, drowsiness or insomnia and problems with vision (seeing yellow 'halos' around lights, blurred or double vision or photophobia – increased sensitivity to light). The blood pressure often becomes low and irregular beating of the heart occurs often accompanied by palpitations and chest pain. Convulsions may occur.

The case of accidental ingestion mentioned earlier illustrates many aspects of foxglove toxicity. A 53-year-old woman presented with persistent nausea and vomiting. The nausea was of acute onset the previous evening followed by vomiting and lightheadedness. The vomiting had occurred every hour for 18 hours. She also had mild discomfort in the chest and abdomen. On physical examination, the heart rate was 36 beats per minute with a regular rhythm. She had minimal postural hypotension. Investigations revealed an elevated serum potassium level (5.2 mmol/L) and the magnesium was 1.6 mg per decilitre. The bradycardia responded to atropine. However, the bradycardia and non-specific electrocardiographic changes persisted for two days after admission. The patient and her partner reaffirmed that the patient had not taken digoxin despite the blood analysis revealing a digoxin level of 1.3 ng/ml. However, the patient's partner reported that he was growing foxglove in his garden and that the patient had picked dandelion leaves for her salad from the location where he was growing foxglove. The digitoxin level measured on the third hospital day was 43 ng/ml (therapeutic range 10–32 ng/ml). This patient's heart rate remained slow at an average of 40 beats per minute and on the seventh day the rate increased to high 40s.

A 55-year-old female in Turkey ingested two bulbs of *Urginea maritime* (squill) plant as a folk remedy for her arthritic pains. Her past history was significant as she suffered from Hashimoto's thyroiditis. She was hypothyroid on presentation. Her main symptoms were nausea, vomiting and seizures and she was found to have an elevated blood potassium level (hyperkalaemia) and serious heart rhythm abnormalities such as atrio-ventricular block and ventricular arrhythmias. These features were similar to those of digoxin toxicity. The serum digoxin level was 1.59 ng/ml. Despite supportive treatment and pacing, the patient died due to a ventricular arrhythmia, 30 hours after ingestion of the two squill bulbs[121].

Ingestion of oleander seeds or leaves is a common cause of accidental poisoning worldwide, particularly among children. Cases have been reported from places as diverse as Hawaii, the Solomon Islands, Southern Africa, Australia, Europe, the Far East and the US. The oleanders have been used for suicide, homicide, abortion and as herbal remedies in India, Thailand, Brazil and elsewhere. A study in Sri Lanka showed clear differences between the abnormal heart rhythms that follow digitalis poisoning and those that follow oleander poisoning[120].

Patients with cardiac glycoside toxicity from plant or herbal sources can be treated initially with activated charcoal, and if toxicity is life-threatening administration of digoxin-specific antibody Fab fragments should be considered for rapid reversal of cardiac effects. However, the efficacy of Fab fragments in plant poisoning has been doubted by some clinicians.

LIVER TOXICITY (HEPATOTOXICITY) OF PLANTS[122,123]

There is a greater risk of hepatotoxicity with herbal medicines than with allopathic medicines. Because the hepatotoxic effects of the former are less well documented, and less familiar to allopathic practitioners and subjects taking such medications, clinicians are less likely to take precautions to minimize the risk.

Allopathic physicians need to have a high index of suspicion in investigating and managing liver dysfunction of uncertain origin and consider the possibility that herbal medications might be the cause. It is important to be aware that several herbal medicines, particularly those in which the ingredients are not accurately displayed on labels, have the potential to cause liver cell damage and liver disease.

The diagnosis of herbal hepatotoxicity remains a challenging area. A report from the California Poison Control System[123] provides an overview of herb-related hepatitis. A Medline search for English language case reports, case series, case–control studies and clinical reviews published from 1996 to 2002 found very few reported cases of liver toxicity. Only three involved use of Chinese herbs: these were herbs used in the treatment of eczema[124].

Hepatotoxicity of plant medications containing pyrrolizidine alkaloids has been discussed in the section under PAs. Reports of liver reactions to kava preparations have also been discussed.

Pennyroyal oil contains pulegone which depletes hepatic glutathione and is metabolized to menthofuran which is toxic to the hepatic cells. Restoration of hepatic glutathione by administration of N-acetylcysteine is now recommended in all instances of ingestion of more than 10 ml of pennyroyal oil.

Levo-tetrahydropalmatine is the main active substance of *Corydalis decumbens* and has been used for its sedative and analgesic effects[140]. It has also been found in the products an shu ling and jin bu huan. Both products are associated with hepatitis[126].

A single acute ingestion of jin bu huan anodyne tablets by three children, rapidly produced life-threatening neurological and cardiovascular manifestations[125].

Breynia officinalis, a species of Euphorbiaceae, is used in Chinese medicine to treat convulsions, heart failure, venereal diseases, growth retardation and conjunctivitis. It was mistaken for a similar plant *Securinega suffruticosa* and cooked in a soup used for the treatment of muscle soreness, lumbago and as a tonic. Nineteen patients consumed an average of 130 ml of the soup: 14 patients developed diarrhoea; 10 experienced nausea and chilly sensations; 9 had sensations of abdominal fullness; and 7 suffered from vomiting. Dose-related toxic effects included gastrointestinal symptoms and signs and hepatotoxicity. Hepatocellular injury rather than cholestatic jaundice was observed; marked jaundice did not occur and with supportive treatment, the majority of the abnormalities in 14 of the cases resolved within six months[127].

Some plants reported to cause liver toxicity are indicated at the end of the chapter in Appendix VI.

SOME HERBS CAUSING TOXICITY IN THE KIDNEY (NEPHROTOXIC HERBS)[128–133]

Direct renal toxicity

Many traditional medicines and foods especially in the tropical regions of Africa and Asia contain plants that can cause renal toxicity. The djenkol bean, a pungent smelling edible fruit of the hardwood tree *Pithecolobium lobatum*, contains the toxic compound djenk. Djenk when fed to monkeys, rats and mice produced severe necrosis of the renal tubules. A traditional remedy in South Africa called impila, made from the roots of *Callilepis laureola*, has marked liver and kidney toxicity.

Kidney toxicity due to oxalic acid content

Some herbs high in oxalic acid content such as rhubarb (*Rheum officinale*) may increase the formation of kidney stones if the oxalic acid combines with calcium. There has also been a report of acute oxalate nephropathy following the ingestion of star fruit (*Averrhoa carambola*).

Herbs that cause changes in electrolyte (e.g. sodium and potassium) exchange in the kidney

Liquorice root (*Glycyrrhiza glabra*) in high doses for prolonged periods causes retention of sodium, which has the potential to increase blood pressure, and a loss of potassium, which leads to hypokalaemia and possibly symptoms such as muscle weakness. It also increases the toxicity of allopathic drugs such as digoxin. These effects are due to the metabolites of liquorice acting on the enzyme systems that regulate electrolyte balance in the kidneys.

Herbs with high potassium content

The juice from the noni fruit (*Morinda citrifolia*) can cause an increase in blood and body potassium due to its high potassium content[133]. Dandelion (*Taraxacum officinale*), stinging nettle (*Urtica dioica*), horsetail (*Equisetum arvense*) and alfalfa (*Medicago sativa*) are also high in potassium.

Herbs that cause an increase in volume of urine (diuresis)

Juniper berry (*Juniperus communis*), parsley (*Petroselenium crispum*), dandelion (*Taraxacum officinale*), horsetail (*Equisetum arvense*), asparagus root (*Asparagus officinalis*), lovage root (*Levisticum officinale*), goldenrod (*Solidago virgaurea*), uva ursi (*Arctostaphylos uva ursi*), stinging nettle leaf (*Urtica dioica*) and alfalfa (*Medicago sativa*) have been used traditionally as diuretics. These drugs should be used cautiously by patients who have compromised kidney function, particularly by those patients who require frequent renal dialysis.

Herbs in patients with renal transplants

The success of renal transplants could be compromised by drugs such as St John's wort, which decrease the effectiveness of immunosuppressants such as ciclosporin. It should not be used by patients who have received a kidney transplant and are on allopathic immunosuppressants. Echinacea (*Echinaceae purpurae*), is an immune system modulator and caution is required in patients using immunosuppressants.

PESTICIDES AND OTHER TOXIC CONTAMINANTS[134–137]

A study conducted by Japan's Ministry of Health, Labour and Welfare found residual agricultural chemicals in samples from 11 types of herbs used in herbal medicines, including the banned pesticide DDT. A Japanese newspaper (the *Asahi Shimbun*, a subsidiary of the *Herald Tribune*) reported that synthetic pyrethroids were found in 31 samples of herbal medicines. The government study was done in response to a report published in June 2004 by the National Confederation Movement on farm chemicals being used on traditional herbal plants.

The 2004 Annual Report of the Government Laboratories in Hong Kong reported that about 1% of the Chinese herbal medicine samples were found to contain levels of pesticides that were of concern. Contamination with pesticides such as quintozene and hexachlorobenzene may have resulted from improper use of pesticides during cultivation or from environmental pollution. In early 2004 some ginseng powder products imported from Taiwan were found to be contaminated with an organochlorine pesticide. Since then, all ginseng powder products imported from Taiwan have been screened for the presence of pesticide residues. Contamination of ginseng was also reported in 2002 on the ConsumerLab.com website. Of the 21 ginseng products tested, two had levels of pesticides 20 times more than allowed levels[129].

Cumin is commonly used in Egypt for childhood coughs, aches or itching. A sample of seeds purchased from a local Egyptian market was found to contain the organophosphorus insecticide profenofos at a concentration of 0.37 g/kg, which was nearly twice the residue the WHO and Codex Alimentarius Commission permit in vegetables. This finding was of concern as children's low body weights may make them vulnerable to the toxicity from the pesticide.

APPENDIX I: SOME SIGNS AND SYMPTOMS OF HEAVY METAL POISONING

Lead poisoning[138–141]

The harmful effects of lead have been recognized for centuries and have been even reported as a contributing factor to the downfall of the Roman Empire. Lead does not have any specific historical medicinal purpose although it has been historically used as an ingredient in cosmetic products.

Lead is present in both inorganic and organic forms. Lead and calcium are used interchangeably by bone. Lead has an affinity for bone and acts by replacing calcium and is deposited in growing bone, hence children are more sensitive to the toxic effects of lead than adults. In adults, 20–70% of ingested lead and nearly 100% of inhaled lead enters the blood. Children under three years are more vulnerable because they absorb lead 5–10 times more effectively than adults and have greater exposure because of their exploratory behaviour and frequent hand-to-mouth activity. Further the developing nervous system in children is much more vulnerable to damage than the nervous system in adults. Other high-risk groups include pregnant women. The intake of lead containing herbal medicines during pregnancy and breastfeeding is not recommended. There is not only increased risk of toxicity to the mother, but there is risk of toxicity to the foetus both during and after birth. As lead follows similar metabolic pathways to calcium in the body, it can pass through the placenta and infants can also be exposed during lactation. There has been at least one case report involving the mother and unborn child being poisoned by an Ayurvedic remedy adulterated with lead[22].

The association of lead poisoning with poor cognition (thinking, knowledge) is well established and provided sound evidence for the removal of lead from gasoline, paint and food cans.

Acute poisoning

Acute poisoning follows exposure to high levels of lead and/or lead compounds and causes abdominal pain which may be diffuse or colicky in nature and may be associated with vomiting. In addition patients may complain of lethargy and constipation. Lead colic was first described by Hippocrates and may be mistaken for an acute surgical disorder of the abdomen; frequently these patients are referred to surgical units due to insufficient information on exposure to lead-containing compounds. These symptoms may be followed by fits (seizures), mania, delirium and coma – a group of symptoms referred to as lead encephalopathy which is more commonly seen in children.

Chronic poisoning

Mild chronic poisoning may give rise to non-specific symptoms such as occasional abdominal discomfort and lethargy.

Chronic poisoning gives rise to symptoms and signs listed below:

- Gastrointestinal (stomach and intestines) disturbances – constipation, abdominal pain and tenderness occur at blood lead levels above 45–60 μg/dl.
- Blood – anaemia (microcytic: small red blood cells) and basophilic stippling of red cells is seen under the microscope. Usually seen at blood lead levels above 45 μg/dl.
- Nervous system – insomnia (inability to sleep) and mental tiredness (fatigue) occurring at blood lead levels 45 μg/dl. In severe cases (blood lead levels above 75 μg/dl) hallucinations, convulsions (fits) and coma. Chronic poisoning may be associated with foot drop (due to damage to nerves supplying muscles of the leg) and later wrist drop.
- Muscles – muscle weakness.
- Kidney – damage to kidneys (nephropathy). Glucose, proteins and phosphates may be detected on examining the urine (Fanconi syndrome). Progressive kidney damage may lead to high blood pressure (hypertension).
- Metabolic – gout.
- Gums – bluish discolouration of gum margins.

The blood lead levels should be less than 10 μg/dl. However, there is recent evidence of impaired development and intellectual performance in children at lead levels below 10 μg/dl.

Mercury poisoning[141,142]

Mercury has been used as an ingredient in diuretics, antibacterial agents, antiseptic skin ointments, laxatives, hair conditioning agents and dentistry for many centuries. Mercurous (calomel) salts were also historically used as a purgative. Mercuric salts (e.g. mercuric chloride) were used as disinfectants and, because of their high solubility and acute toxicity, have been used as homicidal agents in the past.

Mercury exists in three forms – inorganic, organic and elemental. Both inorganic and organic mercury salts are absorbed from the gastrointestinal tract. Elemental mercury, as present in mercury thermometers, is not absorbed through the gastrointestinal tract. However, it could be absorbed through inhalation as it is highly lipid soluble. Inorganic mercury, as found in batteries, is poorly lipid soluble and 10% of an ingested dose would be absorbed. Inorganic mercury is concentrated in the kidney tissues. Organic mercury is readily absorbed through the gastrointestinal system and is concentrated in brain, kidney, liver, hair and skin. Organic mercury also crosses the blood–brain barrier and the placenta. Mercury poisoning is generally misdiagnosed as the symptoms are non-specific and insidious in nature. The gastrointestinal system, nervous system and kidneys are the commonest organ systems affected following mercury poisoning.

Acute poisoning

Acute inhalation of elemental mercury mainly gives rise to respiratory symptoms such as shortness of breath, chest pain and cough. Additionally, patients may develop headache, poor vision, excessive salivation and ataxia. These symptoms may recover with no sequelae. However, there may be complications such as acute respiratory distress syndrome. Rarely patients may develop interstitial fibrosis of the lungs. Heavy acute exposure may give rise to neurological abnormalities as well.

Ingestion of inorganic mercury mainly gives rise to symptoms of the gastrointestinal tract. Due to its corrosive properties, patients develop abdominal pain, nausea, vomiting and gastrointestinal bleeding that may lead to hypovolaemic shock. Several hours to days later, systemic features such as pain in the mouth, foul breath and a metallic taste in the mouth followed by renal failure may follow.

Poisoning due organic mercury generally gives rise to chronic symptoms of the nervous system.

Chronic poisoning

Chronic exposure to elemental mercury can give rise to abnormalities in the nervous system. The classic triad of tremor, gingivitis and erythrism (neuropsychiatric findings such as insomnia, shyness, memory loss, emotional instability, depression and anorexia) may sometimes be seen following chronic exposure.

Chronic ingestion of inorganic mercury, generally due to occupational exposure, leads to dementia, renal failure and acrodynia. Acrodynia, known as Pink disease, presents with redness of the palms and soles, swelling of the hands and feet, desquamating rash, hair loss and pruritus.

Poisoning due to organic mercury gives rise to symptoms of the nervous system. These may appear several days after ingestion and they include ataxia, paraesthesia (abnormal skin sensation) and visual disturbances. In addition, patients may develop hearing loss, mental deterioration, dysarthria (disorganized speech), muscle tremor, movement disorders and, with severe exposure, paralysis and even death.

The normal blood level of mercury should be less than 10 μg/L and less than 20 μg/L in urine.

Arsenic poisoning[139,141,143]

Arsenic compounds were historically commonly used as medications for various disorders such as syphilis, acne, malaria and anaemia. In addition arsenic has been used as a poison since the 15th century and was considered the perfect poison because it is odourless, tasteless and resembles sugar. Fowler's solution composed of 1% potassium arsenite was used for over 150 years for the treatment of various ailments including psoriasis, rheumatism, asthma, cholera and syphilis. Arsenicals are still used in the treatment of African trypanosomiasis (sleeping sickness) and in the treatment of rare forms of leukaemia.

Arsenic exists in both organic and inorganic forms and is absorbed by ingestion, inhalation and across the skin. Arsenic is often referred to as a metalloid as it has properties of both metals and non-metals. It binds to specific groups of chemicals which are essential for enzyme function, e.g. sulphydryl groups, and thus the activity of many enzymes in the body are inhibited. Hence, very few organs escape the toxic effects of arsenic. Arsenic also replaces inorganic phosphorus in enzymes and thus prevents certain metabolic reactions (e.g. inhibits oxidative phosphorylation). Arsenic is present in most food items and the average daily intake of arsenic is 400 to 1000 μg.

Acute poisoning

Patients with acute exposure present mainly with gastrointestinal symptoms characterized by nausea, vomiting, abdominal pain and profuse watery or bloody diarrhoea. Patients often have hypotension and may complain of a metallic taste in their mouth, and their breath may have a garlic odour. Patients frequently exhibit signs of delirium following acute exposure. In severe poisoning they may develop encephalopathy and fits. Frequently, they may have biochemical changes of the liver and renal function tests. An ECG may show changes (QT prolongation and ventricular arrhythmias).

Chronic poisoning

Chronic poisoning may give rise to the signs and symptoms of many organ systems listed below:

- Gastrointestinal: diarrhoea, abdominal pain.
- Skin: hyperpigmentation and hyperkeratosis of skin (dew drops on a dust road appearance), especially palms and soles, are early features. Brittle nails with white transverse discolorations (Mee's lines) and itching (pruritus).
- Mouth, nose and throat: sore throat, salivation, lachrymation (tearing), garlic odour, bleeding gums, ulceration and perforation of nasal septum.
- Hair: alopecia (loss of hair).
- General: weakness, loss of appetite, weight loss, low grade fever, increased risk of cancer (e.g. lung).
- Neurological: hearing loss, psychological impairment and changes in electroencephalogram (EEG) and loss of sensation of limbs.
- Chronic renal failure and liver damage.

The blood level of arsenic should not exceed 50 µg/L. However, blood arsenic concentrations correlate poorly with exposure. Arsenic concentrations in hair and nails have been used to indicate chronic systemic absorption.

Chromium poisoning[131]

Chromium exists in varying states and virtually all natural sources are in the trivalent form. All forms of hexavalent chromium are produced during the manufacturing processes.

Inhaled soluble chromium compounds such as sodium and potassium chromate and dichromate are highly irritant to mucous membranes.

Acute poisoning

Accidental or deliberate ingestion of highly soluble hexavalent chromium compounds leads within minutes to nausea, vomiting, abdominal pain, diarrhoea and a burning sensation in the mouth, throat and stomach which may lead to bleeding from the gastrointestinal tract. Inhalation of chromium compounds leads to irritation of the nose, nasal ulcers and perforation of the nasal septum. Chromium has also been implicated in developmental defects such as neural tube defects and foetal deaths in animals.

Chronic poisoning

'Chrome ulcers', which have a well-defined circular margin with raised edges and a central cavity filled with exudate or tenacious crust, may develop after repeated topical exposure to hexavalent chromium compounds. Chronic exposure has also been associated with the development of lung cancer.

Copper poisoning[132]

Copper sulphate is used as a fungicide, an algicide and in some fertilizers. Approximately a third of ingested copper is absorbed. Copper can cross the placental barrier. Copper sulphate used as an antiseptic on open wounds may also be absorbed causing systemic toxicity.

Acute poisoning

Acute copper poisoning occurs following intake of contaminated food. Copper poisoning mainly gives rise to symptoms of the gastrointestinal system such as profuse vomiting, abdominal pain, diarrhoea, bleeding and a metallic taste in the mouth. In addition headache and dizziness may be experienced. Notably, severe poisoning can give rise to anaemia, renal and liver failure.

Chronic poisoning

Chronic poisoning is difficult to diagnose and symptoms are non-specific. There have been reports of anaemia, malaise, loss of appetite (anorexia), nausea and vomiting as the presenting features.

Silver poisoning[144]

Colloidal silver is a mixture of silver nitrate, sodium hydroxide, gelatine and water. It is used both topically and orally for a variety of conditions. Because inorganic silver is germicidal, it is often used to treat infections. Oral or topical use of colloidal silver can produce an irreversible bluish discoloration of the skin, especially on areas exposed to sun, known as argyria. Bluish discoloration of the eyes is known as argyrosis. Excessive use of silver can produce diffuse silver deposition in visceral organs leading to kidney damage and neurological deficits such as vertigo, gait disturbances, hyperaesthesia and weakness. The evidence for efficacy of silver taken orally for any disorder is at best contentious.

APPENDIX II: SOME HERBAL MEDICINES FOUND TO CONTAIN HEAVY METALS

Some samples of the herbal medicines analysed	Heavy metals identified
Azarcon (alarcon, coral, luiga, Maria Luisa, rueda (Hispanic)	Lead (95%)
Ba-Baw-San (Chinese)	Lead
Baochiwanying-san (Chinese)	Mercuric sulphide (cinnabaris)
Bao ying dan (Chinese)	Lead
Bint al zahab (Iran)	Lead
Bint dahab (Saudi Arabia)	Lead
Bokhoor (Kuwait)	Lead
Bola (Indian)	Lead
Eurycoma madu (Malaysia)	Lead
Fufang luhuijiaonang (Chinese)	Mercury
Ghasard (Indian)	Lead
Goli (Indian)	Lead
Greta (Mexico)	Lead
Hai ge fen (clamshell powder)	Copper, chromium, arsenic, lead
Jierezhenluesan (Chinese)	Mercuric sulphide (cinnabaris)
Jin bu huan (China)	Lead
Jufangniuhuang-qingxinwan (Chinese)	Mercuric sulphide (cinnabaris), realgar, (arsenic sulfide)
Kandu (Indian)	Lead
Karela capsules (Himalaya Drug Co (Ayurveda))	Lead, mercury, arsenic
Liushenwan	Arsenic, mercury
Maha sudarshan churna powder (Ayurveda Zandu Pharmaceuticals)	Possibly lead, arsenic and mercury
Mahayogaraj guggulu (Ayurveda)	Lead, mercury, arsenic
Mahayograj guggulu (Indian)	Lead
Niu huang qing fei-san (Chinese)	Mercuric sulphide (cinnabaris), realgar, (arsenic sulfide)
Niu huang jie du pian (Chinese)	Arsenic
Pay-loo-ah (Vietnam)	Lead
Po ying tan (China)	Lead
Qianjinsan (Chinese)	Mercuric sulphide (cinnabaris)

Continued on following page

Some samples of the herbal medicines analysed	Heavy metals identified
Qing fen	Mercurous chloride (calomel)
SAFI (Hamdard)	Arsenic
Santrinj (Saudi Arabia)	Lead
Shugan wan (Chinese)	Mercuric sulphide (cinnabaris)
Shang han lun (Chinese)	Lead
Shilajit capsules (Dabur)	Possibly lead, arsenic and mercury
Sukarno (Malaysia)	Lead
Super pill tongkat ali (Malaysia)	Lead
Surma (India)	Lead
Tibetan herbal vitamin (Tibet)	Lead
Tiewadan (Chinese)	Mercuric sulphide (cinnabaris)
Tongkat (Malaysia)	Lead
Tongkat ali (Malaysia)	Lead
Tse koo choy	Mercurous chloride (calomel)
Xiaoerqifengsan (Chinese)	Mercuric sulphide (cinnabaris)
Xiaoerqiyingwan (Chinese)	Mercuric sulphide (cinnabaris), arsenic
Yingerbaofeining (Chinese)	Mercuric sulphide (cinnabaris)
Yingerle (Chinese)	Mercuric sulphide (cinnabaris)

APPENDIX III: SOME HERBAL MEDICINES FOUND TO CONTAIN ALLOPATHIC MEDICATIONS

Samples of herbal preparation analysed	Synthetic or allopathic medication/s detected	Some adverse effects of the allopathic medicine/s
Active Rheuma Plus	Dexamethasone	Dyspepsia, osteoporosis, menstrual irregularities, hirsuitism, weight gain, euphoria, infections
Boyjoy (NZ)	Sildenafil	Dyspepsia, vomiting, headache, flushing, dizziness, nasal congestion
Chaso	Fenfluramine and nitrofenfluramine	Drowsiness, diarrhoea, dizziness, headache, irritability, anxiety, palpitations, impotence, valvular heart disease
Dr Tong Shap Yee's Asthma Pills	Theophylline	Tachycardia, palpitations, nausea, headache, insomnia
Gan mao qing	Moroxydine, paracetamol, chlorphenamine	Rashes, blood disorders, liver damage, drowsiness, tinnitus
Gan mao tong pian	Phenylbutazone	Nausea, vomiting, diarrhoea, salt retention, headache, gastric irritation, bone marrow suppression

Continued on following page

Samples of herbal preparation analysed	Synthetic or allopathic medication/s detected	Some adverse effects of the allopathic medicine/s
Hua fo	Sildenafil	Dyspepsia, vomiting, headache, flushing, dizziness, nasal congestion
Keepfitlin	Fenfluramine and nitrofenfluramine	Drowsiness, diarrhoea, dizziness, headache, irritability, anxiety, palpitations, impotence, valvular heart disease
Li da dai dai hua	Sibutramine	Constipation, dry mouth, nausea, taste disturbances, palpitations, high blood pressure, anxiety, seizures
Liqiang 4 dietary supplement capsules	Glyburide – glibenclamide	Nausea, vomiting, diarrhoea, constipation, weight gain, dangerous lowering of blood sugar (hypoglycaemia)
Lee Pui Kee cough pills	Bromhexine	Gastrointestinal upset, altered liver function tests
Manup capsules (NZ)	Tadalafil	Dyspepsia, vomiting, headache, flushing, dizziness, nasal congestion
Ma zin dol	Fenfluramine and nitrofenfluramine	Drowsiness, diarrhoea, dizziness, headache, irritability, anxiety, palpitations, impotence, valvular heart disease
Meizitang	Sibutramine	Constipation, dry mouth, nausea, taste disturbances, palpitations, high blood pressure, anxiety, seizures
Nan Lien Chuifong Toukuwan	Aminopyrine, phenacetin, phenylbutazone, indometacin, mefenamic acid, diazepam, hydrochlorothiazide, dexamethasone, cinnabar	Life-threatening blood disorders, abdominal pain and ulcers, sedation, euphoria, water and electrolyte imbalances
Onshido	Fenfluramine and nitrofenfluramine	Drowsiness, diarrhoea, dizziness, headache, irritability, anxiety, palpitations, impotence, valvular heart disease
Ox Head Brand tong shui wan	Diazepam, mefenamic acid, diclofenac	Drowsiness, diarrhoea, dizziness, headache, irritability, anxiety, palpitations, impotence
Phu Chee	Dexamethasone	Dyspepsia, osteoporosis, menstrual irregularities, hirsuitism, weight gain, euphoria, infections

harmful constituents

Continued on following page

Samples of herbal preparation analysed	Synthetic or allopathic medication/s detected	Some adverse effects of the allopathic medicine/s
Pil ajaib cap emas	Corticosteroids, indometacin	Dyspepsia, osteoporosis, menstrual irregularities, hirsuitism, weight gain, euphoria, infections
Platinum Plus (NZ)	Sildenafil	Dyspepsia, vomiting, headache, flushing, dizziness, nasal congestion
Prostate Cancer Hope (PC-SPES)	Warfarin, indometacin, diethylstilboestrol and ethinylestradiol	Bleeding, oestrogenic activity, which would be dangerous for breast cancer and contraception, fluid retention
Qian er/Quian er	Fenfluramine and nitrofenfluramine	Drowsiness, diarrhoea, dizziness, headache, irritability, anxiety, palpitations, impotence, valvular heart disease
Qing zhi san tain shou	Sibutramine	Constipation, dry mouth, nausea, taste disturbances, palpitations, high blood pressure, anxiety, seizures
Qing zi su	Fenfluramine and nitrofenfluramine	Drowsiness, diarrhoea, dizziness, headache, irritability, anxiety, palpitations, impotence, valvular heart disease
SB slimming capsules	Fenfluramine and nitrofenfluramine	Drowsiness, diarrhoea, dizziness, headache, irritability, anxiety, palpitations, impotence, valvular heart disease
Shubaojiafeijiaolang	Fenfluramine and nitrofenfluramine	Drowsiness, diarrhoea, dizziness, headache, irritability, anxiety, palpitations, impotence, valvular heart disease
Slim 10	Fenfluramine and nitrofenfluramine	Drowsiness, diarrhoea, dizziness, headache, irritability, anxiety, palpitations, impotence, valvular heart disease
Tongyi Tang Diabetes Angel Pearl Hypoglycaemic Tablets	Glyburide	Severe lowering of blood sugar (hypoglycaemia)
Tung shueh (Black ball)	Diazepam, mefenamic acid	Drowsiness, light-headedness, confusion, ataxia, amnesia, rashes, blood disorders, gastrointestinal disturbances
Wei ge wang (NZ)	Sildenafil	Dyspepsia, vomiting, headache, flushing, dizziness, nasal congestion

Continued on following page

Samples of herbal preparation analysed	Synthetic or allopathic medication/s detected	Some adverse effects of the allopathic medicine/s
Xiaoke/Xiaoke wan	Glibenclamide	Nausea, vomiting, diarrhoea, constipation, weight gain, dangerous lowering of blood sugar (hypoglycaemia)
Xiao pang mei	Methylphenidate	Sleep disturbances, night terrors, confusion, rash, fever, joint pains, loss of appetite
Xin xue kang jiao naing	Fenfluramine and nitrofenfluramine	Drowsiness, diarrhoea, dizziness, headache, irritability, anxiety, palpitations, impotence, valvular heart disease
Yin chiao chieh tu pien	Paracetamol, chlorpheniramine, caffeine	Rashes, blood disorders, liver damage, drowsiness/stimulation, tinnitus
Yuzhitang jian fei jiao nang	Fenfluramine and nitrofenfluramine	Drowsiness, diarrhoea, dizziness, headache, irritability, anxiety, palpitations, impotence, valvular heart disease
Zhen qi (Malaysia)	Glibenclamide	Nausea, vomiting, diarrhoea, constipation, weight gain, dangerous lowering of blood sugar (hypoglycaemia)
Zhong Gan Ling	Aminopyrine, chlorphenamine	Blood disorders, rashes, drowsiness, tinnitus
Zhui feng tou gu wan (Black pills for arthritis) – Black pearls, San kee	Phenylbutazone, aminopyrine, indometacin, prednisone, chlordiazepoxide, paracetamol, mefenemic acid, dexamethasone, diazepam	A very serious and life-threatening group of adverse effects including bone marrow depression, risk of infections, drowsiness, amnesia

APPENDIX IV: SOME HERBAL/TRADITIONAL MEDICINES FOUND TO CONTAIN ANIMAL OR HUMAN PARTS

Product name	Manufacturer's name	Toxic ingredients
Chan Su		Toad glycosides
Compound kangweiling	Wo Zhou Pharmaceutical Factory (Lanzhou, China)	Centipede (*Scolopendra*) 10%
Da huo loud an	Beijing Tun Jen Tang (Beijing, China)	Centipede (*Scolopendra*)
Kyushin Heart Tonic	Kyushin Seikyaku Co Ltd (Tokyo, Japan)	Toad venom
Laryngitis pills	China Dzechuan Provincial Pharmaceutical Factory (Chengtu Branch, China)	Toad cake 10% Borax 30
Love stone		Colorado river toad and cane toad glycosides
Lu-shen-wan	Shanghai Chinese Medicine Works (Shanghai, China)	Toad secretion
Nasalin	Kwangchow Pharmaceutical Industry Co (Kwangchow, China)	Centipede 5%
Pak Yuen Tong Hou Tsao powder	Kwan Yung Pak Yuen Tong Main Factory (Hong Kong)	Scorpion 10%

Adapted from Goldfrank LR, Flomenbaum NE, Lewin NA, Weisman RS, Howland MA and Hoffman RS. *Goldfrank's Toxicological Emergencies*, 7th edn. McGraw-Hill, 2002.

APPENDIX V: PYRROLIZIDINE ALKALOIDS (PAs)

Toxic effects of PAs

The toxic PAs may cause the following liver reactions when ingested in doses of 10–20 mg:

- Enlargement of liver cells and their nuclei.
- Disturbances of liver cell metabolism resulting in functional losses, areas of cell destruction and fatty degeneration.
- Long-term administration of smaller doses, 10 μg or less per day, may cause liver cirrhosis.
- In both acute and long-term responses, veno-occlusive liver disease may occur.
- May have effects on other organs and systems, e.g. nervous system.
- Mutagenicity.

Clinical signs of PA toxicity[145]

Clinically patients present with nausea, vomiting, hepatomegaly, portal hypertension, ascites, jaundice (rare) and only moderately elevated liver transaminases.

Common sources of pyrrolizidine alkaloids

- *Adenostyles alliariae* – used in the Alps to treat lung disorders.
- *Alkanna tinctoria* also known as *Lithospermum tinctorium* (Alkanet) – Used topically for skin disorders, sometimes internally, also for diarrhoea.
- *Anchusa officinalis* (bugloss) – used to pro-

mote removal of secretions from the lung and upper airways or as a diuretic.

- *Borago officinalis* – a Western herb used as blood purifier and diuretic.
- *Crotalaria* spp.; *C. juncea*, *C. nana*, *C. retusa*, *C. fulva* (rattlebox) – used in Chinese medicine to dispel heat and promote urination.
- *Cynoglossum officinale* (hound's tongue) – used in Africa as a medicinal herb.
- *Emilia sonchifolia* (tassel flower or emilia) – used to treat fever, cough and bronchitis.
- *Eupatorium cannabinum* (hemp agrimony), *E. perforatum* (boneset), *E. purpureum* (Joe Pye weed) – used to induce sweating to bring down fever.
- *Heliotropium arborescens* (white heliotrope) – used in Africa as a medicinal herb.
- *Lappula intermedia* (stickseed) – used topically for sores.
- *Lithospermum officinale* (gromwell) and *Lithospermum erythrorhizon*.
- *Myosotis scorpioides* (forget-me-not) – used as a sedative and tonic and externally as an eye wash.
- *Petasites hybridus* (pestilence wirt or butter bur) – used in Europe to treat several causes of abdominal pain; also: *P. spurious*.
- *Pulmonaria officinalis* (lungwort or Jerusalem cowslip) – used for treating coughs.
- *Senecio aureus* (golden ragwort) – used for injuries; *S. bicolor* – used to treat cataract; *S. doronicum*, *S. jacobaea*, *S. nemorensis*, *S. vulgaris*, *S. illiciformis*, *S. longilobus*, *S. douglasii*; several species used in Chinese medicine to treat fever, dysuria, diarrhoea and cataracts.
- *Symphytum officinale* – also: *S. asperum*, *S. caucasicum*, *S. tuberosum*, and *S. peregrinum*.
- *Tussilago farfara* (coltsfoot) – used in Europe to treat lung disorders and diarrhoea.
- Bees honey – eating honey collected by bees frequenting PA-containing plants (e.g. *Senecio*).
- Drinking milk and eating eggs of animals feeding on plants rich in PAs (e.g. unregulated grain feed containing *Heliotropium*).

Arsecularatne et al. studied the medicinal plants used in Sri Lanka for the presence of PAs. They screened 50 medicinal plants and obtained positive results with three species, namely *Crotalaria verrucosa* L, *Holarrhena antidysenterica* L Br and *Cassia auriculata* L. Feeding trials in rats with materials from these three species produced liver lesions, compatible with the toxicity of PAs.

APPENDIX VI: SOME CARDIOTOXIC CONSTITUENTS OF PLANTS AND HERBAL MEDICINES

Cardiac glycosides are found in a diverse group of plants including:

- foxgloves (*Digitalis purpurea*, *Digitalis lanata*)
- common oleander (*Nerium oleander*)
- yellow oleander (*Thevetia peruviana*)
- lily-of-the-valley (*Convallaria majalis*)
- squill (*Urginea maritima*, *Urginia indica*)
- ouabain (*Strophanthus gratus*)
- dogbane (*Apocynum cannabinum*)
- wallflower (*Cheiranthus cheiri*).

The herbal sources of cardiac glycosides may be detected by serum immunoassays for digoxin and digitoxin.

APPENDIX VII: SOME HEPATOTOXIC PLANTS

The following may cause liver damage:

Germander (*Teucrium chamaedrys*)
Chapparal leaves
Kava kava
Cycad
Camphor
Mediterranean glue thistle
Impila
Cascara (uncertain)
Greater celandine
Prostata
Comfrey
Celandine
Breynia officinalis
Atractylis gummifera
Callilepsis laureola
Pulegium

REFERENCES

1. Ernst E. Toxic heavy metals and undeclared drugs in Asia herbal medicines. *Trends in Pharmacological Science* 2002; 23: 136–139.
2. Deng JF, Lin TJ, Kao WF, Chen SS. The difficulty in handling poisonings associated with Chinese traditional medicine: a poison control center experience for 1991–1993. *Vetinerary and Human Toxicology* 1997; 39: 106–114.
3. Kasilo OM, Nhachi CF. A pattern of acute poisoning in children in urban Zimbabwe: ten years experience. *Human Experimental Toxicology* 1992; 11: 335–340.
4. Kasilo OM, Nhachi CF. The pattern of poisoning from traditional medicines in urban Zimbabwe. *South African Medical Journal* 1992; 82: 187–188.
5. Chibwana C, Mhango T, Molyneux EM. Child poisoning at the Queen Elizabeth Central Hospital, Blantyre, Malawi. *East African Medical Journal* 2001; 78(6): 292–295.
6. Caldas ED, Machado LL. Cadmium, mercury and lead in medicinal herbs in Brazil. *Food Chemical Toxicology* 2004; 42: 599–603.
7. Chan K. Some aspects of toxic contaminants in herbal medicines. *Chemosphere* 2003; 52: 1361–1371.
8. Ko RJ. Adulterants in 260 Asian patent medicines. *New England Journal of Medicine* 1998; 339: 847.
9. van Schalwyk J, Davidson J, Palmer B, Hope V. Ayurvedic medicines: patients in peril from plumbism. *New Zealand Medical Journal* 2006; 119: U1958.
10. Haq I, Ashgar M. Lead content of some traditional preparations – 'Kushtas'. *Journal of Ethnopharmacology* 1989; 26: 287–291.
11. Zhang QF, Zhang QD, Ye ZX, Liu T. Study of cardiovascular and cerebrovascular disease in Chinese traditional medicines on Pb, Cr, Cd by AAS. *Guang Pu Xue Yu Guang Fen Xi* (Chinese) 2001; 21: 865–867.
12. Ernst E. Heavy metals in traditional Indian remedies. *European Journal of Clinical Pharmocology* 2002; 57: 891–896.
13. Itankar PR et al. Estimation of arsenic content in some Ayurvedic formulations. *Hamdard Medicine* 2001; 19: 95–97.
14. Saper RB, Kales SN, Paquin J, Burns MJ, Eisenberg DM, Davis RB, Phillips RS. Heavy metal content of Ayurvedic herbal medicine products. *JAMA* 2004; 292: 2868–2873.
15. Ang HH, Lee EL, Matsumoto K. Analysis of lead content in herbal preparations in Malaysia. *Human Experimental Toxicology* 2003; 2: 445–451.
16. Koh HL, Woo SO. Chinese proprietary medicines in Singapore. Regulatory control of toxic heavy metals and undeclared drugs. *Drug Safety* 2000; 23: 351–362.
17. Sun RX, Zhou LM, Xue WG, Sun JH. Determination of trace elements in Chinese traditional medicines by atomic absorption spectrometry. *Guang Pu Xue Yu Guang Pu Fen Xi* (Chinese) 2002; 22: 853–855.
18. Mino Y, Yamada Y. Detection of high levels of arsenic and mercury in some Chinese traditional medicines using X-ray fluorescence spectrometry. *Journal of Health Science* 2005; 51: 607–613.

19. Illinois Department of Public Health. Preventing and screening for Childhood Lead Poisoning. A reference Guide for Physicians and Health Care Providers. Accessed at www.idph.state.il.us/HealthWellness/lead_ref_guide.htm on 9th July 2007.
20. McNeil JR, Rheinhard MC. Lead poisoning from home remedies. *Clinics in Pediatrics* (Phila) 1967; 6: 150–156.
21. Hardy AD, Sutherland HH, Vaishnav R, Worthing MA. A report on the composition of mercurials used in traditional medicines in Oman. *Journal of Ethnopharmacology* 1995; 49: 17–22.
22. Rahman H, Al Khayat A, Menon N. Lead poisoning in infancy – unusual causes in the UAE. *Annals of Tropical Paediatrics* 1986; 6: 213–217.
23. Moore C, Adler R. Herbal vitamins: lead toxicity and developmental delay. *Paediatrics* 2000; 106: 600–602.
24. Worthing MA, Sutherland HH, al-Riyami K. New information on the composition of Bint al Dahab, a mixed lead monoxide used as a traditional medicine in Oman and the United Arab Emirates. *Journal of Tropical Paediatrics* 1995; 41: 246–247.
25. Bose A, Vashistha K, O'Loughlin BJ. Azracon por empach – another cause of lead toxicity. *Paediatrics* 1983; 72: 106–108.
26. Yanez L, Batres L, Carrizales L, Santoyo M, Escalante V, Diaz-Barriga F. Toxicological assessment of azarcon, a lead salt used as folk remedy in Mexico. Oral toxicity in rats. *Journal of Ethnopharmacology* 1994; 41: 91–97.
27. Espinoza EO, Mann MJ, Bleasdell B. Arsenic and mercury in traditional Chinese herbal balls (letter). *New England Journal of Medicine* 1995; 333: 803–804.
28. Shaw D, House I, Kolev S, Murray V. Should herbal medicines be licensed? *British Medical Journal* 1995; 311: 451–452.
29. Medicines and Health Regulatory Agency. Press release: Arsenic and mercury found in Ayurvedic and Traditional Chinese Medicines. 17 November 2005. Accessed at www.mhra.gov.uk on 9th July 2007.
30. Medicines and Healthcare Regulatory Agency. Arsenic and mercury in Ayurvedic and traditional Chinese medicines. 9 November 2005. Accessed at www.mhra.gov.uk on 9th July 2007.
31. Sheerin NS, Monk PN, Aslam M, Thurston H. Simultaneous exposure to lead, arsenic and mercury from Indian ethnic remedies. *British Journal of Clinical Practice* 1994; 48: 332–333.
32. Healy MA, Aslam M, Banmgboye OA. Traditional medicine and lead containing preparations in Nigeria. *Public Health* 1984; 98: 26–32.
33. Wood R, Mills PB, Knobel GJ, Hurlow WE, Stokol JM. Acute dichromate poisoning after use of traditional purgatives. A report of 7 cases. *South African Medical Journal* 1990; 77: 640–642.
34. Mojdehi GM, Gurtner J. Childhood lead poisoning through kohl. *American Journal of Public Health* 1996; 86: 587–588.
35. Ali AR, Smales OR, Aslam M. Surma and lead poisoning. *British Medical Journal* 1978; 2: 915–916.
36. Cartwright-Jones C. Tap Dancing Lizard publications 2005. www.harquus.com
37. Steenkamp V, Stewart MJ, Curowska E, Zuckerman M. A severe case of multiple metal poisoning in a child treated with a traditional medicine. *Forensic Science International* 2002; 128: 123–126.
38. Lynch E, Braithwaite R. A review of the clinical and toxicological aspects of traditional (herbal) medicines adulterated with heavy metals. *Expert Opinion. Drug Safety* 2005; 4: 769–778.
39. Tay CH, Seah CS. Arsenic poisoning from anti-asthmatic herbal preparations. *Medical Journal of Australia* 1975; 2: 424.
40. Roche AS, Florkowski C, Walmsley T. Lead poisoning due to ingestion of Indian herbal remedies. *New Zealand Medical Journal* 2005; 118: U 1587.
41. Kanen BL, Perenboom RM. Chronic lead intoxication associated with Ayurvedic medication. *Ned Tijdschr Geneeskd* 2005; 149: 2893–2896.
42. Schilling U, Muck R, Heidemann E. Lead poisoning after ingestion of Ayurvedic drugs (article in German). *Medizinische Klinik* (Munich) 2004; 99: 476–480.
43. Perharic L, Shaw D, Colbridge M, House I, Leon C, Murray V. Toxicological problems resulting from exposure to traditional remedies and food supplements. *Drug Safety* 1994; 11: 284–294.
44. Venter CP, Joubert PH. Aspects of poisoning with traditional medicines in Southern Africa. *Biomedical Environmental Science* 1988; 1: 388–391.

45. Centers for Disease Control and Prevention – Lead poisoning associated with the use of traditional ethnic remedies. California 1991–1992. *MMWR* 1993; 42 (27): 521–524.
46. Centers for Disease Control and Prevention. Lead poisoning associated with Ayurvedic medications – five states, 2000–2003. CDC. *MMWR* 2004; 53 (26): 582–584.
47. Woolf DA. Aetiology of acute lead encephalopathy in Omani infants. *Journal of Tropical Medicine* 1990; 36: 328–330.
48. Abu Melha A, Ahmed NA, el Hassan AY. Traditional remedies and lead intoxication. *Tropical Geographic Medicine* 1987; 39: 100–103.
49. Centers for Disease Control and Prevention. Lead poisoning associated with use of litargirio – Rhode Island 2003. *MMWR* 2005; 53 (9): 227–229.
50. US Food and Drug Administration – FDA Talk Paper October 2, 2003.
51. Prpic-Majiic D, Pizent AS, Jurasovic J, Pongracic J, Restek-Samarzija N. Lead poisoning associated with the use of Ayurvedic metal-mineral tonics. *Journal of Toxicology and Clinical Toxicology* 1996; 34: 417–423.
52. Fernando NP, Healy MA, Aslam M, Davis SS, Hussein A. Lead poisoning and traditional practice: the consequences for world health. A study in Kuwait. *Public Health* 1981; 95: 250–260.
53. Kang-Yum E, Oransky SH. Chinese patent medicine as a potential source of mercury poisoning. *Vetinerary and Human Toxicology* 1992; 34: 235–238.
54. Wong HCG. Acute generalized maculopapular eruption, abnormal liver function and elevated blood mercury level associated with Chinese herbal medicine. *Canadian Journal of Allergy and Clinical Immunology* 2002; 7: 92–96.
55. Kew J, Morris C, Alhie A, Fysh R, Jones S, Brooks D. Arsenic and mercury intoxication due to Indian ethnic remedies. *British Medical Journal* 1993; 306: 507–508.
56. Centers for Disease Control and Prevention. Non fatal arsenic poisoning in three Hmong patients. *MMWR* 1984: 33(24): 347–349.
57. Werner M, Knobeloch LM, Erbach T, Anderson HA. Use of imported folk remedies and medications in the Wisconsin Hmong Community. *Wisconsin Medical Journal* 2001; 100: 32–34.
58. Wu MS, Hong JJ, Lin JL, Yang CW, Chien HC. Multiple tubular dysfunction induced by mixed Chinese herbal medicines containing cadmium. *Nephrology Dialysis and Transplantation* 1996; 11: 867–870.
59. Drugs in imported Chinese herb products, November 1996, Subhuti Dharmananda, Ph.D., Director, Institute for Traditional Medicine, Portland, Oregon.
60. Wooltorton E. Hua Fo tablets tainted with sildenafil-like compound. *CMAJ* 2002; 166: 1568.
61. De Smet PAGM. Perspectives in clinical pharmacology. Health risks of herbal remedies: An update. *Clinical Pharmacology and Therapeutics* 2004; 76: 1–17.
62. Annual Report of National Laboratories of Foods and Drugs, Taiwan 1990 and 1991.
63. Huang WF, Wen KC, Hsiao ML. Adulteration by synthetic therapeutic substances of traditional Chinese medicines in Taiwan. *Journal of Clinical Pharmacology* 1997; 37: 344–350.
64. Government Laboratory Annual report. http:/www.govetlab.gov.hk/ar2004/text/English/ChineseMeds.html
65. Ries CA, Sahud MA. Agranulocytosis caused by Chinese herbal medicines. Dangers of medications containing aminopyrine and phenylbutazone. *JAMA* 1975; 231: 352–355.
66. Keane FM, Munn SE, du Vivier AW, Taylor NF, Higgins EM. Analysis of Chinese herbal creams prescribed for dermatological conditions. *British Medical Journal* 1999; 318: 563–564.
67. Gupta SK, Kaleekal T, Joshi S. Misuse of corticosteroids in some of the drugs dispensed as preparations from alternative systems of medicine in India. *Pharmacoepidemiology and Drug Safety* 2000; 9: 599–602.
68. Adachi M, Saito H, Kobayashi H, Horie Y, Kato S, Yoshioka M et al. Hepatic injury in 12 patients taking the herbal weight loss AIDS Chaso or Onshido. *Annals of Internal Medicine* 2003; 139: 488–492.
69. Corns C, Metcalfe K. Risks associated with herbal slimming remedies. *Journal of R Soc Health* 2002; 122: 213–219.
70. Newman LS, Feinberg MW, LeWine HL. A bitter tale. *New England Journal of Medicine* 2004; 351: 594–599.
71. Saewright AA. Directly toxic effects of plant chemicals which may occur in human and animal foods. *Natural Toxins* 1995; 3: 227–232.

72. Czerwiecki L. Plants as a source of natural harmful substances. *Rocz Panstw Zakl Hig* (Polish) 2005; 56: 215–227.
73. Deinzer ML, Thomson PA, Burgett DM, Isaacson DL. Pyrrolizidine alkaloids: their occurrence in honey from tangsy ragwort (*Senecio jacobaea*). *Science* 1977; 195: 497–499.
74. Edgar JA, Roeder E, Molyneux RJ. Honey from plants containing pyrrolizidine alkaloids: a potential threat to health. *Journal of Agriculture and Food Chemistry* 2002; 50 : 2719–2730.
75. McGee J, Patrick RS, Wood CB, Blumgart LH. A case of veno-occlusive disease of the liver in Britain associated with herbal tea consumption. *Journal of Clinical Pathology* 1976; 29: 788–794.
76. Manteiga R, Park DL, Ali SS. Risks associated with consumption of herbal teas. *Reviews of Environmental Contamination and Toxicology* 1997; 150: 1–30.
77. Chan TY, Critchley JA. Usage and adverse effects of Chinese herbal medicines. *Hum Exp Toxicol* 1996; 15: 5–12.
78. Prakash AS, Pereira TN, Reilly PE, Seawright AA. Pyrrolizidine alkaloids in human diet. *Mutation Research* 1999; 443: 53–67.
79. Stegelmeier BL, Edgar JA, Colegate SM, Gardner DR, Schoch TK, Coulombe RA, Molyneux RJ. Pyrrolizidine alkaloid plants, metabolism and toxicity. *Journal of Natural Toxins* 1999; 8: 95–116.
80. Roeder E. Medicinal plants in China containing pyrrolizidine alkaloids. *Pharmazie* 2000; 55: 711–726.
81. Stickel F, Seitz HK. The efficacy and safety of comfrey. *Public Health Nutrition* 2000; 3: 501–580.
82. Bras G, Jeliffe DB, Stuart KL. Veno-occlusive disease of liver with non-portal type of cirrhosis occurring in Jamaica. *Archives of Pathology* 1954; 57: 285–300.
83. Bras G, Hill KR. Veno-occlusive disease of the liver – essential pathology. *Lancet* 1956; 2: 161–163.
84. Mohabbat O, Srivasta RN, Younos MS, Sediq GG, Merzad AA, Aram GN. The outbreak of veno-occlusive disease in North Western Afghanistan. *Lancet* 1976; 1: 269–271.
85. Tandon BN, Tandon RK, Tandon HD, Narendranathan M, Joshi YK. An epidemic of veno-occlusive disease of liver in Central India. *Lancet* 1976; 1: 271–272.
86. Stillman AS, Huxtable R, Consroe P, Kohnen P, Smith S. Hepatic veno-occlusive disease due to pyrrolizidine (*Senecio*) poisoning in Arizona. *Gastroenterology* 1977; 73: 349–352.
87. Rasenack R, Muller C, Kleinschmidt M, Rasenack J, Wiedenfeld H. Veno-occlusive disease in a foetus caused by pyrrolizidine alkaloids of food origin. *Fetal Diagnosis and Therapeutics* 2003; 18: 223–225.
88. Steenkamp V, Stewart MJ, Zuckerman M. Clinical and analytical aspects of pyrrolidizine poisoning caused by South African traditional medicines. *Therapeutic Drug Monitoring* 2000; 22: 302–306.
89. Zuckerman M, Steenkamp V, Stewart MJ. Hepatic veno-occlusive disease as a result of a traditional remedy: confirmation of toxic pyrrolizidine alkaloids as the cause, using an in vitro technique. *Journal of Clinical Pathology* 2002; 55: 676–679.
90. Schulze J, Raasch W, Siegers C-P. Toxicity of kava pyrones, drug safety and precautions – a case study. *Phytomedicine* 2003;10 (Suppl IV): 68–73.
91. Singh YN. Kava toxicity. *US Pharmacist* 2003: 28: 05. Accessed at www.uspharmacist.com on 9th July 2007.
92. Clouatre DL. Kava kava: examining new reports of toxicity. *Toxicology Letters* 2004; 150: 85–96.
93. Gold LS, Slone TH. Aristolochic acid, a herbal carcinogen, sold on the Web after FDA alert. *New England Journal of Medicine* 2003; 349: 1576–1577.
94. Vanherweghem JL, Depierreux M, Tielmans C, Asbramowicz D, Dratwa M, Jadoul M et al. Rapidly progressive interstitial renal fibrosis in young women: Associations with slimming regimen including Chinese herbs. *Lancet* 1993; 341: 387–391.
95. Violon C. Belgian (Chinese herb) nephropathy: why? *Pharm Belg* 1997; 52: 7–27.
96. Norier JL et al. Urothelial carcinoma associated with the use of a Chinese herb (*Aristolochia fangchi*). *New England Journal of Medicine* 2000; 23(342): 1682–1692 (see also: editorial by former FDA Director, Kessler DA; p. 1742).
97. Tanaka A, Shinkai S, Kasuno K, Maeda K, Murata M, Seta K, Okuda J, Sugawara A, Yoshida T, Nishida R, Kuwahara T. Chinese herbs nephropathy in the Kansai area: a warning

report. *Nippon Jinzo Gakkai Shi* 1997; 39: 438–440.

98. Lord GM, Tagore R, Cook T, Gower P, Pusey CD. Nephropathy caused by Chinese herbs in the UK. *Lancet* 1999; 354: 481–482.
99. Stengel B, Jones E. End-stage renal insufficiency associated with Chinese herbal consumption in France. *Nephrologie* 1998; 19: 15–20.
100. Hansson A, Zelada JC, Noriega HP. Reevaluation of risks with the use of *Ficus insipida* latex as a traditional antihelmintic remedy in the Amazon. *Journal of Ethnopharmacology* 2005; 98: 251–257.
101. Hamouda C, Hedhili A, Zhioua M, Amamou A. A review of acute poisoning from *Atractylus gummifera* L. *Vetinerary and Human Toxicology* 2004; 46: 144–146.
102. Santi R, Cascio G. Richerche farmacologiche sul principo attivo dell *Atractylis gummifera*. *Arch Ital Sci Farmacol* 1955; 5: 354.
103. Larribaud J. Two cases of poisoning by gummy thistle, *Atractylis gummifera* L. *Archives of Institute Pasteur d'Algerie* 1954; 32: 23–29.
104. Daniele C, Dahamna S, Firuzi O, Sekfali N, Saso L, Mazzanti G. *Atractylis gummifera* L. poisoning: an ethnopharmacological review. *Journal of Ethnopharmacology* 2005; 28: 175–181.
105. Hamouda C, Amamou M, Thabet M, Yacoub M, Hedhili A, Bescharnia F, Ben Salah N, Zhioua M, Abdelmoumen S, El Mekki N. Plant poisonings from herbal medication admitted to Tunisian toxicologic intensive care unit, 1983–1998. *Vetinerary and Human Toxicology* 2000; 42: 137–141.
106. Chan TY, Tomlinson BLK, Chan JC, Chan WW, Critchley JA. Aconite poisoning due to Chinese herbal medicines: a review. *Vetinerary and Human Toxicology* 1994; 36: 452–455.
107. Chan TY. Aconite poisoning: A global perspective. *Vetinerary and Human Toxicology* 1994; 36: 326–328.
108. Kolev ST, Leman GC, Kite PC, Stevenson D, Shaw D, Murray VS. Accidental ingestion of *Acotinum* containing Chinese remedy. *Human and Experimental Toxicology* 1996; 15: 839–842.
109. Sato H, Hamada C, Konnno Y, Ohizumi K, Endo Hikino M. Pharmacological actions of aconite alkaloids. *Tohoku Journal of Experimental Medicine* 1979; 128: 175–187.
110. Moher LM, Maurer SA. Podophyllum toxicity: case report and literature review. *Journal of Family Practice* 1979; 9: 237–240.
111. Cassidy DE, Drewry J, Fanning JP. Podophyllum toxicity: a report of a fatal case and a review of the literature. *Journal of Toxicology and Clinical Toxicology* 1982; 19: 35–44.
112. Kao WF, Hung DZ, Tsai WJ, Lin KP, Deng JF. Podophyllotoxin intoxication: toxic effects of Bajiaolian in herbal therapeutics. *Human Experimental Toxicology* 1992; 11: 480–487.
113. Karalambev B. Ocular lesions caused by podophyllin. *Khirurgiia* (Sofia) 1962; 15: 420–423.
114. Frasca T, Brett AS, Yoo SD. Mandrake toxicity. A case of mistaken identity. *Archives of Internal Med* 1997; 157: 2007–2009.
115. Ng TH, Chan YW, Yu YL, Chang CM, Ho HC, Leung SY, But PP. Encephalopathy and neuropathy following ingestion of a Chinese herbal broth containing podophyllin. *Journal of Neurological Science* 1991; 101: 107–113.
116. Conard PF, Hanna N, Rosenblum M, Gross JB. Delayed recognition of podophyllum toxicity in a patient receiving epidural morphine. *Anesthesia and Analgesia* 1990; 71: 191–193.
117. Bonkovsky HL. Hepatotoxicity associated with supplements containing Chinese green tea (*Camellia sinensis*). *Annals of Internal Medicine* 2006; 144: 68–71.
118. E Med – Plant poisoning, Glycosides–Cardia: Article excerpt by Raffi Kapitan.
119. http:/www.emdicine.com/emerg/by name/ plant-poisoning-glycosides…cardiac.htm
120. Eddleston M, Warrell DA. Management of acute yellow oleander poisoning. *Quarterly Journal of Medicine* 1999; 92: 483–485.
121. Tuncok Y, Kozan O, Cavder C, Guven H, Fowler J. *Urginea maritama* (squill) toxicity. *Journal of Toxicology and Clinical Toxicology* 1995; 33: 83–86.
122. Stickel F, Seitz HK, Hahn EG, Schuppan D. Liver toxicity of drugs of plant origin. *Zeitschrift fur Gastroenterologie* (German) 2001; 39: 225–232, 234–237.
123. Haller CA et al. Making a diagnosis of herbal-related toxic hepatitis. California Poison Control System. *Western Journal of Medicine* 2002; 176 (1): 39–44.
124. Harper J. Traditional Chinese medicine for

eczema. *British Medical Journal* 1994; 308: 489–490.

125. Horowitz RS, Feldhaus K, Dart RC, Stermitz FR, Beck JJ. The clinical spectrum of Jin Bu Huan toxicity. *Archives of Internal Medicine* 1996; 156: 899–903.
126. Ko RJA. U.S. Perspective on adverse reactions from traditional Chinese medicines. *Journal of the Chinese Medical Association* 2004; 67: 109–116.
127. Lin TJ, Su CC, Lan CK, Jiang DD, Ttsai MS. Acute poisonings with *Breynia officinalis* – an outbreak of hepatotoxicity. *Journal of Toxicology and Clinical Toxicology* 2003; 41: 591–594.
128. Depierreux M et al. Pathological aspects of a newly described nephropathy related to the prolonged use of Chinese herbs. *American Journal of Kidney Disease* 1994; 24: 172–180.
129. Areekul S, Kirdudom P, Chaovanapricha K. Studies on djenkol bean poisoning (djenkolism) in experimental animals. *South East Journal of Tropical Medicine and Public Health* 1976; 85: 621.
130. Stewart MJ, Steenkamp V, van der Merwe S, Zuckerman M, Crowther NJ. The cytotoxic effects of the traditional Zulu remedy, impila (*Callilepsis laureola*). *Human Experimental Toxicology* 2002; 21: 643–647.
131. Combest W, Newton NM, Combset A, Kosier JH. Effects of herbal supplements on the kidney. *Urological Nursing* 2005; 25: 381–386.
132. Chen CL, Fang HC, Chou KJ, Wang JS, C hung HM. Acute oxalate nephropathy after ingestion of star fruit. *American Journal of Kidney Disease* 2001; 37: 418–422.
133. Mueller B, Scott M, Sowinski K, Prag KA. Noni juice (*Morinda citrifolia*): Hidden potential for hyperkalaemia ? *American Journal of Kidney Disease* 2000; 35: 310–312.
134. Zuin VG, Yariwake JH, Lancas M. Analysis of pesticide residues in Brazilian medicinal plants: matrix solid phase dispersion versus conventional (European Pharmacopoeia) methods. *Journal of the Brazilian Chemical Society* 2003: 14.
135. Beyond Pesticides August 25 2004.
136. Aschwanden C. 2006. World Health Organization.
137. Tuso PJ. The herbal medical update. *Complementary and Alternative Medicine* 2002; 69(4): 22–25.
138. Needleman HL, Schell, Bellinger D, Leviton A, Allred EN. The long-term effects of exposure to low doses of lead in childhood: an 11 year follow up report. *New England Journal of Medicine* 1990; 322: 83–88.
139. Goldfrank LR, Flomenbaum NE, Lewin NA, Weisman RS, Howland MA, Hoffman RS. *Goldfrank's Toxicological Emergencies*, 7th edn. New York: McGraw-Hill, 2002.
140. Why barns are red: the health risks from lead and their prevention. A resource manual to promote public awareness. Toronto: Metropolitan Totonto Teaching Health Units and the South Riverdale Community Health Centre: 1995, Available www.city.toronto.on.ca/health/pubs_index.htm#barns
141. Hathaway GJ, Proctor NH and Hughes JP. *Proctor and Hughes' Chemical Hazards of the Workplace*, 4th edn. New York: Van Nostrand Reinhold, 1996.
142. Mercury Index Sheet, National Poisons Unit (London), Guy's Hospital, London, UK 2005.
143. Arsenic and Compounds Index Sheet. National Poisons Unit (London), Guy's Hospital, London, UK 2005.
144. Fung MC, Bowen DI. Silver products for medical indications: risk-benefit assessment. *Journal of Toxcology and Clinical Toxicology* 1996; 34: 119–126.
145. But PP. Herbal poisoning caused by adulterants or erroneous substitutes. *Journal of Tropical Medicine and Hygiene* 1994; 97: 371–374.

BIBLIOGRAPHY

General

Arsecularatne SN, Gunatilaka AA, Panabokke RG. Studies on medicinal plants of Sri Lanka: occurrence of pyrrolizidine alkaloids and hepatotoxic properties in some traditional medicinal herbs. *Journal of Ethnopharmacology* 1981; 4: 159–177.

Ernst E. Serious adverse effects of unconventional therapies for children and adolescents: a systematic review of recent evidence. *European Pediatrics* 2003, 162: 72–80.

Gilroy W. New study raises questions about safety of herbal supplements. *Newswire* February 27, 2004.

Miller GM, Stripp R. A study of western pharmaceuticals contained within samples of Chinese herbal/patent medicines collected from New York City's Chinatown. *Legal Medicine* 2007; 9(5): 258–264. (Available online 24.7.2007)

Metals

al Khayat A, Menon NS, Alidina MR. Acute lead encephalopathy in early infancy – clinical presentation and outcome. *Annals of Tropical Paediatrics* 1997; 17: 39–44.

Al-Saleh I, Nester M, DeVol E et al. Determinants of blood lead levels in Saudi Arabian school girls. *International Journal of Occupational and Environmental Health* 1999; 5: 107–114.

Centers for Disease Control and Prevention. Lead poisoning-associated death from Asian Indian folk remedies Florida. *MMWR* 1984; 33 (45): 638, 643–645.

Centers for Disease Control and Prevention. Lead poisoning associated with traditional ethnic remedies – California 1991–1992. *MMWR* 1993; 42: 521–524.

Centers for Disease Control and Prevention. Adult lead poisoning from an Asian remedy for menstrual cramps – Connecticut 1997. *MMWR* 1999; 48 (2): 27–29.

Centers for Disease Control and Prevention. Managing elevated blood lead levels among young children: Recommendations from the Advisory Committee on Childhood Lead Poisoning Prevention. Atlanta: CDC; 2002.

Cheng TJ, Wong RH, Lin YP, Hwang YH, Horng JJ, Wang JD. Chinese herbal medicine, sibship and blood lead in children. *Occupational and Environmental Medicine* 1998; 55: 573–576.

Friberg l, Nordberg GF, Vouk VB. *Handbook on the Toxicology of Metals*. Amsterdam: Elsevier, 1989.

Mojdehi GM, Gurtner J. Childhood lead poisoning through kohl. *American Journal of Public Health* 1996; 86: 587–588.

Sanborn MD, Abelsohn A, Campbell M, Weir E. Identifying and managing adverse environmental health effects: 3. Lead exposure. *Canadian Medical Association Journal* 2002; 166.

Tomlinson B, Chan TY, Chan JC, Critchley JA, But PP. Toxicology of complementary therapies: an eastern perspective. *Journal of Clinical Pharmacology* 2000; 40: 451–456.

Kidney diseases

Cosyns JP, Jadoul M, Squifflet JP, Wese FX, van Ypesele de Strihou C. Urothelial lesions in Chinese herb nephropathy. *American Journal of Kidney Disease* 1999; 33: 1011–1017.

Tatu CA, Oren WH, Finkelman RB, Feder GL. The etiology of Balkan endemic nephropathy: more questions than answers. *Environmental Health Perspectives* 1998; 106: 689–700.

Skin diseases

Atherton D et al. Chinese herbs for eczema. *Lancet* 1990; 336: 1254.

Clark AM. Naturally occurring mutagens. *Mutation Research* 1976; 32: 361–364.

Ferguson JE, Chalmers RJ, Rowlands DJ. Reversible dilated cardiomyopathy following treatment of atopic eczema with Chinese herbal medicine. *British Journal of Dermatology* 1997; 136: 592–593.

Latchman Y et al. The efficacy of traditional Chinese herbal therapy in atopic eczema. *International Archives of Allergy and Immunology* 1994; 104: 222–226.

Liao SC, Chiu TF, Chen JC, Lin CC. *Ajuga nipponensis* Makino poisoning. *Clinical Toxicology* (Phila) 2005; 43: 583–585.

Medicines and Healthcare products Regulatory Agency (MHRA) report, 18th November 2005.

New Zealand Director General's Privileged Statement Under Section 98 of the Medicines Act 1981, 22nd October 2004.

Shane-McWhorter. Biological complementary therapies: A focus on botanical products in diabetes. *Diabetes Spect* 2001; 14: 199–208.

Sheehan MP, Atherton DJ. One-year follow up of children treated with Chinese medicinal herbs for atopic eczema. *British Journal of Dermatology* 1994; 130: 488–493.

Sheehan MP et al. Efficacy of traditional Chinese herb therapy in adult atopic dermatitis. *Lancet* 1992; 340: 13–17.

4

Precautions to be Taken in Special Circumstances

Pregnancy, Breastfeeding, Surgery, Extremes of Age and Some Disease States

Age, life events such as pregnancy, or diseases such as heart disease, diabetes and asthma, alter body functioning and may affect its resistance or vulnerability to toxins and medications. Whether you are using herbal medications yourself, or as a physician are recommending them to others, it is very important that you take these factors into account when assessing the safety of a medicine for a specific individual.

It is also important to remember that genetic variations between individuals may be responsible for marked differences in their responses to external substances (e.g. pesticides, or alcohol) and medications. In the past decade it has emerged that genetic variations are responsible for individual differences in resistance or susceptibility to both herbal preparations and allopathic (Western) medications.

In this chapter we consider some of the dangers that may be associated with taking herbal medicines in situations where body functioning (physiology) differs from that of healthy young adults. Those situations include:

- presence of genetic abnormalities
- pregnancy
- breastfeeding (lactation)
- disease states – diabetes mellitus, high blood pressure, liver disease, kidney disease
- infancy and childhood
- old age.

We also consider the possible problems associated with the use of herbal medications by patients awaiting surgical operations.

Finally, we discuss the plant products which may produce effects on mood and behaviour. We must emphasize that such products, despite being of plant origin, are not free of adverse effects and use may lead to dependence and addiction in the same way as synthetic drugs that are commonly abused, and they should be used with caution.

INDIVIDUAL DIFFERENCES – GENETICALLY DETERMINED SUSCEPTIBILITY

As noted above, the way a drug acts in the body is not only determined by the person's environment, diet and state of health, but also and to a greater extent, by their genes.

'Pharmacogenetics' is the study of the influence of heredity on the extent to which an individual metabolizes or processes some drugs (pharmacokinetics) and the response of an individual (sensitivity/resistance) to certain drugs (pharmacodynamics).

Inherited factors appear to determine the effects of several common medications and even substances like alcohol, so that some adverse effects are experienced only by certain population groups. For example, some Japanese people lack an enzyme that metabolizes alcohol and suffer severe discomfort (facial flushing, increase in heart rate, muscle weakness) following alcohol intake. Genetic factors may determine whether some individuals are able to metabolize a particular drug rapidly while others metabolize the same drug slowly. An example is the drug isoniazid, which is used in the treatment of tuberculosis. In anaesthesia, a short-acting muscle relaxant popularly known as scoline (suxamethonium) may paralyse a patient for longer period than usual due to the genetically determined absence of, or an abnormality in, the enzyme (pseudocholinesterase) which metabolizes it. Similarly, in some races, around 10% of individuals may lack the important enzyme glucose-6-phosphate dehydrogenase, which is essential for the metabolism of certain herbal and allopathic medicines, for example herbs such as heartsease (*Viola tricolor*), *Acalypha indica* and *Salix caprea* (used in Ayurvedic medicine), menthol, which is used in many remedies, and chloroquine and primaquine which are used in the allopathic treatment of malaria. Intake of these substances will cause the red blood cells to start to break down (haemolysis) in affected individuals, and there is increased risk of ill-health.

The risk of oral cancer in chewers of betel quid is also genetically determined. Individuals with a deficiency of enzyme CYP2A6 have a lower risk of cancer. This enzyme metabolizes betel quid to toxic cancer-forming metabolites, so individuals with low levels of the enzyme, produce small amounts of the toxic constituent. The risk of cancer is increased, on the other hand, in individuals with genetic variation in the enzyme, known as CYP1A1 exon 7 polymorphism, because this enzyme produces more of the toxic metabolites.

You need to be aware of the significance of differences between individuals. Plant preparations that are used safely by some individuals may produce adverse effects and serious illness in others.

HERBS TO AVOID DURING PREGNANCY

Introduction

Considering that an estimated $3.87 billion is spent annually in the US on herbal products, botanicals and nutritional supplements, the potential for inadvertent exposure to these agents during pregnancy is substantial. The actual incidence of use in pregnancy is unknown, but one expert recently suggested that as many as 4 in 10 women use natural products such as echinacea, ginger or peppermint tea at some time during pregnancy and 1 in 5 opt to continue them throughout the full nine months of gestation in the US.

Significant dilemmas exist when assessing the impact of a drug on the developing foetus, whether it is an allopathic medicine obtained on prescription or purchased over the counter (OTC), or a herbal medication.

It is almost impossible for manufacturers of allopathic drugs to undertake pre-marketing tests of safety in pregnant women to determine effects on the foetus. In general, therefore, information regarding the use of allopathic prescription drugs in pregnancy is either scanty or difficult to interpret. Therefore, most drugs are not licensed for use during pregnancy. Typically, descriptions of drugs that appear in the *Physician's Desk Reference*[1] and similar sources contain statements such as, 'Use in pregnancy is not recommended unless the potential benefits justify the potential risks to the foetus'.

Assessing the risks associated with over-the-counter and herbal medications is even more problematic. Though herbal medicines have been in use for centuries, little has been done to monitor the safety of these preparations (disregarding variations in their constituents or concentrations) and there is rarely enough information to provide useful information on safety in pregnancy.

Usually, the only information on reproductive effects of these drugs comes from studies of animals, where pregnant females have been given doses high enough to cause adverse effects in the adult. However, such animal studies may not accurately indicate human risk.

The German Commission E lists herbs as contraindicated in pregnancy if there are reports in the literature that an agent has been successfully used as an abortifacient, or if there are experimental data proving genotoxic risk. Of the 300 herbs evaluated by this Commission, 26 were considered to be contraindicated in pregnancy.

A review of the *Physicians' Desk Reference for Non-Prescription Drugs*[1] reveals little or no information about reproductive toxicity for most medications. *The Botanical Safety Handbook*[2], published by the American Herbal Products Association, records that 200 out of the 644 botanicals in the handbook are not to be used in pregnancy. However, this review does not include the evidence on which these cautions are based and is intended to be a checklist for industry.

These typical disclaimers, although understandable from a medico-legal standpoint, put large numbers of women and their physicians in difficult situations, because:

1. In many countries, in both the developed and the developing world, at least half of all pregnancies are unplanned, and every year hundreds of thousands of women therefore expose their unborn children to drugs before they know they are pregnant. Such women often interpret the statement 'use during pregnancy is not recommended' as meaning that the drug is not safe during pregnancy. There is evidence that this perception of foetal risk causes many women to consider or even seek termination of otherwise wanted pregnancies.
2. Increasing numbers of women delay having children, and before they have become pregnant many more women have developed conditions that need to be treated with long-term drug therapy. Furthermore, in the past few decades the outcome of pregnancy has improved dramatically for women with conditions once believed to be incompatible with pregnancy, such as systemic lupus erythematosus and heart disease.

Many OTC and herbal agents include multiple constituents, both active and inactive, and it is difficult to determine the impact of several agents in combination. In addition, because most herbal agents are classified in the US as dietary supplements, they are exempt from the pre-marketing safety and efficacy standards that are required for conventional medications and there may be uncertainties regarding purity, dose, efficacy and side-effects.

It is a major concern that many herbal products are used without their physician's knowledge by pregnant women who do not realize they are potentially harmful. Finally, patients may misinterpret dosage instructions and take the agent in larger amounts or more frequently than recommended, resulting in unnecessarily excessive exposures of the fetus.

As a general rule, if drugs are available that are known to be safe for use in pregnancy, it is best to avoid those for which only limited information is available, unless physicians have reason to believe that they will have significant benefits for the mother.

Classification (see page 283)

We have attempted to classify drugs to be avoided during pregnancy as follows:

- Those with a tendency to promote or regulate menstruation (emmenagogues) and also cause abortions (abortifacients).
- Those that either directly or indirectly produce contractions of the smooth muscle of the uterus, e.g. laxatives, essential oils and bitters. These may also cause adverse effects on the developing systems in the foetus such as the nervous system.
- Those that produce hormonal effects which would either cause feminizing of a male foetus or masculinization of a female foetus – oestrogenic and androgenic herbs.
- Those that could cause malformation in the foetus – teratogens or teratogenic drugs.
- Those that could cause changes in the genetic make up of the foetus – mutagens.

Herbs that promote menstruation

Herbs that act as emmenagogues or have 'oxytocic' properties (i.e. make the muscle of the womb or uterus contract) should be avoided at all times during pregnancy. This is because by inducing severe cramping contractions of the uterus they can cause miscarriages. See the Table below for the herbs concerned.

Herbs with laxative properties that stimulate the uterus

Stimulant laxatives often produce an increase in activity of the uterus, which may be harmful to the pregnancy. Anthraquinone laxatives stimulate the uterus and other muscles, and may cause miscarriage. Any known uterine stimulant is best avoided in pregnancy and the use of laxative preparations which are of doubtful purity or concentration are particularly unsuitable.

Although herbal teas in general are encouraged as an alternative to caffeine-containing brews during pregnancy, some herbal teas may contain laxative herbs such as senna, frangula and cascara, and these also should be avoided.

Herbs that have been documented to have a stimulant or spasmolytic action on uterine muscle include blue cohosh, burdock, fenugreek, golden seal, hawthorn, Jamaica dogwood, motherwort, nettle, raspberry and vervain.

Culinary herbs (basil, oregano, etc.) are usually safe if used in small amounts in cooking, but if used in larger doses in teas they may be unsafe.

Essential oils

Essential oils are scented, or 'odorous', plant ingredients that evaporate at room temperature. Most are irritants to the mucous membranes and, more importantly, affect the central nervous system. This means they could harm the developing nervous system of the unborn child. In addition, a number of essential oils are also irritant to the genitourinary tract (kidney, bladder) when taken by mouth and may induce uterine contractions which are harmful during the course of a pregnancy.

Many herbs are traditionally reputed to be abortifacient (induce abortions or miscarriages) and for some, this reputation can be attributed to their essential oil component.

However, several texts (e.g. Tisserand and Balacs[3]) list essential oils that are considered safe to use during pregnancy. These are:

Cardamom	Neroli
Chamomile (German)	Palma rosa
Chamomile (Roman)	Patchouli
Clary	Petit grain
Coriander seed	Rose
Geranium	Rosewood
Ginger	Sage
Lavender	Sandalwood.

Essential oils which are safe to use externally, but should not be administered orally, rectally or vaginally during pregnancy, include:

Anise	Nutmeg
Fennel	Rosemary
Lava din	Spike lavender
Lavandula stoechas	Star anise
Mace	Yarrow (camphor CT).

Bitters

Bitters are plant constituents that stimulate the body's metabolism. They also stimulate 'smooth muscles' as found in the uterus. They may act as emmenagogues and all strong bitters should be avoided during pregnancy.

Herbs with hormonal effects

Several herbs are considered to have hormonal activity. Herbs with effects similar to those of the female hormone oestrogen may cause a male foetus to develop feminizing features. These include agrimony, alfalfa, aniseed, black cohosh, pleurisy root, red clover, saw palmetto and wild carrot.

Fucus and horseradish stimulate thyroid hormone activity, and vervain is considered to inhibit hormones which are associated with production of ova and/or sperm.

Herbs which cause fetal malformations or toxicity to the fetus (teratogenic and embryotoxic herbs)

Impaired development of fetal organs is termed teratogenesis. It may result in defects in structure or function of organs, known as malformations, restricted growth of the fetus, carcinogenesis or death. Malformations vary in severity from those that are so mild as to be unnoticed, i.e. hypospadias, to those that are life-threatening and require major surgery, or have serious cosmetic or functional effects.

Drugs that have teratogenic effects in animals when administered in high doses may not be teratogenic in humans when given in clinically relevant doses. For example, high doses of glucocorticoids (hormones from the adrenal gland) or benzodiazepines (drugs like Valium) can cause oral clefts in animals, but have no such effects in humans at clinically relevant doses. Similarly, salicylates (as found in aspirin) cause cardiac malformations in animals but not in humans. Although studies in animals may identify teratogenic effects, it can be difficult to extrapolate these effects to humans.

Some herbs have been found to be teratogenic in animal studies: for example, the popular eastern European herb *Plectranthus fruticosus* was found to be teratogenic in mice. However, in most cases, little information is available about the effects of herbs on the human embryo and fetus. It is possible that herbal chemicals may be transported across the placenta and cause toxic effects on the sensitive growing fetus. There is evidence from Morocco that fenugreek tea may be associated with malformation at birth if taken in early pregnancy.

Several principles should guide the selection of therapy during pregnancy. Since fetal safety is a major concern, it is preferable to use effective drugs with a long history of use, rather than newer alternatives.

To minimize risk to the fetus, drugs should be prescribed in doses at the lower end of the therapeutic range during pregnancy. Some women, however, may need higher than normal doses of many drugs (e.g. lithium, digoxin and phenytoin) during late pregnancy because of their increased body weight, blood volume and more rapid clearance.

Pregnant women should be discouraged from taking over-the-counter drugs (OTC) without counselling, since many factors, including the stage of pregnancy, can influence the risk to the fetus. For example, there is increasing evidence that although non-steroidal anti-inflammatory drugs (NSAIDs such as ibuprofen) may be taken safely for pain during the first trimester of pregnancy, in some cases they may constrict or even close the fetal ductus arteriosus (a tube that is present between the aorta and the artery to the lungs – pulmonary artery – in the fetus during late pregnancy and for a short period after birth).

In addition to the risk associated with fetal exposure to teratogenic drugs, there is a risk associated with misinformation about the teratogenicity of drugs, which can lead to unnecessary abortions or the avoidance of needed therapy. For example, drugs that have been shown to be teratogenic in animals, although known to be safe in humans, have caused women, their families and physicians unwarranted anxiety and may have contributed to unnecessary terminations of pregnancies. The medical community and drug manufacturers should make a concerted effort to protect women and their unborn babies from both risks. It is important to be aware that abortifacient herbs are highly toxic and can cause renal and liver failure, and ideally these herbal medicines should carry warnings on their labels.

Herbs to be avoided

The table on page 283 gives an alphabetical list of some of the herbal preparations that are recorded as 'to be avoided' during pregnancy. An obvious shortcoming of any list like this is that it does not take into account that effects may depend on dose taken and duration of use. However, in view of their potential to cause harm, it is best to avoid using them until more definite evidence regarding safety becomes available. This list is compiled from the information available to us and is not considered to be comprehensive.

Contaminants in herbal medicines

As indicated in Chapter 3, a major disadvantage of many herbal preparations is the presence of contaminants (e.g. allopathic medicines, heavy metals and toxic alkaloids). Obviously these contaminants, which are potentially toxic to adults, would have adverse effects of possibly greater severity in the unborn child.

Toxic plants and plant components

A 5-day-old Swiss child was diagnosed with veno-occlusive disease of the liver attributed to the consumption of large quantities of herbal tea containing pyrrolizidine alkaloids (PAs) by the mother throughout pregnancy. The child died on the 37th day.

The toxicity of pyrrolizidine alkaloids, including another case of an unborn child being affected by their use, is described in Chapter 3 (see pp. 251–252).

Allopathic medications

Allopathic medicines added to herbal medicines as adulterants can also have adverse effects on the unborn child. Corticosteroids, for example, may be included in some herbal products without being declared on the label or other product literature. These drugs are likely to affect the unborn child.

The Committee on Safety of Medicines documented the following effects of steroids on the fetus:

- Different corticosteroids vary in their ability to cross the placenta from mother to fetus, but prolonged or repeated treatment with corticosteroids during pregnancy increases the risk of fetal

(Continued on page 285)

Herb	Effect
Aloe	Laxative
American mandrake	Uterine stimulant
Arnica	Hormonal effects (oestrogenic)
Barberry	Bitters
Beth root	Uterine stimulant
Betony	Uterine stimulant
Black cohosh	Uterine stimulant
Blood root	Uterine stimulant, bitter
Blue cohosh	Uterine stimulant
Borage	Hepatotoxicity
Broom	Abortifacient
Buckthorn	Laxative
Butterbur	Hepatotoxicity
Calamus	Uterine stimulant, essential oil
Capsicum	Uterine stimulant
Carline thistle	Uterine stimulant
Cascara sagrada	Laxative, emmenagogue
Catnip	Emmenagogue
Cayenne	Uterine stimulant, essential oil
Celandine	Bitters, Embryotoxicity
Chamomile	Abortifacient/teratogenic potential
Chasteberry	Antiandrogenic, uterine stimulant
Cinchona	Bitters
Colt's foot	Carcinogenicity, abortifacient in animals
Cotton root bark	Emmenagogue
Cumin	Abortifacient
Devil's claw	Uterine stimulant
Docks	Laxative
Ephedra	Bitters
Fennel	Uterine stimulant, essential oil
Fenugreek	Contraction of uterus (oxytocic action)
Feverfew	Uterine stimulant
Flax seed	Uterine stimulant
Fucus (kelp)	Abortifacient
Garlic	Contraction of uterus (oxytocic action)
Ginseng – Panax ginseng	Embryotoxicity/fetotoxicity
Goldenrod	Abortifacient
Goldenseal	Uterine stimulant, bitter
Guggul	Emmenagogue
Herbs rich in pyrrolizidine alkaloids	Embryotoxicity/fetotoxicity
Hops	Hormonal effect (oestrogenic)
Horehound white	Laxative, abortifacient
Horehound, black	Laxative, menstrual regulation
Juniper	Essential oils
Lady's mantle	Uterine stimulant, emmenagogue

Continued on following page

Herb	Due to effect as:
Lavender	Essential oil
Liquorice	Uterine stimulant, oestrogenic activity
Madder	Mutagenic potential
Magnolia flower buds	Uterine stimulant
Malefern	Uterine stimulant
Marjoram	Essential oil
Mayapple	Emmenagogue
Meadow saffron	Laxative
Mistletoe	Emmenagogue, uterine stimulant
Motherwort	Uterine stimulant and also hormonal effects
Mugwort	Abortifacient
Nettle	Diuretic and uterine stimulant
Oregano	Essential oil
Oregon grape	Uterine stimulant
Parsley oil	Uterine stimulant
Passion flower	Uterine stimulant, emmenagogue, essential oil
Pennyroyal	Uterine stimulant, emmenangogue
Periwinkle	Uterine stimulant, emmenagogue
Pokeroot	Uterine stimulant, emmenagogue
Rhubarb	Uterine stimulant, emmenagogue
Rosemary	Essential oil
Rue	Emmenagogue
Sage	Uterine stimulant, essential oil
Sassafras	Carcinogenic potential
Senega	Emmenagogue
Senna	Laxative, uterine stimulant, emmenagogue
Shepherd's purse	Emmenagogue
Slippery elm bark	Abortifacient
Sophora japonica (Japanese pagoda tree) – seed pods	Abortifacient
Squaw vine	Emmenagogue
Squill	Cardiotoxicity
Tansy	Uterine stimulant, emmenagogue
Thuja	Uterine stimulant, emmenagogue, essential oil
Thyme	Uterine stimulant, emmenagogue, essential oil
Turmeric	Emmenagogue
Vervain	Emmenagogue
Wild cherry	Bitters, uterine stimulant
Wormwood	Uterine stimulant, emmenagogue
Yarrow	Essential oil, emmenagogue

growth being retarded. If the fetus is exposed to corticosteroids this can lead to suppression of adrenal function in the newborn child, but this usually resolves spontaneously after birth and only rarely leads to complications.

- The corticosteroid prednisolone appears in breast milk. Maternal doses of up to 40 mg daily are unlikely to cause the ill effects known to be associated with corticosteroids, such as 'moon face' (rounded faces similar to the moon which is a sign of steroid overdose), increased risk of infections, diabetes or brittle bones in the newborn, but if mothers receive a higher dose infants should be monitored for adrenal suppression (i.e. decreased output of hormones from the adrenal gland, which are necessary to combat stress and for many other vital functions).

HERBS TO AVOID DURING BREASTFEEDING/LACTATION

Often, a breastfeeding mother wants to increase her milk supply, particularly if she has been separated from her baby because of illness and is unable to nurse her baby at the breast. However, many herbal medicines contain ingredients that pass into breast milk (similar to many allopathic medications) and could be dangerous to the infant. At present, there is little information on the active components of herbs that appear in breast milk.

The herbal literature suggests that some herbs increase milk production. Fenugreek (*Trigonella foenum-graecum*) is reported to have this effect and also to cause low blood sugar (hypoglycaemia). Fenugreek seems to affect milk supply only if taken by the mother in large amounts, of the order of about three capsules three times per day, although the strength of the capsules varies greatly. Such high doses cause the mother's milk and urine, and the baby's as well, to smell like maple syrup. This has led to some babies being misdiagnosed as having 'maple syrup urine disease', a rather serious metabolic disorder. Another danger with fenugreek is that the herb is related to peanuts, a food associated with allergy in some individuals. In addition, coumarin and nicotinic acid found in fenugreek can have potent effects on heart rate, blood pressure, blood sugar and other bodily functions in the mother and infant.

Blessed thistle is another popular herb considered to enhance milk production. It was first described by the monks in the Middle Ages as a cure for smallpox. Today it is most commonly used in herbal medicine as a contraceptive and to treat infections and fever.

Fennel has also gained a reputation for promoting lactation, although oil from the fennel plant is very toxic and can cause fits, convulsions and breathing problems in doses as small as 1–5 ml (less than one teaspoon).

However, there is insufficient scientific evidence associated with the claims of many of these herbs as regards lactation. Many herbs used as herbal teas are safe for breastfeeding mothers in the concentrations that are recommended for use in tea. The major problem is that accurate quantification of ingredients is often lacking, and thus unqualified statements regarding safety cannot be made.

This chapter describes the possible risk to infants based on pharmacological profiles of herbs. A safe policy would be to avoid taking/prescribing a medication, whether herbal or allopathic, that is not clearly safe for the baby, during lactation. Breastfeeding mothers should be advised to avoid using herbal medicines that contain pharmacologically active substances (e.g. ginseng, kava kava, valerian) and also products which do not indicate ingredients in precise amounts or products that are unlabelled.

Herbal remedies best avoided during breastfeeding

As a general rule, breastfeeding mothers should avoid:

1. Remedies containing high doses of herbs containing alkaloids, particularly those that may affect the nervous system e.g. Chinese herbs

coptis, phellodendron (berberine alkaloids), sophora root (oxymantrine), ma-huang (ephedrine) and evodia (rutecarpine).
2. Remedies containing high doses of herbs known to have hormonal effects, e.g. fennel, anise, liquorice.
3. Herbs containing plant alkaloids known to cause liver and/or kidney damage. For example, to avoid some herbs that contain toxic pyrrolizidine alkaloids known to cause liver failure.
4. Strong purgatives, e.g. aloe or rhubarb root, that can cause diarrhoea or colic in the infant.
5. Herbs with a powerful immunosuppressive effect, e.g. tripterygium.

The list below is compiled from the information available at present.

Common name – Botanical name(s)	**Possible effects**
Aloe – *Aloe ferox, Aloe perryi, Aloe vera*	Strong purgative that can produce colic and diarrhoea in infants; however, topical use is considered safe
Anise – *Pimpinella anisum*	May produce hormonal effects in infants
Black snakeroot – *Cimicifuga racemosa*	May cause stomach upsets in infants
Bladderwrack – *Fuscus vesiculosus*	Contains a high amount of iodine which may affect infants
Borage – *Borago officinalis*	May cause liver toxicity
Buckthorn – *Rhamnus catharticus, Rhamnus frangula*	May affect the muscle tone of the uterus
Bugleweed – *Lycopus americanus, Lycopus europaeus, Lycopus virginicus*	Considered to have a hormonal effect which may reduce breast milk (antiprolactin activity)
Cascara sagrada – *Rhamnus purshiana*	Can cause diarrhoea and colic in infants
Coltsfoot – *Tussilago farfara*	Contains pyrrolizidine alkaloids; can accumulate in the liver
Comfrey – *Symphytum officinale*	Contains pyrrolizidine alkaloids; can accumulate in the liver and cause serious liver disease and blood clots in infants – banned in Canada
Cork tree – *Phellodendron amurense* (Huang bai)	Contains alkaloids that may affect the nervous system
Dang gui – Dong quai – *Angelica sinensis*	Can stimulate the nervous system and make skin more sensitive to light
Elecampane – *Inula helenium*	Can cause gastrointestinal upset in infants
Ephedra – *Ephedra* spp. (ma-huang)	May stimulate the nervous system of infants
Evodia danielli (Wu zhu yu)	Contains rutecarpine, an alkaloid that may affect the nervous system

Continued on following page

Common name – Botanical name(s)	Possible effects
Fennel – *Foeniculum vulgare*	Fennel teas are often recommended to breastfeeding mothers of infants with colic. However, essential oil from the fennel is toxic. Can also cause convulsions and respiratory problems in doses as small as 1–5 ml (less than one teaspoon) and may produce hormonal effects in the infant
Fenugreek – *Trigonella foenum-graecum*	Highly likely to cause an allergic reaction in babies (fenugreek is related to peanuts), and associated with increased colic and diarrhoea in babies. Can cause hypoglycaemia in the nursing mother and can raise blood pressure (contains coumarin and nicotinic acid)
Garlic – *Allium sativum*	Can taint the flavour of milk resulting in reduced milk ingestion by infant
Ginkgo biloba leaf	Platelet inhibitor
Ginseng	Oestrogenic effects and platelet changes
Gold thread – *Coptis*	Contains berberine alkaloids that may affect the nervous system
Gravel root – *Eupatorium purpureum*	Contains pyrrolizidine alkaloids which may cause liver toxicity
Kava kava – *Piper methysticum*	May affect nervous system (hypnotic/sedative effects) and damage the infant's liver
Liquorice – *Glycyrrhiza glabra, Glycyrrhiza uralensis*	May produce hormonal effects in the infant
Male fern – *Dryopteris filix-mas*	Nausea and vomiting and diarrhoea may occur even with therapeutic doses. Contraindicated in children under four years
Parsley – *Petroselinum crispum*	May reduce production of breast milk
Rauwolfia – *Rauwolfia serpentina*	May cause changes in blood pressure in the infant
Rhubarb (root) – *Rheum officinale, Rheum palmatum tanguticum*	May cause colic and diarrhoea in the infant
Sage – *Salvia officinalis*	May decrease production of breast milk
Senna – *Senna alexandrina, Senna obtusifolia, Senna tora*	May cause colic and diarrhoea in the infant
Sophora root – *Sophora japonica*	Contains alkaloids that affect the nervous system
Stillingia – *Stillingia sylvatica*	Has laxative properties which may cause diarrhoea, colic in infant

Continued on following page

Common name – Botanical name(s)	Possible effects
St John's wort – *Hypericum perforatum*	Used for postnatal depression and is considered safer than allopathic medications. May interact with any other medications so should only be used if advised by a physician. See Interactions, p. 337–341
Tripterygium	Powerful immunosuppressant
Wormwood – *Artemisia absinthium*	The thujone content of the herb causes vomiting, intestinal cramps and disturbances in the nervous system
Wintergreen – *Gaultheria procumbens*	One of the main components is methyl salicylate which is contraindicated in neonates and in all children under the age of 12 years, as is aspirin

Natural plant toxicants in milk

Although elimination of toxicants in breast milk is a minor route of excretion, the contaminated milk may have an important effect on the health of individuals for whom it is a primary food source, particularly neonates. This needs to be considered when a breastfeeding infant presents with an unusual form of ill-health or when the diagnosis of ill-health in a breastfeeding infant is in doubt.

Among the plant toxicants excreted in milk[4] are:

- Tremetol or tremetone, the toxin in white snake root (*Eupatorium rugosum*) and rayless goldenrod (*Haplopappus heterophyllus*): these plants have been responsible for intoxication of cows and their suckling calves and for many human poisonings.
- Pyrrolizidine alkaloids from *Senecio, Crotalaria, Heliotropium, Echium, Amsinckia, Symphytum* (comfrey), *Cynoglossum* (hound's tongue), *Festuca* (tall fescue).
- Piperidine alkaloids in *Conium*, tobacco.
- Quinolizidine alkaloids in *Lupinus*.
- Sesquiterpene lactones in bitterweed and rubber weed.
- Glucosinolates in *Amoracia* (horseradish), *Brassica* (cabbage, broccoli), *Limanthes* (meadowfoam), *Nasturtium* (watercress), *Raphanus* (radish), *Thlaspi* (stinkweed).

HERBAL MEDICINES TO BE USED WITH CAUTION IN CHILDREN AND ADOLESCENTS

Ingestion of herbal medication among children is high. As many as 30% of children in the US, 33% of children with asthma in the UK, and over 70% of children with some form of cancer have tried at least one form of non-allopathic treatment.

Children differ from adults in their absorption, distribution, metabolism and excretion of most substances. They have relatively large livers and thus in some respects they are more efficient in reducing the toxicity of some substances. However, they also have a developing nervous system and a developing immune system which may make them more sensitive to the adverse effects of some herbs. Thus, infants and children are likely to be physiologically more vulnerable to the adverse effects of certain herbs. For example some herbs such as buckthorn, senna and aloe are known cathartics and some herbal teas and juniper oil contain diuretics. Herbal products are generally considered to be mild diuretics and the use of laxatives or cathartics is likely to be more of a problem. These actions may cause dehydration in a child. Further, disturbances of the salt contents in the blood and body (electrolyte contents) may occur more quickly than in adults and any agent that predisposes to loss of electrolytes in the urine or from the bowel should be used carefully.

Also, as with adults, there may be subpopulations of children who are more susceptible to adverse effects of herbal medications. For example, individuals with allergies may be at increased risk of adverse reactions from herbs or herbal remedies known to contain allergens (substances capable of causing allergies or allergic reactions). The first use of a potentially allergenic herb must be approached with caution since individuals may not be aware that they have an allergy. Some plants cause allergic reactions in the skin (contact dermatitis) whereas others may cause wheezing, runny nose (rhinitis), redness and tearing of the eyes (conjunctivitis), itchy throat and other allergic manifestations. Chamomile for example can cause anaphylaxis in individuals who are allergic to other members of the plant family Compositae (such as ragweed, chrysanthemum). Photosensitization can also occur with herbs such as angelica and rue which contain certain chemicals known as psoralens, especially if used in creams or ointments for topical application. If such creams are used it is advised that exposure of the skin to sunshine is reduced and children should wear long sleeves or trousers. High doses of St John's wort are also capable of photosensitization.

Parents should be aware that herbal remedies may contain combinations of potentially toxic or harmful constituents. As such there is an increased risk of toxicity to a child from preparations that contain combinations of herbs. Parents should not be tempted to give combinations of herbs to children, or to rely on information from advertising magazines or websites or advice from friends and relatives. Such experimentation is not only expensive, but also potentially hazardous.

Woolf[5] has produced guidelines for paediatricians for prescribing for children, adapted from Eisenberg's guidelines for clinicians on the use of allopathic medicines[6] quoted in many textbooks.

It is important for clinicians to find out about the beliefs of the parents and about the alternative therapies, herbs and other remedies used by the family and given to children. In the study by Spigelblatt et al.[7], up to 50% of families that used non-allopathic medications did not reveal this to their primary care physician.

The potential danger associated with medications, both allopathic and herbal due to inadequate tests for ill-effects in the young or in vulnerable population sectors, is illustrated by the case of sulfanilamide. Steinbrook[8] reports this tragedy. The allopathic medication sulfanilamide became available in the 1930s. At that time there was a need for a liquid preparation that could be taken by small children. Because the sulphur drug did not dissolve easily in water, a chemist at the Massengill pharmaceutical company in the US prepared an 'elixir' containing diethylene glycol. At the time medications had to meet standards for purity and truth in labelling, but there was no requirement to establish safety before using them clinically. Tragically, 107 persons, including many children, died of diethylene glycol poisoning as a result. This illustrates the necessity for testing for safety of products particularly to be used in children. Sulfanilamide-related deaths, and the epidemic of birth defects associated with thalidomide in the 1960s, were significant incidents that initiated major changes in the laws and regulations that govern the testing and marketing of new drugs in the US.

However, as Steinbrook[8] points out, testing of medications for safety and effectiveness has mainly benefited adults, who outnumber children and take many more medicines. Allopathic medications, including many that are widely used in children, are rarely tested in children; 'Thus even with allopathic medications in children, educated guesses about doses, safety and effectiveness are in use'. Rigorous testing of herbal medications in adults is rare, so use in children must be approached with a degree of caution.

The following herbal/traditional medicines need to be used with caution or avoided in children and neonates:

1. ***St John's wort.*** There is recent concern that certain allopathic antidepressant medications such as the selective serotonin reuptake inhibitors may have an unfavourable benefit/risk ratio in

children and adolescents with major depression. This raises the question about the benefit/risk ratio of St John's wort in this age group. The available studies of St John's wort in juvenile patients have such limitations that they do not provide an adequate answer to this question.

2. ***Lead-containing herbal medicines.*** Metallic lead is absorbed to a greater degree in the juvenile gut. Chronic low level exposure in children is associated with reduced intellectual capacity and behavioural/learning disorders. Prolonged raised blood lead levels in children are associated with squint, foot drop, passage of protein (albumin) in urine and delayed growth. Lead-induced encephalopathy (brain swelling) is a serious and potentially fatal condition in children. Bint al dhahab (translates as 'daughter of gold') contains mainly lead oxide and is used in the Middle East to treat stomach ailments in neonates and children. It has been associated with encephalitis and neurological deficits due to lead poisoning (see Chapter 3).
3. ***Neem tree (Azadirachta indica).*** Neem oil given orally to neonates and infants has been associated with toxic encephalopathy.
4. ***Blue cohosh (Caulophyllum thalictroides).*** Blue cohosh contains substances (glycosides and alkaloids) that act on the heart and blood vessels in animals. Animal experiments have shown that black cohosh could cause damage to the heart muscle (myocardium). Severe neonatal heart disease has been reported following maternal ingestion of blue cohosh over a period of one month prior to delivery.
5. ***Herbs containing pyrrolizidine alkaloids* (PAS) – *see Chapter 3.*** In adults pyrrolizidine alkaloids present in plants such as *Senecio* and *Symphum* have been known to cause liver disease, particularly veno-occlusive disease. South African authors reported a case series of 20 children suffering from hepatic veno-occlusive disease due to the use of pyrrolizidine alkaloid-containing herbal remedies. The mortality was high and those who survived developed cirrhosis and portal hypertension.
6. ***Germander (Teucrium chamaedrys).*** Ingestion of germander caused liver cell necrosis in a 15-year-old girl which resolved promptly on discontinuing germander, thus confirming liver toxicity (hepatotoxicity) of the herb. *Teucrium* is toxic in adults as well and has been withdrawn from use.
7. ***Thunder God vine (Tripterygium wilfordii).*** A severe birth defect involving the brain and skull in an infant at birth was attributed to the intake of this herb by the mother during early pregnancy for rheumatoid arthritis.
8. ***Asafoetida (Ferula assafoetida).*** Newborns with their higher levels of foetal haemoglobin may be more susceptible to assafoetida, which can cause methaemoglobinaemia[9].
9. ***Jin bu huan.*** Slowing of the heart rate (bradycardia) and respiratory and central nervous system depression developed in children given the product jin bu huan for pain relief[10].
10. ***Topical vinegar.*** Repeated application caused burns.
11. ***Eucalyptus oil* (80–85% Cineole oil).** Australian data bases revealed that eucalyptus oil was a leading cause of hospital admission for childhood poisoning in Victoria. Following topical application the signs of toxicity include slurred speech, unsteady gait and drowsiness leading to unconsciousness.
12. ***Herbs containing allopathic contaminants.*** Presence of medications of uncertain purity and age are a concern in children and more so when found as constituents of herbal medicines. The availability of chloramphenicol, an allopathic medication, from non-Western sources is of particular concern. Chloramphenicol is a prescription antibiotic that can cause serious blood disorders such as aplastic anaemia (reduction of blood cells) and thrombocytopenia (reduction in platelets). Its use in infants is contraindicated except in life-threatening infections, as is its use during pregnancy and lactation. Acetylsalicylic acid in young children has been associated with Reye's syndrome, a potentially fatal condition.

13. ***Herbal enemas.*** Herbal enemas are popular in South Africa where 40% mortality has been reported in children who developed the 'paediatric enema syndrome' – respiratory distress, tachypnoea (increased rate of breathing), abdominal distension, hypotonia (diminished tone in muscles) and loss of consciousness accompanied by hyperglycaemia (elevation of blood sugar) and leucocytosis (increase in white cells in the blood).

HERBAL MEDICINES TO BE USED WITH CAUTION IN OLDER AGE

Older people (aged 65 and over) consume more prescription and over-the-counter medicines than any other age group. They are also more likely to take traditional medicines and to use more of them, particularly in countries where traditional medical practice provides the most affordable and accessible form of medical practice[11]. As a result, drug–drug interactions and drug–herb interactions are more likely[12].

Older people tend to be more sensitive to drugs than younger people due to a deterioration in function of organs such as the heart, lung and kidney, and the loss of muscle mass, which means that for a given dose of drug the blood concentration is higher than it would be in younger people.

Any form of drug therapy in the elderly, whether with allopathic or herbal medicines, is associated with the following risks or dangers, many of which increase the risk of side-effects having more serious consequences:

- The risk of drug interactions is greater as older people tend to suffer from several disease states and are required to take multiple medications.
- Most functions of the vital organs are decreased, and if kidney function is decreased, drugs are likely to be excreted from the body more slowly; there is a risk of accumulation of drugs and thus of adverse effects and toxicity.
- The metabolism of some drugs may be reduced in the elderly.
- Mouth lesions are likely both due to lack of oral hygiene and due to retention of medications in the mouth when there is some difficulty in swallowing.
- Altered mental activity often occurs in old age due to nerve cells having been lost or damaged, or due to some defect in the production and effects of the chemical messengers (neurotransmitters). The loss of nerve cells results in many elderly patients becoming more sensitive to drugs that act on the nervous system, particularly nervous system depressants such as sedatives and painkillers.
- Drugs which affect the heart and blood vessels increase the risk of adverse effects such as low blood pressure and dangerous changes in heart rhythm as a result of their use in the older age group. This is due to loss of elasticity of the blood vessels and the degenerative changes in blood vessel walls and in heart muscle cells that occur with ageing.
- Adverse reactions to drugs may present in the elderly in an unusual manner – vague symptoms should not be ignored. Confusion is often the presenting symptom.
- Since falls are likely to have serious consequences for the elderly, all precautions should be taken to minimize side-effects that might result in falls, such as decrease in blood pressure, sedation or confusion.

The broad principles applicable to use of both allopathic and herbal medicines in old age are:

1. Always start with a lower dose (50%) than that prescribed for healthy young adults – 'Start low and go slow'.
2. Prescribe from a range of drugs whose effects on the elderly are well documented or known.
3. Review patients carefully prior to repeat prescriptions.
4. Explain to relatives/carers the drugs, the side-effects and the manner in which the drugs should be taken. It is always safer to write down instructions. Studies have shown that between 40% and 75% of older people do not

take their medications at the right time or in the right amount.

Older people who experience dizziness, constipation, upset stomach, sleep changes, diarrhoea, incontinence, blurred vision, mood changes, a rash and any other new symptom should consult a physician as soon as possible.

HERBAL MEDICINES TO BE USED WITH CAUTION OR DISCONTINUED PRIOR TO SURGERY

As soon as a date for a surgical operation is known, patients should seek advice from their doctors about when to stop taking herbal medicines. Different herbs remain within the body for different lengths of time, and it may be necessary to stop taking them a week or more before surgery. In a study of 601 patients in Hong Kong, Lee et al[13] found that 80% used self-prescribed traditional Chinese herbal medicines in the two weeks prior to surgery.

Patients may be using herbal medicines chronically for conditions such as eczema. Others may use them as a tonic in preparation for an operation. However, there are few trials to show either the benefits or adverse effects of using herbal medicines prior to surgery. Although the properties of several herbs show that they can theoretically interfere with bleeding or recovery from anaesthesia, the clinical data are weak as they are based on anecdotal reports. Lee et al[13] attempted to investigate whether discontinuation of herbal medicines prior to surgery or anaesthesia would alter outcome, but they could not define any such changes. This lack of effect may indicate limited adverse effects of herbal medicines, but further systematic investigations are required. Herbal medicines may cause adverse effects during anaesthesia and surgery, in the same way as some allopathic medications do. However, the relationship between the dose and duration of therapy and the potential to cause adverse effects during surgery and anaesthesia has not been extensively studied or documented for herbal medicines compared with allopathic medicines.

In a review of the scientific literature, Ang-Lee et al[14] concluded that echinacea, ephedra, garlic, ginkgo, ginseng, kava kava, St John's wort and valerian are commonly used herbal medications that may pose a concern during the period just before and just after surgery. Adverse interactions during surgery may be restricted to a limited list of herbs, but without more extensive studies it is not possible to state which herbs can be safely used. Without clear evidence of safety, it may be prudent for patients to stop taking herbal medicines prior to surgery.

Herbal medicines may produce adverse effects during surgery and anaesthesia in several ways:

- by increasing the tendency to bleed during and after surgery
- by potentiating the drugs used during anaesthesia, thereby delaying recovery from anaesthesia
- by delaying healing of wounds
- by causing electrolyte disturbances that would affect the action of drugs and also the responses of the body to events during the perioperative period
- by decreasing immunity and thus increasing the likelihood of infections
- by producing harmful changes in pulse rate, blood pressure and heart rhythm which may potentiate the cardiovascular toxicity of some of the drugs used during anaesthesia
- by causing anxiety, restlessness and insomnia and increasing the mental discomfort associated with surgical procedures
- by producing changes in metabolism (e.g. lowering of blood sugar – hypoglycaemia) which may cause complications during and after surgery
- by producing changes in drug metabolizing enzymes (e.g. CYP450 enzymes) which would cause unpredictable changes in activity of drugs used during and after surgery
- by causing abdominal discomfort, heartburn and distension and thus increasing discomfort during the postoperative period

- by interfering with immune mechanisms and promoting the rejection of organs after transplant surgery.

If surgery is scheduled at short notice, patients should bring the herbal medicines they are using to the hospital in their original containers. The surgeon and anaesthetist can then review the dosage and strength of the herbal drugs and provide the necessary guidelines. By discontinuing herbs for a period before surgery and informing the doctor of all herbs and medications that are being taken, the number of complications that may accompany the surgical procedure may be minimized.

There are some herbs which should not be withdrawn abruptly but by gradually reducing the dose. For example, if feverfew is withdrawn suddenly, this can cause 'post-feverfew syndrome' – characterized by rebound headaches. Withdrawal of guarana, which contains caffeine (consumed daily in many parts of South America), after regular daily consumption may cause anxiety, headache and irritability.

The following herbal medicines have been reported to produce adverse effects during or after surgery and to interfere with the safety of the anaesthesia. These considerations have also been considered to be applicable to pets undergoing surgery (Holly Nash DVM MS, Veterinary Services Department, Drs Foster and Smith Inc).

Herbal drug	Effect	Advice
Alfalfa	Prolongs coagulation time.	Be aware.
Black cohosh	Can cause slowing of the heart rate and a drop in blood pressure. Also active ingredients have oestrogen-like hormonal activity. Also contains salicylates.	May potentiate effects of anaesthetic drugs that lower blood pressure. Discontinue for two weeks before surgery.
Chamomile	Can increase bleeding. Apigenin, one of its active components, inhibits effect of benzodiazepines (e.g. Valium).	Titrate doses of benzodiazepines (e.g. Valium) carefully.
Dang gui – Dong quai – *Angelica sinensis*	May cause bleeding.	Discontinue prior to surgery.
Danshen	May cause bleeding.	Discontinue prior to surgery.
Echinacea	Stimulates immune system and could therefore interfere with immunosuppressant therapy, anabolic steroids, amiodarone, methotrexate, ketoconazole and ciclosporin. NOTE: to be avoided particularly in transplant surgery.	Discontinue as soon as transplant surgery is decided as there is a possible risk of transplant rejection. For other forms of surgery discontinue at least a week beforehand. If treatment continued for more than eight weeks there is a risk of immunosuppression (suppression of normal immune responses in the body).

Continued on following page

precautions in special circumstances

Herbal drug	Effect	Advice
Ephedra	Raises blood pressure and heart rate and causes arrhythmias (irregular heart beats), may block blood supply to the heart muscle. Central nervous system stimulation when used with decongestants (e.g. pseudo ephedrine hydrochloride) which can interfere with anaesthesia and sedation. Interaction between ephedra and anaesthesia may cause life-threatening high blood pressure, bleeding into the brain and coma.	Discontinue at least 24 hours before surgery. Extreme caution in patients with high blood pressure (hypertension), other cardiovascular diseases (heart disease) and hyperthyroidism (increased activity of the thyroid gland).
Evening primrose oil	Reduces platelet aggregation, may interact with anticoagulants and/or antiplatelet drugs. Use cautiously with drugs that lower threshold for seizure.	Discontinue prior to surgery and anaesthesia.
Feverfew	Bleeding, nervousness, insomnia and tiredness before and after surgery. Can inhibit platelet aggregation. Suggested may cause release of serotonin, hence caution when given in combination with serotonergic drugs (e.g. fluoxetine, sumitriptan).	Discontinue before surgery and anaesthesia.
Garlic	Reduces blood clot formation, increases risk of operative bleeding. Gastrointestinal effects – abdominal distension.	Discontinue 7 days before surgery.
Ginger	Heartburn. May relieve anaesthesia-induced nausea.	Be aware.
Ginkgo biloba	Reduces platelets and blood clotting. Additive anticoagulant effect with aspirin, clopidogrel, ticlopidine, dipyridamole, warfarin. Increases intraoperative and postoperative bleeding. NOTE: coagulation studies may be normal.	Discontinue *Ginkgo biloba* at least 7 days before surgery.
Ginseng	Increases bleeding and anticoagulant effect of warfarin, increases incidence of arrhythmias (irregular heart beat), increases blood pressure and heart rate, causes hypoglycaemia (low blood sugar). Trembling, headache and manic behaviour if taken with phenelzine. If taken with digoxin makes it difficult to monitor the response to digoxin.	Discontinue at least 7 days before surgery.

Continued on following page

Herbal drug	Effect	Advice
Goldenseal	Increases blood pressure.	Be aware. Monitor blood pressure closely.
Kava kava	Prolongs coagulation time. Interacts with alcohol, hypnotics (drugs that induce sleep) and antipsychotics (drugs used to treat psychiatric disorders) to increase the sedative effect. Interacts with alprazolam to produce deep sedation/ coma. With general anaesthetics has an additive effect.	Discontinue at least 24 hours before surgery. Taper off dose over several weeks prior to surgery if used to aid sleep. NOTE: Should not be used with benzodiazepines, e.g. Valium.
Kudzu	Report of bleeding after surgery.	Be aware and avoid administration in patients awaiting surgery or after surgery.
Liquorice	Prolongs coagulation time, increases blood pressure and causes water retention and electrolyte imbalance. May cause hypokalaemia (decreased body potassium) induced arrhythmias.	Most liquorice candy contains no herbal liquorice. Monitor serum potassium and other electrolytes prior to surgery and anaesthesia.
Psyllium and fibre	Used in constipation. May cause adverse effects in patients with intestinal obstruction.	Monitor serum potassium prior to surgery if on long-term laxatives.
St John's wort	Interacts with many drugs metabolized in the liver. Affects warfarin and lidocaine (a local anaesthetic) therapy. Interacts with preoperative and postoperative medications including narcotic drugs and anaesthetic agents. Can raise blood pressure and also cause confusion, agitation and drowsiness in surgical patients. When taken in combination with sertraline may cause serotonin syndrome. Possibly associated with rejection of transplanted organs. May cause increased metabolism of a wide range of drugs that may be used in the treatment of the patient prior to, during and after surgery due to the induction of drug-metabolizing enzymes.	Discontinue as soon as transplant surgery is decided. Discontinue for at least 5 days before other forms of surgery.
Valerian	Increases sedative effects of anaesthetics, painkillers (analgesics) and sleeping tablets (hypnotics). Long-term use may reduce the effects of these drugs.	Taper dose as soon as surgery is planned – weeks before surgery.

Another group of drugs that need to be considered prior to surgery and anaesthesia in some patients, are those which increase the formation and flow of urine (diuretics). The following herbs have been traditionally used as diuretics:

Alfalfa (*Medicago sativa*)
Asparagus root (*Asparagus officinalis*)
Dandelion (*Taraxacum offinale*)
Goldenrod (*Solidago virgaurea*)
Horsetail (*Equisetum arvense*)
Juniper berry (*Juniperus communis*)
Lovage root (*Levisticum officinale*)
Parsley (*Petroselinum crispum*)
Stinging nettle leaf (*Urtica dioica*)
Uva-ursi (*Arctostaphylos uva-ursi*)

The study by Anna Lee et al.[13] revealed that the following herbs were considered to have been possibly associated with preoperative hypokalaemia (reduction in potassium levels) which necessitated oral potassium chloride supplementation in one patient:

Achyranthes root	Cinnamon twig
Atractylodes	Loranthus

These herbs vary in their diuretic activity, though generally herbs are weakly diuretic. However, all have the potential, particularly with prolonged use, to cause disturbances in electrolyte balance within the body. They may cause depletion of potassium, which may adversely affect the activity of muscle relaxants that are used during anaesthesia. Thus it is necessary for clinicians to ask patients about their use of diuretic drugs or drugs related to kidney disease, in addition to the herbs that are better documented as having the potential to cause unwanted reactions during surgery and anaesthesia.

Health professionals need to be aware of the use of herbal and other traditional medicines by their patients prior to surgery or anaesthesia. It is likely that there are unrecorded resources of knowledge in countries where traditional and orthodox medicine have been used together in hospital settings (e.g. China). Given the paucity of information on the safety of individual herbs, systematic research and investigation is required to improve on this knowledge, and this applies to all herbal medicine, regardless of origin, whether Ayurvedic, Chinese, Unani, African or South American.

As doctors learn more about herbal supplements and their effects, other herbs may be added to the list of those causing concern. Ask your doctor about any herbal product you are taking, even if it is not on this list.

HERBAL MEDICINES TO USE WITH CAUTION IN DIABETIC PATIENTS ON ALLOPATHIC MEDICATION

Over 400 plants have been identified as being hypoglycaemics (capable of lowering blood sugar). These include rehmannia, ginseng, vanadium and ubiquinone. Hypoglycin in the young Jamaican akee fruit can cause profound hypoglycaemia.

Similarly, elecampane, *Panax gingseng*, *Hydrocotyle*, liquorice and rosemary have been reported to have hyperglycaemic (increasing blood sugar) effects.

Before insulin was developed, diabetes was treated worldwide with a multitude of traditional medicines. American ginseng was shown to lower blood sugar levels after an oral glucose challenge when compared with a placebo, and many considered ginseng as being capable of lowering blood sugar after a meal.

Unripe bitter melon was a traditional Asian remedy for diabetes as was gymnema, an ancient Ayurvedic remedy. In an animal experiment, gymnema was shown to double the density of insulin-producing beta cells in the pancreas.

Fenugreek, the popular Middle Eastern and Indian spice was also considered to have antidiabetic properties.

Of the Hispanic foods, the pads and fruits of the

prickly pear cactus or nopal was a traditional antidiabetic remedy. Nopal was shown to contain substances that increased the sensitivity to insulin in the human body.

In the Arabian Peninsula, aloe vera was used to treat diabetes. A Polynesian cure for diabetes was noni juice (*Morinda citrifolia*). Native Americans used devil's club, barberry, *uva-ursi*, Canada and daisy fleabane, alum root, Joe Pye weed, red trillium, wild ginger, clintonia, bugleweed and flowering spurge for treating diabetes.

Other herbal or related substances used in the treatment of diabetes were cinnamon, jambul (Ayurvedic) and stevia, a popular sugar substitute isolated from a South American shrub.

There is insufficient evidence at present to either dismiss or accept the claims for the many herbal preparations that have been used for centuries by diverse communities in the world to treat diabetes.

However, the concern is that herbal products for treatment of diabetes may be adulterated with allopathic prescription drugs that interact with allopathic medicines used to treat diabetes. In 2000, the FDA issued a healthcare warning about the following herbal products that contained adulterants:

- Diabetes hypoglucose capsules
- Pearl hypoglycaemic capsules
- Tongyi Tang Diabetes Angel Pearl hypoglycaemic capsules
- Tongyi Tang Diabetes Angel hypoglycaemic capsules
- Zhen qi capsules

A cautious, but possibly necessary approach would be to assume that most traditional medicines would have had some effect on the control of blood sugar in humans.

Therefore any diabetic patient on allopathic medication should inform their physician if they are using any of the traditional antidiabetic herbal medicines, so that the possibility of harmful effects from the concomitant intake of allopathic and herbal antidiabetic medications can be assessed. Also, individuals who are using only herbal medications should use the available facilities for monitoring urine and blood sugar to ensure that blood sugar is adequately controlled, and to reduce the risk of the multitude of well-documented and serious complications associated with diabetes mellitus.

HERBAL MEDICINES TO BE USED WITH CAUTION OR AVOIDED BY PATIENTS WITH HEART DISEASE

In patients with heart disease, herbal remedies may produce dangerous complications such as an increase in blood pressure, disturbances in heart rhythm and an increase in the activity of the sympathetic nervous system[15]. All these effects can adversely affect the wellbeing of these patients.

Herbal medicines that have the potential to cause harm to patients with heart disease can be classified as follows:

Herbal medicines that increase heart rate and/or blood pressure

Belladona alkaloids increase the heart rate due to their atropine content.

Ginger, ginseng, yohimbine and liquorice may increase blood pressure. Ginger increased blood pressure in animal experiments. When used for long periods ginseng produces an abuse syndrome which includes high blood pressure. However some studies show that ginseng has a tendency to lower blood pressure. Yohimbine is a stimulant of the sympathetic nervous system which leads to an increase in blood pressure. The herb causes an increase in the levels of the chemical messengers of the sympathetic nervous system such as adrenaline and noradrenaline, and this may also lead to dangerous disturbances in the heart rhythm (arrhythmias). Patients with autonomic failure or bipolar depression are particularly sensitive to the autonomic and central side-effects of yohimbine[16].

Liquorice causes retention of sodium and water (mineralocorticoid activity) which leads to an increase in blood pressure, and sometimes fluid may accumulate in the lungs and cause severe difficulty in breathing (pulmonary oedema).

As noted above in the section on use of herbal drugs prior to surgery, ephedra raises blood pressure, due to its action on the sympathetic nervous system, which is similar to activity of the body's chemical messengers. Ephedra is a constituent of ma huang, which has been reported to cause disturbances in the heart beat/rhythm and even heart attack (myocardial infarction) and stroke.

Herbal medicine that decreases blood pressure and heart rate

Hellebore has been reported to cause a slowing of the heart rate and a fall in blood pressure.

Herbal medicines that increase the tendency to bleed

Danshen, feverfew, garlic, ginger, ginkgo and kava increase the tendency to bleed, due to their effect on the activity of the blood platelets, which usually stop bleeding by forming a platelet plug.

Herbal medicines that may cause disturbances in heart rhythm

Oleander contains substances similar to the cardiac drug digoxin and so excessive intake may produce disturbances in heart rhythm and arrhythmias. Other agents that act like oleander are foxglove (*Digitalis purpurea*), dogbane (*Apocynum cannabinum*), lily-of-the-valley (*Convallaria majalis*), wallflower (*Cheiranthus cheiri*), red squill (*Urginea maritima*). Aconite contained in monkshood or wolfsbane should also be avoided, though it has been used in herbal cardiac medications.

The activity and toxicity of many drugs used in the treatment of heart disease are affected by the concentrations of electrolytes such as sodium and potassium in the body fluids. The activity of digoxin is markedly affected by the concentration of potassium in the body and in the blood. The toxicity of digoxin may be increased in patients who have been using laxatives such as senna, cascara sagrada and buckthorn for a long period, because these drugs significantly reduce the amount of potassium in the blood.

HERBAL MEDICINES TO BE USED WITH CAUTION OR AVOIDED BY PATIENTS WITH JAUNDICE

Coptis chinensis/japonica and *Artemisia scoparia* are highly effective in displacing bilirubin from its serum protein binding and for this reason should not be used in patients with elevated serum bilirubin (jaundice).

Huang lian (*Coptis chinensis*) causes kernicterus in pre-term infants with neonatal jaundice, which is thought to be mainly due to the activity of its major ingredient, berberine, a potent bilirubin displacer and an inhibitor of bilirubin metabolism.

Non-infectious hepatitis has been associated with the use of blue-green algae (microcystins), chaparral (*Larrea tridentata*), germander (*Teucrium chamaedrys*), jin bu huan (*Stephania sinica*), lobelia (*Lobelia inflate*), mistletoe (*Phoradendron flavescens*), penny royal (*Hedeoma pulegiodes*), fo-ti, ho shou wu (*Polygonum multiflorum*).

HERBAL MEDICINES TO BE USED WITH CAUTION OR AVOIDED BY INDIVIDUALS WITH ALLERGIES

The term allergy is used to describe exaggerated responses to external substances. These 'allergic' reactions are mediated by immune mechanisms within the human body. Although up to 20% of the population perceive themselves as suffering from food allergies, it is probable that only 1–2% really have genuine food allergies.

Clinical effects following exposure to an allergic substance occur immediately. The clinical reactions may range from trivial symptoms such as itchiness (pruritus), rash, flushing and sneezing, to life-threatening effects such as fall in blood pressure, severe breathing difficulties and dangerous changes in heart rate and heart rhythm.

In view of the unpredictability of the severity of an allergic response and the life-threatening consequences that may follow exposure to allergens, caution is a necessity and it is best to avoid or prevent exposure.

There are several herbs that are reported to cause allergic reactions. These include:

Agnus castus	Dandelion
Angelica	Elecampane
Anise	Euphorbia
Apricot	Feverfew
Arnica	Ginkgo
Artichoke	Gravel root
Asafoetida	Guaiacum
Calendula	Juniper
Cassia	Meadowsweet
Celery	Tansy
Chamomile	Vornsilk
Cinnamon	Yarrow
Cowslip	

(Adapted from Barnes et al.[17])

HERBAL MEDICINES TO BE USED WITH CAUTION OR AVOIDED BY PATIENTS WITH BOWEL DISEASE

Symptoms of diarrhoea, constipation or an alteration of bowel habit should be considered as meriting medical attention or advice, particularly if the symptoms have been persistent for more than two weeks.

Senna, buckthorn, cascara and rhubarb are anthraquinone laxatives which have constituents that are activated in the bowel to stimulate motility of the bowel. They also act as bulk forming agents promoting the accumulation of water and electrolytes in the gut lumen and can produce fluid shifts which may be life-threatening. Chronic use can be harmful, resulting in a form of dependency on laxatives causing fluid and electrolyte imbalance in the blood, fall in blood pressure and a certain degree of dysfunction of the cardiovascular system. Melanosis coli, a black pigmentation pattern of the mucosa of the colon, is pathognomonic of chronic anthraquinone use and has an epidemiological association with carcinoma.[18]

Pokeweed (*Phytolacca americana*) contains phytolaccine which is a potent gastrointestinal irritant capable of producing haemorrhagic gastritis, hypotension and death[19].

HERBAL MEDICINES TO BE USED WITH CAUTION OR AVOIDED BY INDIVIDUALS LIKELY TO SUFFER FROM SUNBURN

Herbal preparations rich in psoralens (e.g. fruit of *Psoralea corylifolia* and celery root[20,21]) may produce phototoxic burns in visitors to sun parlours or patients undergoing therapy with a psoralen and ultraviolet A (PUVA).

HERBS THAT HAVE PRODUCED CANCERS IN LABORATORY ANIMALS

Aristolochia fangchi – urothelial carcinoma
Betel (*Areca catechu*)
Borage
Calamus (*Acorus calamus*)
Coltsfoot
Comfrey
Croton oil (*Croton tiglium*)
Khat (*Catha edulis*)
Life root
Rue (*Ruta graveolens*)
Sassafras (*Sassafras albidum*)

HERBS AFFECTING THE FUNCTION OF THE NERVOUS SYSTEM

Herbal medications and individual herbs may affect the nervous system, either as stimulants or depressants, and many tend to be abused for these specific effects, e.g. hallucinogenic effect. Almost all of these plant products have rather severe and discomforting side-effects such as nausea and vomiting, and it is certainly not recommended that they are used solely for their effects on mood.

Ephedra or ma huang. One of the best known stimulants of the nervous system is ephedra or ma huang, which has been used to treat narrowing of the breathing tubes (bronchoconstriction) for centuries. Ephedra may increase body temperature and cause symptoms such as agitation and, as has already been noted above, may increase heart rate and blood pressure.

***Khat* (*Catha edulis*)** is widely used in the Arabian Peninsula and East Africa for its stimulant and fatigue-decreasing effects (amphetamine-like effects)[22]. Khat contains over 30 compounds including norpseudoephedrine (cathine) and cathinone, the latter being the main psychoactive ingredient. The cathinone content is higher in red khat which is more potent than white khat. It releases chemical messengers (neurotransmitters e.g. dopamine) in the brain. Physical dependence has not been reported, but psychological dependence is common in chronic users. Norpseudoephedrine is found in the urine and breast milk of women who use khat. Chronic use is associated with oral cancers, constipation and high blood pressure. Severe adverse effects include myocardial infarction, cerebral (brain) haemorrhage and pulmonary oedema. Cirrhosis, decreased libido and impotence have also been reported.

***Betel nut* (*Areca catechu*)** is chewed worldwide for its stimulant effect in the nervous system. One of its constituents, arecoline, causes diarrhoea, vomiting, salivation and seizures. It also narrows the small breathing tubes in the lung (bronchoconstriction) and may exacerbate spasm of these tubes in asthmatics. Chronic use is associated with oral cancer[23].

Kava kava is often enjoyed as a social drink in the South Pacific Islands because it induces a pleasant sense of tranquillity, sociability and euphoria. It is not considered to be a hallucinogen. It does not appear to cause physiologic dependence, but the risk of psychological dependence exists.

***Arnica* (*Arnica montana*)** also contains toxic ingredients like arecoline and its oral ingestion can be lethal.

***Wormwood* (*Artemesia absinthium*)** acts on the nervous system to produce sedation, seizures and hallucinations. It is believed to act like camphor. The active component thujone is thought to produce hallucinations by acting on the same receptor as the active ingredient in cannabis. Thujone may also cause seizures and rhabdomyolysis which may be followed by kidney disease[24]. Absinthism is a psychotic disorder which is accompanied by some intellectual impairment. Vincent Van Gogh and Edgar Degas were reputed to be absinthe drinkers. Van Gogh is thought to have eaten paint and camphor and drunk turpentine for its terpene content when craving for absinthe[25]. Use of absinthe has now been restricted.

Herbs affecting mood and thinking

The following herbs have been used for their effects on mood and thinking (psychoactive effect) and may carry the risk of abuse and some degree of dependence.

Hallucinogens	Euphoriants	Stimulants	Sedatives/ tranquillizers
Ibogaine *(Tabernanthe iboga)*	California poppy *(Eschscholtzia californica)*	Cinnamon *(Cinnamomum camphora)*	Broom *(Cytisus* spp.*)*
Juniper *(Juniper macropoda)*	Catnip *(Nepeta cataria)*	Damiana *(Turnera diffusa)*	Hops *(Humulus lupulus)*
Kava kava *(Piper methysticum)*	Cloves *(Syzygium aromaticum)*	Hydrangea *(Hydrangea paniculata)*	Snake root *(Rauwolfia serpentina)*

Continued on following page

Hallucinogens	Euphoriants	Stimulants	Sedatives/ tranquillizers
Mandrake *(Mandragora officinarum)*	Lobelia *(Lobelia inflate)*	Kola nut *(Cola* spp.*)*	Wormwood *(Artemesia absinthium)*
Morning Glory *(Ipomoea violacea)*		Mate *(Ilex parguayensis)*	Valerian *(Valeriana officinalis)*
Nutmeg *(Myristica fragrans)*		Mormon tea *(Ephedra nevadensis)*	
Periwinkle *(Catharanthus roseus)*		Passion flower *(Passiflora incarnata)*	
Thorn apple *(Datura stramonium)*			
Yohimbe *(Pausinystalia yohimbe)*			

Adapted from Hung OL et al.[26]

REFERENCES

1. *Physicians' Desk Reference for Non-Prescription Drugs*. Montvale, New Jersey: Thomson PDR, 2005.
2. McGuffin M (Ed.). *American Herbal Products Association's Botanical Safety Handbook*. Boca Raton, Florida: CRC Press, 1997.
3. Tisserand R, Balacs T. *Essential Oil Safety*. Edinburgh: Churchill Livingstone, 1995.
4. Panter KE, James LF. Natural plant toxicants in milk: a review. *Journal of Animal Science* 1990; 68: 892–904.
5. Woolf A D. Herbal remedies and children: Do they work? Are they harmful? *Paediatrics* 2003; 112: 240–246.
6. Eisenberg DM. Advising patients who seek alternative medical therapies. *Annals of Internal Medicine* 1997; 127: 61–69.
7. Spigelblatt L, Laine-Ammara G, Pless IB, Guyer A. The use of alternative medicine by children. *Pediatrics* 1994; 94: 811–814.
8. Steinbrook R. Testing medications in children. *New England Journal of Medicine* 2002; 347: 1462–1470.
9. Kelly KJ, Neu J, Camitta BM, Honig GR. Methemoglobinaemia in an infant treated with the folk remedy glycerated asafoetida. *Pediatrics* 1984; 73: 717–719.
10. Centers for Disease Control and Prevention. Jin bu huan toxicity in children, Colorado 1993. *MMWR* 1993; 42: 633–636.
11. Bruno JJ, Ellis JJ. Herbal use among US elderly: 2002 National Health Interview Survey. *Annals of Pharmacotherapy* 2005; 39: 643–648.
12. Dergal JM, Gold JL, Laxer DA, Lee MS, Binns MA, Lanctot KL, Freedman M, Rochon PA. Potential interactions between herbal medicines and conventional drug therapies used by older adults attending a memory clinic. *Drugs and Aging* 2002; 19: 879–886.
13. Lee A, Chui PT, Aun CS, Lau AS, Gin T. Incidence and risk of adverse perioperative events among surgical patients taking traditional Chinese herbal medicines. *Anesthesiology* 2006; 105: 454–461.
14. Ang-Lee MK, Moss J, Yuan CS. Herbal medicines and perioperative care. *JAMA* 2001; 286: 208–216.
15. Valli G, Giardina EG. Benefits, adverse effects and drug interactions of herbal therapies with cardiovascular effects. Review article. *Journal of the American College of Cardiologists* 2002; 39: 1083–1095.
16. Onrot J, Goldberg MR, Biaggioni I, Wiley RG, Hollister AS, Robertson D. Oral yohimbine in human autonomic failure. *Neurology* 1987; 37: 215–220.
17. Barnes J, Anderson LA, Phillipson JD. *Herbal Medicines*, 2nd edn. London: Pharmaceutical Press, 2002.

18. Siegers CP, Von Hertzberg-Lottin E, Otte M et al. Anthranoid laxative abuse – a risk for colorectal cancer. *Gut* 1993; 34: 1099–1101.
19. Roberge R, Brader E, Martin ML et al. The root of evil – pokeweed intoxication. *Annals of Emergency Medicine* 1986; 15: 470–473.
20. Ljunggren B. Severe phototoxic burn following celery ingestion. *Archives of Dermatology* 1990; 126: 1334–1336.
21. Boffa MJ, Gilmour E, Ead RD. Celery soup causing severe photosensitivity during PUVA therapy. *British Journal of Dermatology* 1996; 135: 334.
22. Loqman W. Danowskie TS. The use of khat (*Catha edulis*) in Yemen, social and medical observations. *Annals of Internal Medicine* 1976; 85: 246–249.
23. Taylor RF, al-Jarad N, John LM et al. Betel nut chewing and asthma. *Lancet* 1992; 339: 1134–1136.
24. Weisbord SD, Soule JB, Kimmel PL. Brief report: Poison on line – acute renal failure caused by oil of wormwood purchased through the internet. *New England Journal of Medicine* 1997; 337: 825–827.
25. Arnold WN. Vincent Van Gogh and the thujone connection. *JAMA* 1988; 260: 3042–3044.
26. Hung OL, Lewin NA, Howland MA. Herbal preparations. In: Goldfrank LR, Flomenbaum NE, Lewin NA, et al. (Eds) *Goldfrank's Toxicologic Emergencies*, 7th edn. New York: McGraw-Hill, 2002:1129–49.

BIBLIOGRAPHY

General

De Smet PAGM. Perspectives in Clinical Pharmacology. Health risks of herbal remedies: an update. *Clinical Pharmacology and Therapeutics* 2004; 76: 1–17.

Ko RJ. A U.S. perspective on the adverse reactions from traditional Chinese medicines. *Journal of the Chinese Medical Association* 2004; 67: 109–116.

Pregnancy

Koren G, Pastuszak A, Ito S. Drugs in pregnancy. *New England Journal of Medicine* 1998; 338: 1128–1137.

Breastfeeding

Lawrence RA. Herbs and breastfeeding. http://www.breastfeeding.com/reading_room/herbs.htm

Dharmananda S. On taking herbs while breastfeeding. Portland, Oregon: Institute for Traditional Medicine, 2001. http://www.itmonline.org/arts/breast.htm.

Anaesthesia

Hodges PJ, Kam PCA. The perioperative implications of herbal medicines. *Anaesthesia* 2002; 57: 889–899.

Jayasekera N, Moghal A, Kashif F, Karalliedde L. Herbal medicines and postoperative haemorrhage. *Anaesthesia* 2005; 60: 725–726.

Crowe S, Lyons B. Herbal medicine use by children presenting for ambulatory anaesthesia and surgery. *Pediatric Anaesthesia* 2004; 14: 916–919.

Critchley LA, Chen DQ, Chu TT, Fok S, Yeung C. Preoperative hepatitis in a woman treated with Chinese medicines. *Anaesthesia* 2003; 58: 1096–1100.

Cheng B, Hung CT, Chiu W. Herbal medicine and anaesthesia. *Hong Kong Medical Journal* 2002; 8: 123–130.

Mayo Clinic. Herbal supplements and surgery: What you need to know. www.mayoclinic.com

The American Association of Nurse Anesthetists (AANA). Guide for those awaiting surgery. www.aana.com

Diabetes

Johnston L. Nutritional and botanical approaches to diabetes. http:/www.healingtherapies.info/DIABETES.htm accessed 2006

Werner M, Knobeloch LM, Erbach T, Anderson HA. Use of imported folk remedies and medications in the Wisconsin Hmong Community. *Wisconsin Medical Journal* 2001; 100: 32–34.

Medicines Healthcare Products Regulatory Agency. Department of Health, UK. www.mhra.gov.uk

Price LH, Charney DS, Heninger GR. Three cases of manic symptoms following yohimbine administration. *American Journal of Psychiatry* 1984; 1267–1268.

Shepherd C. Sleep disorders. Liver damage warning with insomnia remedy. *British Medical Journal* 1993; 306: 1477.

5

Drug–Herb and Herb–Herb Interactions

Research on herbal medicines is not as advanced as research on pharmaceutical drugs. Although manufacturers, prescribers, users and nationally appointed authorities have established procedures and systems for monitoring the safety, adverse effects and interactions associated with the use of allopathic medicines, none of these groups monitors herbal medicines to the same extent.

In addition, the lack of regulatory control over the production of herbal medicines has compounded the problem. There may be significant variations in the composition and strengths of components of identically marketed herbal medicines. This is likely to occur more frequently if the medicines come from different sources, but may occur even if the medicines are from the same source. These differences make interpretation of interactions very difficult.

Descriptions of drug–herb interactions are often unspecific and imprecise because there are no sophisticated systems for monitoring such interactions and reports are often poorly and inconsistently documented. Information on the management of drug–herb interactions is also sparse and anecdotal and often published in languages that are not globally understood, resulting in errors in translation. There have been very few studies of drug–herb interactions by scientific bodies.

The following account of drug–herb interactions has been compiled from a variety of sources. It does not claim to be comprehensive, but aims to provide an overview including both interactions that are known to occur and those that are considered likely based on knowledge and presumptions about the possible actions of components of herbal drugs on vital organs, drug-metabolizing enzymes and transport systems.

However, there are some important considerations that are necessary when studying or reading the list of interactions we have provided.

For example, many herbs contain the constituent coumarins. Though it is widely believed that this constituent is likely to interfere with blood clotting, in all instances this may not necessarily be so. The same applies to the salicylic acid content of herbs. As to whether the salicylic acid content would produce effects similar to aspirin when administered in the doses used in herbal practice is uncertain in all instances. Thus some interactions associated with coumarin and salicylic acid contents in particular are indicated with the assumption that the products do produce effects similar to their allopathic counterparts.

As regards induction or inhibition of the cytochrome P450 metabolizing enzymes in the liver and or intestine, there is little information available as to what doses of the herbs are associated with specific degrees of inhibition or induction of these metabolizing enzymes. This is important as some of the herbs known to cause effects on the metabolizing enzyme systems are widely used as antidepressants (e.g. St John's wort) and in the treatment of HIV infections (e.g. *Sutherlandia frutescens*). The same applies to effects on drug transport systems such as P-gp. Some herb–herb interactions are also included at the end of the chapter for completion and to raise awareness that interactions are just as much a risk even when only herbal medications are used.

It is very important for allopathic physicians to consider the possibility that drug–herb interactions may be the cause of unusual reactions following administration of allopathic medicines.

In general, drug interactions including drug–herb interactions lead to an alteration of the blood levels of the drug. Some drugs have a narrow range of blood levels within which they produce the desired therapeutic response. If the upper limit of therapeutic range is exceeded, adverse effects and toxicity are likely. Similarly if the blood level is lowered below the therapeutic range, lack of response or therapeutic failure is likely.

Additionally, drug–drug interactions become important when the disease that is being treated is serious or life-threatening.

In general, interactions that are clinically important occur with:

- oral anticoagulants – blood thinning agents
- oral hypoglycaemic agents – drugs that lower blood sugar
- antibiotics – drugs used to treat infections
- antiepileptic agents – drugs used to control or prevent fits in epilepsy
- anti-arrhythmic agents, cardiac glycosides – drugs that act on the heart to prevent or treat disturbances in the rhythm of the heart and heart failure
- oral contraceptives
- antiviral HIV drugs – drugs used in the treatment of AIDS and HIV infections.

Mechanisms of drug–herb interactions, similar to drug–drug interactions, can be broadly classified as 'pharmacokinetic' and 'pharmacodynamic' interactions. To find out what this means, read on.

PHARMACOKINETIC INTERACTIONS

Pharmacokinetic interactions change the way the body absorbs, distributes, metabolizes and excretes a drug.

Interactions during drug absorption

- A drug that alters the acidity of the stomach contents could either decrease or increase the absorption of the co-administered drug. Herbal medications are more likely to form complexes with, for example, metal cations such as calcium.
- A drug that chelates (forms a strong bond with) a co-administered drug will prevent its absorption.
- A drug that increases or decreases the muscular movement of the gut will affect the rate at which co-administered drugs move through the gut and the time available for their absorption, and therefore the amount absorbed.
- Intestinal transport mechanisms are required by certain drugs for either their absorption and/or secretion (excretion) back in to the gut. There are many drugs that either inhibit or induce these intestinal transport mechanisms. Thus drugs inhibiting or inducing the transport mechanisms can alter the absorption/excretion and consequently the blood levels of the co-administered drug.

Interactions during protein binding

Once absorbed from the gut, drugs enter the blood. A proportion of the absorbed amount of some drugs binds to proteins in the blood, forming molecules that are unable to pass into the tissues, so have no therapeutic activity. The proportion of the drug bound to proteins may be altered if another drug is taken that forms a stronger bond with the same proteins. The first drug is displaced, and the blood concentration of unbound active drug increases. A given dose of the first drug may have a greater toxic or therapeutic effect when taken with the second drug than when taken on its own.

Interactions during metabolism

Most drugs undergo chemical changes in the liver and gut. The rate at which these changes take place may be increased or decreased by other drugs, herbal medicines, foods or drinks such as grapefruit. Changes in the rate at which drugs are made active or inactive by metabolic processes, the speed of onset and the duration of its therapeutic activity will occur if the associated processes or their particular constituents such as enzymes are affected by other medications. Drug interactions may also affect chemical breakdown of a drug in the body by changing the nature of the chemical reactions, and these altered processes may produce toxic end products.

Interactions during excretion (elimination of drug from body)

Most drugs are eliminated (cleared) from the bloodstream by the kidney and the liver. Drugs that alter the pH (acidity or alkalinity) of the urine or alter the concentration of certain ions necessary for interchange with the drug in the filtering systems (nephrons) of the kidney will interfere with the excretion of some drugs.

Another important interaction can occur between two drugs which use a common excretory pathway. If one drug is excreted in preference to the other, the second drug may accumulate in the body, increasing the likelihood of toxicity. Some drugs inhibit the enzymes in the kidney that are necessary for excretion of other drugs.

PHARMACODYNAMIC INTERACTIONS

Pharmacodynamic interactions are changes in the pharmacological effect of one drug caused by another drug.

Pharmacodynamic interactions occur at the site of action of a drug or herbal medicine. Two drugs that produce a similar effect when given alone may, if taken together, produce an effect that is a summation of the normal effect of each drug, or a synergistic effect that is greater than the summation of their individual effects. When medications have opposing effects at the target site, co-administration is likely to cause reduced effect of one of them.

TABLE OF INTERACTIONS

The evidence found in the scientific literature for interactions between natural products and drugs is often contradictory. There is evidence from *in vitro*, *in vivo* and clinical studies that herbals and other dietary supplements interact with many drugs, but drug–herbal interactions are difficult to evaluate because of the lack of reliability of these products[1]. The interactions often involve drug-metabolizing enzymes and drug transporter systems, although pharmacodynamic interactions could also be involved. It is often difficult to predict potential interactions because knowledge of the pharmacokinetic and pharmacodynamic characteristics of most herbal and other dietary supplements is incomplete.

Fugh-Berman and Ernst[2] developed a rubric for determining the reliability of case reports of drug–herb interactions. The probability of an interaction is scored using a 10-point scale, where one point is given for each of 10 items such as patient's medical history and event chronology. We were unable to use this system to evaluate reliability of drug–herb interactions as access to the related scientific literature was inconsistent.

The following table is a summary of the information about potential drug–herb interactions available to us.

We have attempted to present the level of evidence for each of the interactions. Our experience was similar to that reported by Chavez et al[1]: we found the experimental data in the field of drug–herb interactions was limited, case reports were scarce and case series even rarer. Nevertheless, we considered it would be most useful to provide an overview of potential drug–herb interactions that *have* been reported in the scientific literature, although they are based on varying degrees of evidence, in order that prescribers and users should be aware of the possible risks.

At the end of this chapter is a paragraph on the effects of herbal remedies on clinical laboratory tests. Be aware that a blood test, for example, may produce inaccurate results if certain herbal remedies are being taken.

Herbal drug	Allopathic drug	Probable cause/s of interaction	Clinical effects	Precautions
Adonis	Digoxin	Additive inotropic actions of the constituent cardiac glycosides	May cause an increase in adverse effects of digoxin	Be aware
	Quinidine	Additive inotropic effects of the constituent cardiac glycosides	May cause an increase in adverse effects of quinidine	Be aware
Aloe	Cardiac glycosides, e.g. digoxin	Causes decreased blood levels of potassium. Can also cause a diarrhoea which decreases the absorption of drugs with a narrow therapeutic index	Potentiates toxicity of cardiac glycosides	Monitor serum potassium and administer potassium supplements orally if indicated. Take drugs 1 hour before or 2 hours after herbal products
	Diuretics	Increases potassium loss from the gut	Low body potassium – may give rise to lethargy and muscle weakness	Provide potassium supplements orally
	Tolbutamide	Prolongs presence of drug in the plasma	Risk of low blood sugar (hypoglycaemia)	Monitor blood glucose regularly, inform physicians
	Warfarin	Unknown	May cause an increased effect of warfarin (blood test INR is prolonged)	Be aware, inform physicians
Angelica dahurica	Tolbutamide	Angelica extracts reduced the elimination of tolbutamide in animal experiments	May interfere with control of blood sugar	Be aware
Anise	Iron	May enhance absorption of iron from the gut	None	Be aware
Arnica	Warfarin	Coumarin components may increase bleeding tendency	May cause bleeding	Be aware

Continued on following page

Herbal drug	Allopathic drug	Probable cause/s of interaction	Clinical effects	Precautions
Ashwagandha	Barbiturates and benzodiazepines (e.g. Valium)	Unknown	Potentiates sedative effects	Be aware, avoid concomitant use
Asian ginseng	Hexobarbital	Unknown	May prolong sleep	Be aware and inform physicians
	MAO inhibitors (e.g. phenelzine, tranylcypromine, selegiline)	Unknown	Hallucinations and psychosis	Be aware, inform physicians
	Warfarin	Unknown	May decrease the effect of warfarin–decreased INR (a measure of the anticoagulant effect of warfarin)	Inform physicians, avoid concomitant use
	Antidiabetic agents	Enhances the blood sugar lowering effect (hypoglycaemic)	Increases risk of hypoglycaemia (low blood sugar)	Monitor blood glucose regularly and warn patients
Astralagus	Immunosuppressants – ciclosporin/ azathioprine, methotrexate	Impairs immunosuppressant activity	Possibility of graft rejection	Stop astralagus treatment
Avocado	Warfarin	Reduces absorption and possibly induces increased metabolism	Decreased anticoagulant effect	Inform physician, monitor INR closely and avoid concomitant use if possible
Baizhi	Tolbutamide	Inhibits CYP2E1 isoenzymes which prolong presence of drug in the blood (half life is prolonged)	Hypoglycaemia (low blood sugar)	Inform physicians, monitor blood sugar closely

Continued on following page

Herbal drug	Allopathic drug	Probable cause/s of interaction	Clinical effects	Precautions
Baizhi (*cont'd*)	Diazepam	Reduces metabolism by the liver	Potentiates CNS effects of diazepam (e.g. drowsiness)	Warn patients, inform physicians
	Insulin and other anti-diabetic drugs	Unknown	Risk of low blood sugar (hypoglycaemia)	Monitor blood sugar closely, inform physicians
Betel nut	Flupentixol	Unknown	Slowness of movement (bradykinesia), rigidity,	Inform physicians, avoid concomitant use
	Fluphenazine	Unknown	Tremor, stiffness	Inform physicians, avoid concomitant use
	Prednisolone and salbutamol	Arecoline challenge caused dose-related bronchoconstriction	Poor control of asthma	Inform physicians, be aware
	Procyclidine	Unknown, possibly antagonistic action on some (anticholinergic) properties of betel nut	Slowness of movement (bradykinesia), rigidity	Inform physicians, avoid concomitant use
	Beta-blockers, calcium channel blockers digoxin	Unknown	Has been shown to worsen bradycardia (slow heart rate)	None, be aware
Bilberry leaf	Warfarin	Decreases platelet aggregation	Increases potential for bleeding	Inform physician, monitor for increased tendency to bleed (petechiae, bruising and bleeding), avoid concomitant use
	Aspirin	Decreases platelet aggregation	Increases potential for bleeding	Inform physician, be aware

Continued on following page

Herbal drug	Allopathic drug	Probable cause/s of interaction	Clinical effects	Precautions
Black and long pepper (*Piper nigrum* L, *Piper longum* L)	Amoxicillin, cefotaxime	Unknown	Increased blood levels	None
	Phenytoin	Inhibition of transport (P-gp) and metabolizing enzymes (CYP2C9 and 3A4)	Increased blood levels of phenytoin	Inform physicians, avoid if side-effects worsen
	Propranolol	Inhibition of metabolizing enzymes (CYP1A1, CYPA2)	Increased blood levels of propranolol	Inform physicians, be aware
	Rifampicin	Inhibition of transport (P-gp) proteins	Increased plasma levels of rifampicin	Inform physicians, avoid concomitant use
	Theophylline	Inhibition of CYP	Increased plasma level of theophylline	Inform physicians, frequent monitoring if used concomitantly
Black cohosh	Aspirin	Black cohosh contains coumarin constituents	Increased risk of bleeding due to aspirin	Inform physician, monitor for increased bleeding tendency, be aware
	Cisplatin	Unknown	Decreased effectiveness of cell killing (cytotoxicity)	Inform physicians, avoid concomitant use
	Clopidogrel	Contains coumarin constituents	Increased risk of bleeding	Inform physician, monitor for increased bleeding tendency, be aware
	Dipyridamole	Contains coumarin constituents	Increased risk of bleeding due to dipyridamole	Inform physician, monitor for increased bleeding tendency, be aware
	Docetaxel	Unknown	Increased effects of docetaxel (cytotoxicity)	Inform physicians, avoid concomitant use

Continued on following page

Herbal drug	Allopathic drug	Probable cause/s of interaction	Clinical effects	Precautions
Black cohosh (*cont'd*)	Doxorubicin	Unknown	Increased cytotoxicity	Inform physicians, avoid concomitant use
	Heparin	Contains coumarin constituents	Increased risk of bleeding due to heparin	Inform physician, monitor for increased bleeding tendency, be aware
	Ticlopidine	Contains coumarin constituents	Increased risk of bleeding due to ticlopidine	Inform physician, monitor for increased bleeding tendency
	Warfarin	Contains coumarin constituents	Increased risk of bleeding due to warfarin	Inform physician, monitor for increased bleeding tendency, avoid concomitant use
	Anaesthetics	Unknown	Increases hypotensive effects of anaesthetics	Discontinue black cohosh two weeks before surgery
	Antihypertensives	Unknown	Increased hypotensive effects of antihypertensives – increased risk of low blood pressure (hypotension)	Be aware, monitor blood pressure, inform physicians if symptomatic
Boldo	Warfarin	Has anticoagulant properties	Increased risk of bleeding due to warfarin	Inform physicians, avoid concomitant use
Broom	Digoxin	Unknown	Potentiation of action of digoxin	Inform physicians, avoid concomitant use
	Beta adrenergic blockers e.g. propranolol, atenolol	Unknown	May enhance therapeutic effects of beta adrenergic blockers	Be aware, avoid concomitant use

Continued on following page

Herbal drug	Allopathic drug	Probable cause/s of interaction	Clinical effects	Precautions
Broom (*cont'd*)	Tricyclic antidepressants	Unknown	May develop cardiac arrhythmias (disturbances in heart rhythm)	Avoid concomitant use
Caffeine	Clozapine	Unknown	Elevated blood clozapine levels	Be aware, inform physicians
	Lithium	Unknown	Decreased blood lithium levels with decreased clinical effects	Be aware, inform physicians
	Theophylline	Unknown	Increased theophylline blood levels with increased risk of toxicity	Be aware, inform physicians
Capsicum spp. (Chilli pepper)	ACE inhibitors (e.g. captopril)	Capsicum depletes substance P	Increased risk of cough	Be aware and avoid concomitant use
	Theophylline	Likely to cause increased absorption and bioavailability	May increase risk of toxicity of theophylline	Be aware
Cascara	Laxative activity	May decrease absorption of drugs	May produce a poor response to many drugs	Be aware
Catnip	Central nervous system depressants (e.g. benzodiazepines)	May have additive sedative action	Risk of central nervous system depression (e.g. drowsiness)	Avoid concomitant use with alcohol, sedatives, hypnotics
Chamomile	Aspirin	Contains coumarin constituents	Increased risk of bleeding due to aspirin	Inform physician, monitor for increased bleeding tendency
	Clopidogrel	Contains coumarin constituents	Increased risk of bleeding due to clopidogrel	Inform physician, monitor for increased bleeding tendency

Continued on following page

Herbal drug	Allopathic drug	Probable cause/s of interaction	Clinical effects	Precautions
Chamomile (*cont'd*)	Dipyridamole	Contains coumarin constituents	Increased risk of bleeding due to dipyridamole	Inform physician, monitor for increased bleeding tendency
	Heparin	Contains coumarin constituents	Increased risk of bleeding due to heparin	Inform physician, monitor for increased bleeding tendency
	Ticlopidine	Contains coumarin constituents	Increased risk of bleeding due to ticlopidine	Inform physician, monitor for increased bleeding tendency
	Warfarin	Contains coumarin constituents	Increased risk of bleeding due to warfarin	Inform physician, monitor for increased bleeding tendency
Chaste tree	Metoclopramide	Chaste tree constituents are possibly dopamine agonists	Decreases the effect of dopamine antagonists such as metoclopramide	Theoretical possibility
Condurango	Carbamazepine, paroxetine, ritonavir, sertraline and other drugs metabolized by liver isoenzymes – CYP2A6	Contains 7-hydroxy coumarin, which is metabolized by liver isoenzymes CYP2A6	May produce unpredictable blood levels	None, be aware
Cowslip	Antihypertensives	Has been shown to have hypotensive effects in animals	None	Be aware
Cranberry juice	Melatonin	Unknown	Vitamin B_{12} influences melatonin secretion. Low levels of vitamin B_{12} will produce low levels of melatonin	Be aware

Continued on following page

Herbal drug	Allopathic drug	Probable cause/s of interaction	Clinical effects	Precautions
Cranberry juice (*cont'd*)	Omeprazole	Additive decrease in acidity may increase absorption of vitamin B_{12}	None	Be aware
	Warfarin	May inhibit metabolizing enzymes	Increased risk of bleeding due to warfarin	Inform physicians, avoid if possible
Cucurbita	Warfarin	Unknown	Increased anticoagulation effects of warfarin	Be aware
Dandelion	Diuretics (e.g. furosemide)	Constituents have diuretic action *in vivo*	May potentiate action of diuretics	Be aware, monitor electrolytes if symptomatic (weakness) and increased passing of urine (polyuria)
	Antidiabetic drugs Antihypertensives Quinolone antibiotics (e.g. ciprofloxacin, norfloxacin, nalidixic acid)	Because of high mineral content absorption is decreased	None	Be aware
Dang gui (Dong quai) (*Angelica sinensis*)	Warfarin	Unknown, possibly through inhibition of metabolizing enzymes – CYP3A4 and CYP1A. Also contains coumarins	Prolonged INR	Caution, inform physician if INR is deranged and avoid concurrent use
Danshen (*Salvia miltiorrhiza*)	Warfarin	Additive anticoagulant effects, probably displaces from protein binding	Enhanced anticoagulation with bleeding	Avoid concomitant use, inform physicians
	Digoxin	Digoxin level may be either falsely elevated or falsely decreased (interferes with the assay)	None	Be aware

Continued on following page

Herbal drug	Allopathic drug	Probable cause/s of interaction	Clinical effects	Precautions
Devil's claw	Digoxin	Constituents of devil's claw are cardioactive *in vivo*	Potentiation of effect of digoxin	Watch for enhanced effect/toxicity of cardiac glycosides, be aware
Echinacea	Anabolic steroids, methotrexate, amiodarone, ketoconazole	Unknown	Potentiates hepatotoxicity	Inform physician, avoid concomitant use
	Azathioprine	Unknown	Decreased immunosuppressant by azathioprine – risk of graft rejection	Avoid concomitant use, inform physician
	Corticosteroids	Unknown	Decreased immunosuppressant by corticosteroids – risk of graft rejection and therapeutic failure	Avoid concomitant use, inform physicians
	Ciclosporin	Unknown	Decreased immunosuppression by ciclosporin – risk of graft rejection	Avoid concomitant use, inform physician
	Tacrolimus	Unknown	Decreased immunosuppression by tacrolimus – risk of graft rejection	Avoid concomitant use, inform physician
Elder	Diuretics (e.g. furosemide)	Constituents have diuretic action *in vivo*	None, may potentiate action of diuretics	Be aware, monitor electrolytes if symptoms develop (weakness, polyuria)

Continued on following page

Herbal drug	Allopathic drug	Probable cause/s of interaction	Clinical effects	Precautions
Ephedra	Antihypertensive medications	Opposing pharmacological actions – (causes an increase in blood pressure)	Poor and unpredictable blood pressure response	Avoid concomitant use, inform physicians
	Beta-blockers (e.g. atenolol)	Has opposite pharmacological properties	Poor and unpredictable blood pressure response	Avoid concomitant use, inform physicians
	Caffeine	Additive cardiovascular effects (faster heart rate and palpitations)	Additive stimulation. At high dose, ephedra–caffeine interaction has been cited as a cause of death	Avoid concomitant use
	Decongestants (e.g. nasal decongestants)	Additive effects (faster heart rate and palpitations)	Sedation, heart attacks, seizures and rarely death	Avoid concomitant use, discontinue before elective surgery
	Green tea (*Camellia sinensis*) a caffeine-containing herb	Additive cardiovascular effects, (faster heart rate and palpitations). At high dose, ephedra–caffeine interaction has been cited as a cause of death	Additive stimulation may develop palpitations	Avoid concomitant use, be aware
	Guarana – caffeine-containing herb	Additive cardiovascular effects (faster heart rate and palpitations). At high dose, ephedra–caffeine interaction has been cited as a cause of death	Additive stimulation	Avoid concomitant use
	MAO inhibitors (MAOI)	Increased ephedrine levels as MOAI decrease metabolism of ephedrine	Hypertension (high blood pressure) due to decreased metabolism of ephedrine	Avoid concurrent use

Continued on following page

Herbal drug	Allopathic drug	Probable cause/s of interaction	Clinical effects	Precautions
Mate (*Ilex paraguariensis*) – caffeine-containing herb	Ephedrine	Additive cardiovascular effects (faster heart rates and palpitations). At high dose, ephedra–caffeine interaction has been cited as a cause of death	Additive stimulation	Avoid concomitant use
	Theophylline (aminophylline) Phenothiazines	Additive cardiovascular effects	Additive effects (faster heart rates and palpitations)	Be aware, avoid concomitant use
Evening primrose oil	Anticonvulsant drugs (e.g. barbiturates, phenytoin)	Lowers seizure threshold	Increased tendency for seizures	Avoid concurrent use, Warn patients
	Fluphenazine	Lowers seizure threshold	Can induce seizures	Inform physicians, avoid concurrent use
Fenugreek	Warfarin	Has coumarin-like properties (additive effects)	Increased anticoagulant effect of warfarin	Inform physicians, monitor INR, observe for bleeding tendency, avoid if possible
Feverfew	Warfarin	Unknown	Increased anticoagulant effect of warfarin – increased INR	Inform physicians
Frangula	Several drugs	May decrease absorption of drugs due to its laxative action	May produce a poor response to many drugs and alter blood levels	Be aware
Garlic	Chlorpropamide	Unknown	Enhances blood sugar lowering (hypoglycaemic) effects	Inform physician if the blood sugar fluctuates
	Ritonavir	Additive gastrointestinal effects	Increased incidence of gastrointestinal symptoms	Be aware

Continued on following page

Herbal drug	Allopathic drug	Probable cause/s of interaction	Clinical effects	Precautions
Garlic (*cont'd*)	Saquinavir	Induction of CYP3A4 metabolizing enzymes and/or induction of P-gp	Diminished blood levels of saquinavir, may reduce effects	Avoid concomitant therapy. Garlic does not affect metabolism of ritonavir
	Warfarin and antiplatelet agents (e.g. aspirin)	Inhibition of platelet aggregation by constituents of garlic has been demonstrated both *in vitro* and *in vivo*	Prolongs INR, increased risk of spontaneous bleeding (e.g. spontaneous spinal epidural haematoma), prolonged postoperative bleeding	Inform physicians. Warn of increased risk of bleeding. Stop 4–8 weeks before surgery
German chamomile	Hypnotics and anxiolytics	Sedative activity *in vivo*. May inhibit metabolizing enzymes – CYP3A4	May potentiate effects of hypnotics and anxiolytics	Be aware, avoid concomitant use if side-effects appear
Ginger	Cardiac glycosides	Constituents are cardioactive *in vivo*	Potentiates effect of cardiac glycosides	Watch for increased effect/toxicity of cardiac glycosides, be aware
	Phenprocoumon	Ginger inhibits platelet aggregation	Potentiates anticoagulation due to phenprocoumon	Inform physicians and be aware
	Saquinavir	Unknown	Decreased blood levels of saquinavir	Avoid concomitant use
	Warfarin	Antiplatelet activity *in vitro* (conflicting data in humans)	Increased INR	Patients on warfarin should avoid consuming large amounts of ginger
Ginkgo biloba	Aspirin	Potentiates antiplatelet action. Ginkgosides are potent inhibitors of platelet activating factor	Enhanced bleeding due to aspirin	Inform physicians, be aware, avoid concomitant use

Continued on following page

Herbal drug	Allopathic drug	Probable cause/s of interaction	Clinical effects	Precautions
Ginkgo biloba (*cont'd*)	Alprazolam	Unknown	Concentrations of alprazolam in the blood may be decreased slightly	Be aware
	Digoxin	Unknown	Increased levels of digoxin	Closely monitor digoxin level if used concomitantly
	Diltiazem	Inhibition of metabolizing enzymes – CYP3A4	Increased blood diltiazem levels, with enhanced blood pressure lowering effect	Be aware
	Haloperidol	Ginkgo may scavenge free radicals produced by hypodopaminergic activity	Increased effectiveness and decrease in extrapyramidal effects	Be aware, monitor doses carefully
	Ibuprofen	Possible additive/synergistic inhibitory effects on platelet aggregation	Increased risk of bleeding	Avoid concurrent use
	Trazodone	Unknown	Increased risk of sedation	Monitor effects of trazodone closely
	Nicardipine	Induction of metabolizing enzymes – CYP3A2	Poor blood pressure control	Be aware
	Nifedipine	Possible inhibition of CYP3A4	Elevated plasma concentrations of nifedipine and increased risk of pharmacological and adverse effects	Avoid concurrent administration or decrease dose of nifedipine
	Omeprazole	Probably induction of metabolizing enzymes – CYP2C19	Unknown, possibly reduced efficacy of omeprazole	Be aware

Continued on following page

Herbal drug	Allopathic drug	Probable cause/s of interaction	Clinical effects	Precautions
Ginkgo biloba (*cont'd*)	Thiazide diuretics (e.g. bendroflumethiazide)	Unknown	Raised blood pressure, poor blood pressure control	Avoid concomitant therapy, be aware
	Ticlopidine	Unknown	Enhanced bleeding tendency due to ticlopidine	Inform physicians
	Tolbutamide	Increases metabolism of tolbutamide	Poor control of blood sugar	Be aware
	Valproate	Uncertain	Increased risk of seizures/tonic clonic seizures	Avoid concurrent use
	Warfarin	Additive/synergistic anticoagulant effects most likely	Enhanced bleeding tendency due to warfarin	Patients on warfarin therapy should be advised to avoid concurrent use of *Ginkgo biloba*
	Trazodone	Enhanced GABA activity in the brain, may increase formation of an active metabolite via metabolizing enzymes – CYP3A4	Enhanced sedation and perhaps coma	Inform physicians, avoid concomitant use
Gingseng (*Panax ginseng*)	Alcohol	In mice, gingseng increases the activity of alcohol dehydrogenase and aldehyde dehydrogenase	Reduced blood concentrations of alcohol	Be aware
	Bumetanide	Mechanism uncertain	Decreased diuretic effect	Be aware
	Digoxin	Possibly a pharmacokinetic interaction, exact basis uncertain	Falsely elevated digoxin serum assay or elevated digoxin plasma levels	Be aware, inform physicians
	Ethacrynic acid	Mechanism uncertain	Decreased diuretic effect	Be aware

Continued on following page

Herbal drug	**Allopathic drug**	**Probable cause/s of interaction**	**Clinical effects**	**Precautions**
Gingseng (*cont'd*)	Furosemide	Mechanism uncertain	Decreased diuretic effect	Be aware
	Isocarboxazid	Unknown mechanism	Increased risk of occurrence of central nervous system effects (e.g. manic-like symptoms, headache, insomnia, tremors)	Be aware and inform physicians
	Nifedipine	Possibly due to inhibition of metabolism of nifedipine by CYP3A4	Increased plasma levels of nifedipine with increased pharmacological effects and adverse effects	Be aware and avoid concomitant use
	Oestrogens, corticosteroids	Additive effects	None	Be ware
	Phenelzine	Most probably has similar biological effects	Untoward side-effects (manic-like symptoms headache, tremor, sleeplessness)	Be aware, inform physicians
	Torasemide	Mechanism uncertain	Decreased diuretic effect	Be aware
	Tranylcypromine	Unknown mechanism	Increased risk of occurrence of central nervous system effects (e.g. manic-like symptoms, headache, insomnia, tremors)	Be aware and avoid concomitant uses
	Warfarin	Antiplatelet action, induction of metabolizing enzymes (CYP induction), thrombotic events could occur	International Normalized Ratio (INR) decreases; antagonism of effect of warfarin	Patients on warfarin treatment should avoid ginseng

Continued on following page

Herbal drug	Allopathic drug	Probable cause/s of interaction	Clinical effects	Precautions
Ginseng (cont'd)	Antidiabetic agents	Constituents have hypoglycaemic activity *in vitro* and *in vivo*	May develop low blood sugar (hypoglycaemia)	Monitor blood sugar closely and be aware
Ginseng – Siberian	Digoxin	Siberian ginseng contains eleutherosides which may interfere with digoxin assay	Elevated serum digoxin levels with no known clinical sequelae	Be aware
Glycyrrhizin	ACE inhibitors	Pseudoaldosteronism	Due to interaction of the renin–angiotensin system with glycyrrhizin. ACE-1 inhibitor retarded the development of pseudoaldosteronism	Watch for metabolic alkalosis with severe hypokalaemia in patients treated with glycyrrhizin
Goldenseal	Aspirin	Unknown	Decreases antiplatelet effects of aspirin	Inform physician, be aware
	Clopidogrel	Unknown	Decreases antiplatelet effects of clopidogrel	Inform physician, be aware
	Dipyridamole	Unknown	Decreases anticoagulation effects of dipyridamole	
	Fexofenidine	Known to inhibit metabolizing enzymes (CYP3A4)	None	Be aware
	Heparin	Unknown	Decreases anticoagulation effects of heparin	Inform physician, monitor clotting indices
	Ketoconazole	Known to inhibit metabolizing enzymes (CYP3A4)	None	Be aware
	Lovastatin	Known to inhibit metabolizing enzymes (CYP3A4)	None	Be aware

Continued on following page

Herbal drug	Allopathic drug	Probable cause/s of interaction	Clinical effects	Precautions
Goldenseal *(cont'd)*	Ticlopidine	Unknown	Decreases antiplatelet effects	Inform physician
	Triazolam	Known to inhibit metabolizing enzymes (CYP3A4)	None	Be aware
Grapefruit juice	Amiodarone	Known to have an effect on CYP450 drug metabolizing systems	Elevated amiodarone blood levels	Avoid concomitant use
	Amlodipine	Known to have an effect on CYP450 drug metabolizing systems	Elevated blood levels of amlodipine	Avoid concomitant use, those who had been on long-term grapefruit juice and amlodipine should not stop grapefruit juice abruptly
	Atorvastatin	Known to have an effect on CYP450 drug metabolizing systems	Increased blood levels of atorvastatin with increased risk of side-effects (e.g. muscle pain)	Avoid concomitant use
	Benzodiazepines (e.g. diazepam)	Known to have an effect on CYP450 drug metabolizing systems	Increased blood levels of benzodiazepines, enhanced sedation	Inform physicians, be aware
	Buspirone	Known to have an effect on CYP450 drug metabolizing systems	Elevated blood levels of buspirone	Avoid concomitant use, be aware
	Carbamazepine	Known to have an effect on CYP450 drug metabolizing systems	Elevated blood levels of carbamazepine	Be aware, avoid concomitant use
	Cisapride	Known to have an effect on CYP450 drug metabolizing systems	Elevated blood levels of cisapride	Avoid concomitant use (contraindicated)

Continued on following page

Herbal drug	Allopathic drug	Probable cause/s of interaction	Clinical effects	Precautions
Grapefruit juice (*cont'd*)	Clomipramine	Known to have an effect on CYP450 drug metabolizing systems	Elevated blood levels of clomipramine	Avoid concomitant use
	Ciclosporin	Known to have an effect on CYP450 drug metabolizing systems	Elevated blood levels of cyclosporin	Avoid concomitant use
	Digoxin	Known to have an effect on CYP450 drug metabolizing systems	Marginal elevation of blood levels of digoxin	Be aware
	Erythromycin	Known to have an effect on CYP450 drug metabolizing systems	Elevated blood levels of erythromycin, increased side-effects	Avoid concomitant use
	Ethinylestradiol	Known to have an effect on CYP450 drug metabolizing systems	Elevated blood levels of ethinylestradiol	Avoid concomitant use
	Fluvoxamine	Known to have an effect on CYP450 drug metabolizing systems	Elevated blood levels of fluvoxamine	Be aware, avoid concomitant use
	Indinavir	Known to have an effect on CYP450 drug metabolizing systems	Delayed peak plasma concentrations of indinavir, possibly delays onset of effect of indinavir	Avoid concomitant use
	Losartan	Known to have an effect on CYP450 drug metabolizing systems	Unpredictable blood levels of losartan, may cause poor control of high blood pressure	Be aware and avoid concomitant use if possible
	Lovastatin	Known to have an effect on CYP 450 drug metabolizing systems	Elevated blood levels of lovastatin – may increase side-effects of lovastatin	Avoid concomitant use

Continued on following page

Herbal drug	Allopathic drug	Probable cause/s of interaction	Clinical effects	Precautions
Grapefruit juice (*cont'd*)	Nicardipine	Known to have an effect on CYP450 drug metabolizing systems	Elevated blood levels of nicardipine – may increase blood pressure lowering effect of nicardipine	Avoid concomitant use
	Nisoldipine	Known to have an effect on CYP450 drug metabolizing systems	Elevated blood levels of nisoldipine may increase blood pressure lowering effect of nisoldipine	Avoid concomitant use
	Praziquantel	Known to have an effect on CYP450 drug metabolizing systems	Elevated blood levels praziquantal – may increase side-effects of praziquantel	Avoid concomitant use
	Quinidine	Known to have an effect on CYP450 drug metabolizing systems	Delayed onset of therapeutic effects of quinidine	Avoid concomitant use
	Simvastatin	Known to have an effect on CYP450 drug metabolizing systems	Increased blood levels of simvastatin – may increase side-effects of simvastatin	Avoid concomitant use
	Sildenafil	Known to have an effect on CYP450 drug metabolizing systems	May increase blood levels of sildenafil	Be aware
	Verapamil	Known to have an effect on CYP450 drug metabolizing systems	Blood levels of verapamil may be elevated and may increase effects of verapamil	Avoid concomitant use

Continued on following page

Herbal drug	Allopathic drug	Probable cause/s of interaction	Clinical effects	Precautions
Green tea (*Camellia sinensis*)	Clozapine	Unknown, possibly induction of metabolizing enzymes (CYP1A2)	Low clozapine blood levels	Be aware
	Theophylline	Additive effect due to caffeine	Increased stimulation. palpitations and tachycardia (increased heart rate)	None
	Warfarin	Has vitamin K which may antagonize warfarin	Decreased anticoagulation with warfarin and risk of thrombosis	Patients on warfarin therapy should not consume large quantities of green tea
Guar gum	Digoxin	Slows absorption of digoxin	Unpredictable blood levels of digoxin, may produce poor response to digoxin	Inform physicians, be aware
	Metformin	Decreases absorption of metformin	Reduced blood levels of metformin, may lead to poor control of diabetes	Be aware
	Bumetanide	Slows absorption of bumetanide	May produce ineffective blood levels of bumetanide	Be aware
	Phenoxymethyl-penicillin	Decreases absorption of phenoxymethylpenicillin	May produce ineffective blood concentrations of antibiotic	Be aware
	Glibenclamide	Decreases absorption of some formulations of glibenclamide	May lead to poor control of diabetes mellitus	Be aware

Continued on following page

Herbal drug	Allopathic drug	Probable cause/s of interaction	Clinical effects	Precautions
Guarana	Theophylline	Additive effect due to caffeine	Increased stimulation, palpitations and tachycardia (increased heart rate)	Be aware
Hawthorn	Cardiac glycosides (e.g. digoxin)	Constituents act on heart muscle and heart rate control centres (cardioactive) *in vivo*	Potentiates effect of cardiac glycosides	Watch for increased effect/toxicity of cardiac glycosides
	Antihypertensives	Unknown	Increased blood pressure lowering effect of antihypertensives with risk of low blood pressure (hypotension)	Be aware
	Nitrates	Unknown	Increased blood pressure lowering effect of nitrates with risk of low blood pressure (hypotension)	Be aware
Herbal diuretics	Lithium	Unknown	Decreased lithium blood levels and risk of poor therapeutic response to lithium	Avoid concomitant use
Hops	Hypnotics and anxiolytics and alcohol	Hops show sedative activity *in vivo*	May potentiate effects of hypnotics and anxiolytics	Be aware. Warn patients re driving and handling machinery
	Phenothiazine-type antipsychotics	Unknown	Risk of increased body temperature (hyperthermia)	Be aware
Horse chestnut	Aspirin	Coumarin constituents in horse chestnut enhance anticoagulant effect	Increased risk of bleeding due to aspirin	Be aware

Continue on following page

Herbal drug	Allopathic drug	Probable cause/s of interaction	Clinical effects	Precautions
Horse chestnut (*cont'd*)	Warfarin	Coumarin constituents in horse chestnut enhance anticoagulant effect	Increased risk of bleeding due to warfarin	Monitor INR
Huang qin	Irinotecan	Multifactorial	Beneficial effects (reduced irinotecan-induced diarrhoea)	Be aware
Hypoxis hemerocallidea (African potato)	All drugs dependent on CYP3A4 metabolism and P-gp transport	*Hypoxis* has been shown to inhibit up to 86% of the normal CYP3A4 isoform activity Mildly inhibits P-gp A two-fold increase in pregnane receptors	Due to inhibition of CYP3A4 which is a major metabolizing enzyme for several important drugs, the blood concentrations and thus the risk of adverse effects and toxic effects of this wide group of drugs would be increased	Be aware
Ispaghula	Several drugs e.g. warfarin, calcium, iron, lithium, zinc, vitamin B_{12}, digoxin	Has laxative activity, may decrease absorption of drugs by increasing the time of passage of intestinal contents (increasing intestinal transit time)	Reduced blood levels of several drugs	Separate dosing with concomitant medications by at least 1 hour
Kangen – karyu	Ticlopidine	Unknown	Augmented anti-thrombotic effect of ticlopidine	Inform physicians, be aware
Karela or bitter melon	Chlorpropamide	Karela decreases loss of glucose in urine	May interfere with blood glucose control	Be aware

Continued on following page

Herbal drug	Allopathic drug	Probable cause/s of interaction	Clinical effects	Precautions
Kava kava	Alprazolam, benzodiazepines and pentobarbital	Kavapyrones – active ingredients have a pharmacological action resembling benzodiazepines by binding to gamma aminobenzoic acid (GABA) receptors – which are the same receptors to which benzodiazepines bind	Increased blood levels of benzodiazepines, pentobarbital and additive or synergistic pharmacological effects (sedative), rarely coma	Warn patients re. driving, handling machinery. Inform physicians, be aware and avoid concomitant use
	Acetaminophen (paracetamol)	Increases likelihood of liver and kidney damage	Unknown	Be aware
	Anaesthetic agents	Unknown. Possibly due to effects of kavapyrones on the central nervous system	Lengthens effects of anaesthetics	Inform the anaesthetist before the procedure
	Ethanol	Uncertain. Possibly due to effects of kavapyrones on the central nervous system	Enhanced hypnotic effect of ethanol in mice, not confirmed in humans	Be aware
	Haloperidol	Uncertain. Possibly due to effects of kavapyrones on the central nervous system	Increases side-effects	Be aware
	Risperidone	Uncertain. Possibly due to effects of kavapyrones on the central nervous system	Increases side-effects	Be aware
	Metoclopramide	Uncertain	Increases side-effects	Be aware
	Levodopa	Antagonistic pharmacological effects	Reduced efficacy of levodopa, flare up of disease	Inform physicians, avoid concomitant use
Kelp (Fucus)	Thyroxine and antithyroid drugs (carbimazole)	Contains iodine which has an important role in production of thyroid hormones	May interfere with thyroid replacement	Inform physician, be aware

Continued on following page

Herbal drug	Allopathic drug	Probable cause/s of interaction	Clinical effects	Precautions
Khat	Penicillin, ampicillin and amoxicillin	Unknown. Possibly reduced absorption due to the formation of a tannin–antibiotic complex in the stomach	Reduced blood levels of antibiotics which may produce a decreased response to the antibiotics	Avoid concomitant use
Kudzu	Verapamil	Possibly additive effect on calcium channels	Adverse reactions reported during co-administration – possibly additive hypotensive effects	Avoid co-administration
	Triptans, e.g. sumitriptan	Possibly additive effects on neurotransmitters (chemical messengers)	Adverse reactions reported with co-administration	Avoid co-administration
	Methotrexate	Reduced metabolism and higher blood levels of methotrexate	Increases toxic reactions following methotrexate administration	Findings are from rat experiments. Necessary to be aware
Lavender	Barbiturates	Additive nervous system sedative effects	Theoretically may enhance sleepiness	Be aware
	Chloral hydrate	Additive nervous system sedative effects	Theoretically may enhance sleepiness	Be aware
Liquorice	Digitalis glycosides	Unknown	Low potassium blood levels increase sensitivity to digitalis	Be aware, avoid concomitant use
	Oral contraceptives	Oral contraceptive use may increase sensitivity to glycyrrhizin acid	May increase adverse effects (hypertension, hypokalaemia, oedema) of liquorice	Be aware

Continued on following page

Herbal drug	Allopathic drug	Probable cause/s of interaction	Clinical effects	Precautions
Liquorice (*cont'd*)	Prednisolone	Glycyrrhizin decreases the removal (plasma clearance) of prednisolone and increases the concentrations in the blood	May increase adverse effect of prednisolone	Be aware
	Spironolactone	Unknown	Antagonism of diuretic effect of spironolactone	Avoid concurrent use
	Thiazide and loop diuretics	Unknown	Additive potassium loss from the body	Monitor blood potassium levels closely. Avoid concurrent use
	Tolbutamide	Unknown	Unknown	Be aware
	Loratidine, procainamide, quinidine	Unknown	Several ECG changes (prolonged QT interval) and risk of adverse effects due to the cardiac drugs	Be aware, avoid concomitant use
Lycium barbarum (Chinese wolfberry)	Warfarin	Inhibits metabolizing enzyme system (CYP450)	Increases blood levels of warfarin	Inform physicians, self-monitoring for bleeding tendency
Milk thistle	Amiodarone	Unknown Preliminary evidence suggests that milk thistle inhibits metabolizing enzymes (CYP3A4)	Enhanced anti-arrhythmic activity	None, be aware
	Indinavir	Unknown	Reduces indinavir levels insignificantly	None, be aware
Neem	Azathioprine	Not known	May decrease immunosuppressant effect and produce a poor response to azathioprine	Be aware

Continued on following page

Herbal drug	Allopathic drug	Probable cause/s of interaction	Clinical effects	Precautions
Neem (*cont'd*)	Imuran	Not known	May decrease immunosuppressant effect and produce a poor response to Imuran	Be aware
	Glimepiride	Possibility of additive blood sugar lowering effects	May cause lowering of blood sugar (hypoglycaemia)	Be aware
	Glucotrol	Possibility of additive blood sugar lowering effects	May cause lowering of blood sugar (hypoglycaemia)	Be aware
	Micronase	Possibility of additive blood sugar lowering effects	May cause lowering of blood sugar (hypoglycaemia)	Be aware
	Orinase	Possibility of additive blood sugar lowering effects	May cause lowering of blood sugar (hypoglycaemia)	Be aware
	Prednisolone	Not known	May decrease immunosuppressant effect and produce a poor response to prednisone	Be aware
	Tolinase	Possibility of additive blood sugar lowering effects	May cause lowering of blood sugar (hypoglycaemia)	Be aware
	Zenapax	Not known	May decrease immunosuppressant effect and produce a poor response to Zenapax	Be aware

Continued on following page

Herbal drug	Allopathic drug	Probable cause/s of interaction	Clinical effects	Precautions
Nettle	Diuretics (e.g. furosemide)	Constituents have diuretic action *in vivo*	Potentiates action of diuretics	Watch for enhanced effect/toxicity of diuretics, monitor fluid and electrolyte balance
Oleander	Digoxin	Has similar pharmacological properties on the heart	Increased risk of toxicity and fatal outcomes	Avoid concomitant use
Papaya	Warfarin	Unknown	Increased anticoagulant effect of warfarin	Inform physician, monitor for bleeding tendency and be aware
Passion flower	Hypnotics and anxiolytics	Shown to have a sedative activity *in vivo*	May potentiate effects of hypnotics and anxiolytics	Warn patients re driving, handling machinery. Be aware, inform physicians
Pineapple	ACE inhibitors	Unknown	May antagonize effects of bradykinin	Be aware
Plantain	Carbamazepine	Psyllium seed reported to inhibit gastrointestinal absorption of carbamazepine	None	Be aware
	Lithium	Psyllium seed reported to inhibit gastrointestinal absorption of lithium	None	Be aware
	Digoxin	Unknown	None/or increased digitalis effects	Be aware
Psyllium (*Plantago ovata*)	Lithium	Decreases blood concentrations of lithium	May produce a poor therapeutic response to lithium	Be aware. Monitor lithium levels closely

Continued on following page

Herbal drug	**Allopathic drug**	**Probable cause/s of interaction**	**Clinical effects**	**Precautions**
Rhubarb (da huang)	Cardiac glycosides (e.g. digoxin)	Causes lowering of body potassium (hypokalaemia). Can also cause diarrhoea which decreases absorption of drugs with a narrow therapeutic index	Potentiates toxicity of cardiac glycosides	Monitor serum potassium and administer potassium supplements orally if indicated. Take drugs 1 hour before or 2 hours after herbal products
	Diuretics (e.g. furosemide, bendroflumethiazide)	Increases potassium loss from the gut	Low body potassium – risk of lethargy, muscle weakness	Provide potassium supplements orally if symptomatic
Rosemary	Antidiabetic agents	Hyperglycaemic activity *in vitro*	Antagonises blood sugar lowering effects of hypoglycaemics	Monitor blood sugar closely, be aware
Salboku-to (Asian herbal mixture)	Prednisolone	Increased blood levels of prednisolone	Increased risk of adverse effects of prednisolone	Be aware
Saw palmetto	Finasteride	Inhibition of 5-alpha-reductase, inhibition of dihydrotestosterone binding to cellular and nuclear receptor sites	Affects levels of male sex hormones (androgens)	Avoid concurrent use
	Flutamide	Inhibition of 5-alpha-reductase, inhibition of dihydrotestosterone binding to cellular and nuclear receptor sites	Affects levels of male sex hormones (androgens)	Avoid concurrent use
	Oral contraceptives/ hormone replacement therapy	Unknown	Affects levels of oestrogens	Be aware
	Disulfiram	Unknown	Nausea and vomiting	Avoid concurrent use
	Warfarin	Unknown	Increased anticoagulant effect	Monitor effects of warfarin therapy regularly

Continued on following page

Herbal drug	Allopathic drug	Probable cause/s of interaction	Clinical effects	Precautions
Saw palmetto (*cont'd*)	Ibuprofen	Inhibits cyclo-oxygenase and 5-lipoxygenase	Risk of serious bleeding	Avoid concurrent use
	Naproxen	Inhibits cyclo-oxygenase and 5-lipoxygenase	Risk of serious bleeding	Avoid concurrent use
	Metronidazole	Unknown	Increased risk of nausea and vomiting	Be aware
Scopolia (*Scopolia carniolica*)	Tricyclic antidepressants	Unknown	Increased effectiveness of tricyclic antidepressants	Be aware
	Amantadine	Unknown	Increased effectiveness of amantadine	Be aware
	Quinidine	Unknown	Increased effectiveness of quinidine	Be aware
Scutellaria baicalensis (huang qin)	Irinotecan	Uncertain	Ameliorates irinotecan-induced gastrointestinal toxicity	May be beneficial in cancer patients
Sea buckthorn	Cyclophosphamide	Not known	May decrease cell destroying effects – produce poor response to cyclophosphamide	Be aware
	Farmorubicin	Not known	May decrease cell destroying effect – produce poor response to farmorubicin	Be aware

Continued on following page

Herbal drug	Allopathic drug	Probable cause/s of interaction	Clinical effects	Precautions
Senna	Several drugs	Decreases absorption of drugs due to its laxative effects	Poor absorption of several drugs may lead to low blood levels and poor response to several drugs	Be aware
Shankhapushpi (Ayurvedic herbal syrup)	Phenytoin	Aqueous extract has convulsive effects; decreases blood concentrations of phenytoin	May cause loss of seizure control with phenytoin	Do not administer in patients with fits; be aware and warn patients
Soy/Soya	Warfarin	Animal experiments show induction of CYP3A and CYP2 isoenzymes	Decreased anticoagulation of warfarin	Patients on anticoagulant therapy should be cautioned against use of large amounts of soya products
	Tamoxifen	Phyto-oestrogens in soy may counteract effects of tamoxifen	May reduce drug levels of tamoxifen which may cause a poor response to tamoxifen	Be aware
Squill	Quinidine	Cardioactive glycosides increase force of cardiac contraction and slow the rate of cardiac contractions	Increased effectiveness and risk of adverse effects. Increased risk of arrhythmias	Avoid concomitant use
	Calcium	Cardioactive glycosides increase force of cardiac contraction and slow the rate of cardiac contractions	Increased effectiveness and risk of adverse effects	Avoid concomitant use
	Digoxin	Cardioactive glycosides increase force of cardiac contraction and slow the rate of cardiac contractions	Increased effectiveness and risk of adverse effects	Avoid concomitant use

Continued on following page

Herbal drug	Allopathic drug	Probable cause/s of interaction	Clinical effects	Precautions
Squill (*cont'd*)	Sympathomimetics (e.g. adrenaline, noradrenaline, isoprenaline)	Unknown	Increased risk of arrhythmias	Avoid concomitant use
	Methylxanthines (e.g. aminophylline, theophylline)	Unknown	Increased risk of arrhythmias	Avoid concomitant use
	Phosphodiesterase inhibitors (e.g. sildenafil, tadalafil, vardenafil)	Unknown	Increased risk of arrhythmias	Avoid concomitant use
St John's wort	Alprazolam	Induction of metabolizing enzymes (CYP3A4)	None	Inform physicians
	Amitryptyline Nortriptyline	Due to induction of metabolizing CYP3A4 enzymes and P-gp transport proteins	Low blood amitryptyline levels (<20%) Nortriptyline levels may be decreased by 50%	Inform physicians and patients/carers. Watch for poor therapeutic response to antidepressant, may need dose increases
	General anaesthetics	Uncertain	Delayed emergence from anaesthesia	Be aware
	Anti-HIV drugs (indinavir, lamivudine, amprenavir, saquinavir, nelfinavir, lopinavir, efavirenz, nevirapine)	Probably induction of metabolizing enzymes CYP3A4	Reduced drug levels of these antiviral drugs – with increased viral load and possibility of development of resistance	Avoid concomitant use, inform physicians

Continued on following page

Herbal drug	Allopathic drug	Probable cause/s of interaction	Clinical effects	Precautions
St John's wort (*cont'd*)	Anticonvulsants – phenytoin, phenobarbital, carbamazepine	Induction of metabolizing enzymes – CYP3A4 which metabolize these anticonvulsants	Loss of seizure control	Be aware. Avoid concomitant use, monitor blood levels of anticonvulsants when possible
	Benzodiazepines (alprazolam)	Due to induction of metabolizing enzymes (CYP3A4) which metabolize midazolam and alprazolam	Low benzodiazepine blood levels	Inform physicians
	Buspirone	Synergistic effects on 5-hydroxytryptamine receptors	Hypomania	Inform physicians
	Ciclosporin	St John's wort preparations decrease bioavailability by decreasing intestinal absorption through induction of multidrug resistance transporter P-gp at low clinically relevant concentrations and induction of CYP3A4 iso-enzymes	Risk of transplant rejection due to low ciclosporin blood levels	Avoid concomitant use, inform physicians
	Digoxin	Intestinal P-gp induction which decreases blood levels of digoxin	Reduced digoxin level by 25% which is important as digoxin has a narrow therapeutic index	Avoid concomitant use, inform physicians
	Fenoxfenadine	Induction of metabolizing enzymes (CYP3A4) which metabolize fenofexadine	Plasma levels of fenofexadine may fall by 35–45%, reducing antihistaminic activity	Be aware
	Imatinib mesylate	Unknown	Reduced imatinab blood levels, may produce a poor response to imatinab	Avoid concomitant use, may need to increase imatinab dose

Continued on following page

Herbal drug	Allopathic drug	Probable cause/s of interaction	Clinical effects	Precautions
St John's wort (*cont'd*)	Irinotecan	Unknown	Reduced blood level of irinotecan with reduced therapeutic effects	Avoid concomitant use, inform physicians
	Iron	Tannic acid may inhibit iron absorption	Poor response to iron	Avoid concomitant use
	Loperamide	Induction of metabolizing enzymes	Increased risk of serotonin syndrome	Be aware
	Methadone	Induction of metabolizing enzymes (CYP enzymes)	Reduced methadone blood levels which may lead to withdrawal symptoms	Avoid concomitant use, inform physicians
	Midazolam	Induces metabolizing enzymes (CYP3A4)	Decreased plasma levels, decreased effect	None
	Nifedipine	Induction of metabolizing enzymes (CYP3A4) which metabolize nifedipine	Plasma concentrations of nifedipine may decrease by 50% with failure of blood pressure lowering (antihypertensive) response	Monitor blood pressure regularly, avoid concomitant use
	Oral contraceptive pills	St John's wort preparations induce metabolizing CYP3A4 enzymes and glycoprotein drug transporter	Bleeding in between periods (intermenstrual bleeding), contraceptive failure	Avoid concomitant use, inform physicians
	Serotonin reuptake inhibitors, e.g. paroxetine, setraline, fluoxetine, venlafaxine and nefazodone	Inhibits uptake of serotonin and thereby increases serotonin levels	Increased sedative effects – hypnotic effects (weakness, lethargy, fatigue, slow movements, incoherence) Serotonin syndrome	Avoid concomitant use

Continued on following page

Herbal drug	Allopathic drug	Probable cause/s of interaction	Clinical effects	Precautions
St John's wort (*cont'd*)	Phenprocoumon	Induction of metabolizing enzymes	Decreased anticoagulant effect	Inform physicians, avoid if possible
	Quazepam	Induction of metabolizing CYP3A4 enzymes which metabolize quazepam	Decreased plasma concentrations of quazepam (by 25%) There may be no clinical changes	Be aware
	Simvastatin	Induction of metabolizing CYP3A4 enzymes which metabolize simvastatin	Reduced blood levels of active metabolite simvastatin hydroxy acid and poor cholesterol lowering effect	Be aware. Monitor response to simvastatin closely and inform physicians
	Tacrolimus	Due to induction of metabolizing CYP3A4 enzymes	Decreased plasma concentrations – may be as low as 6–10 μg/L to 1.6 μg/L, increasing risk of rejection of transplants	Avoid concomitant use, may need to increase dose of tacrolimus, inform physicians
	Theophylline	Due to activation of metabolizing CYP1A2 enzymes which metabolizes theophylline	Reduced theophylline levels and risk of therapeutic failure	Inform physicians and discontinue St John's wort if therapeutic effects of theophylline reduce
	Verapamil	Induction of metabolizing (intestinal) CYP3A4 enzymes. Reduced blood levels	May produce a poor response to verapamil	None

Continued on following page

Herbal drug	Allopathic drug	Probable cause/s of interaction	Clinical effects	Precautions
St John's wort (*cont'd*)	Warfarin	Due to induction of metabolizing CYP2C9 enzymes and possibly reduction in intestinal absorption of warfarin	Decreased plasma levels and anticoagulant effect of warfarin	Monitor INR closely and adjust dosages regularly. Inform physicians. Discontinue St John's wort if INR unstable
Sutherlandia frutescens	Drugs metabolized by CYP3A4 and P-gp	Near complete inhibition of metabolizing enzymes (CYP3A4) and inhibition of transport protein (P-gp) activity	Increased risk of toxicity and adverse effects due to decreased metabolism	Be aware
Tamarind	Aspirin	Increases bioavailability of aspirin	May increase adverse effects of aspirin	Be aware
Valerian	Benzodiazepines (e.g. Valium)	Increases concentrations of chemical messenger in the brain (GABA)	Increases sedative effects	Warn patients re driving, handling machinery. Inform physicians. Avoid concomitant use if possible
Willow	Anticoagulants	Salicylate constituents in willow enhance anticoagulant effect	Increase in bleeding likely	Monitor INR, monitor for bleeding tendency
	NSAIDS (e.g. ibuprofen and diclofenac sodium)	Unknown, possibly an additive effect of the salicylic acid and the NSAID on gastric mucosa	May increase risk of gastrointestinal ulceration and bleeding	Be aware
	Phenytoin	Salicylate constituents displace phenytoin from protein binding sites	Increased blood levels of phenytoin	Be aware

Continued on following page

Herbal drug	Allopathic drug	Probable cause/s of interaction	Clinical effects	Precautions
Yohimbine	Tricyclic antidepressants	Increased stimulation of sympathetic nervous system. Yohimbine alone can cause hypertension but lower doses cause hypertension when combined with tricyclic antidepressants	Blood pressure may increase	Be aware, check blood pressure
	Tetracyclines	Chelation with antibiotic	May produce a poor response to tetracyclines	Be aware and watch for poor response to antibiotic. May need to separate oral intake by 2 hours
	Venlafaxine	Unknown	Manic reactions	Be aware, avoid concomitant use

A case report in 2006 highlights the necessity to consider and document drug–herb interactions in all clinical scenarios to caution other clinicians.

An elderly 77-year-old man went to his doctor with limb weakness and long-standing constipation. His hypertensive heart disease had worsened. He was also suffering from hyperuricaemia and allergic rhinitis. For the latter complaint he had used a Chinese herbal remedy for 10 years. He had also used a Chinese medicine for his constipation for about four months. For his hypertension he was taking 20 mg enalapril (an angiotensin-converting enzyme inhibitor). The dosage of enalapril had been reduced to 10 mg daily about one year before his admission. On admission, the laboratory tests revealed metabolic acidosis and a very low serum potassium. His urine showed increased loss of potassium and thus a diagnosis of pseudoaldosteronism was made. Discontinuation of the Chinese remedies, which contained glycyrrhizin, and potassium supplements, corrected the electrolyte disturbances and the patient felt well within a short time. The intake of Chinese herbal medicines containing glycyrrhizin caused pseudoaldosteronism due to its effects on the interaction of the rennin–angiotensin–aldosterone system. It is also of interest that the administration of the angiotensin-converting enzyme inhibitor enalapril, retarded the development of pseudoaldostronism.[3]

It has recently been recognized that herbal medicines could interact with allopathic medicines used in the treatment of HIV[4–6]. Herbal medicines are very frequently used by patients with HIV in some African countries (e.g. Tanzania), particularly since government authorities recommended their use for HIV disease. The incidence of use may be as high as 80%. However, several herbal drugs could potentially alter the activity of the cytochrome enzyme system which metabolizes some of the allopathic medicines used to treat HIV and interact with HIV medications in other ways.

Hypoxis and *Sutherlandia* are two popular remedies which are thought to affect the activity of cytochrome (CYP) enzymes and interact with HIV medications known as non-nucleoside reverse transcriptase inhibitors (NNRTI) and protease inhibitors (PI). *Sutherlandia* is likely to increase the adverse effects of any concomitantly administered allopathic anti-HIV drugs. Other herbs that could interact with HIV medications include echinacea, garlic, ginkgo, milk thistle and St John's wort. These potential drug interactions could influence therapy in millions of HIV patients in Africa, and researchers have called for urgent action to evaluate the risk[4–6].

HERB–HERB INTERACTIONS

1. Neem theoretically might have additive effects with herbs that decrease blood glucose levels such as devil's claw, fenugreek, garlic, guar gum, horse chestnut, *Panax ginseng*, psyllium and Siberian ginseng. Other herbal ingredients reported to cause lowering of blood sugar (hypoglycaemia) include: agrimony, alfalfa, burdock, celery, cornsilk, damiana, dandelion, elecampane, eucalyptus, ispaghula, juniper, myrrh, tansy and senega.
2. Concomitant use of American ginseng can potentiate the stimulant effects of caffeine, guarana, mate and tea.
3. Theoretically, the concomitant use of Siberian ginseng with herbs that have sedative properties (calamus, California poppy, camp, capsicum, catnip, celery, centaury, elecampane, German couch grass, German chamomile, golden seal, hawthorn, hops, Jamaican dogwood, kava, lemon balm, passion flower, sage, scullcap, St John's wort, senega, Shepherd's purse, stinging nettle, valerian) might enhance therapeutic and adverse effects.
4. Concomitant use of herbs with anticoagulant/antiplatelet potential could enhance effects and increase the risk of side-effects. These include angelica, anise, arnica, asafoetida, capsicum, celery, chamomile, clove, fenugreek, feverfew, garlic, ginger, ginkgo, horse chestnut, horseradish, liquorice, onion, passion flower, red clover, turmeric and willow.

5. Plants belonging to the Lamiaceae family (hyssop, basil, mint, sage, lavender) seem to show cross-reactivity on the basis of clinical history and *in vitro* and *in vivo* test results.
6. Safrole is a major constituent of the bark of sassafras. Safrole in large amounts can cause hallucinations lasting for several days. It is also known to cause shakes, vomiting, dilated pupils, abortion and hypertension. It has is also been associated with liver cancer. Concomitant use with other safrole-containing herbs should be avoided due to the potential for additive toxicity. Herbs containing safrole include basil, camphor, cinnamon and nutmeg.
7. Laxative herbal ingredients should not be taken concomitantly. Laxative herbs include aloes, cascara, eyebright, frangula, horehound (in large doses), white ispaghula, plantain, rhubarb, senna and yellow dock.
8. Cardioactive herbal ingredients include broom, calamus, coltsfoot, devil's claw, fenugreek, figwort, fumitory, ginger, ginseng (Panax), golden seal, hawthorn, horehound – white, lime flower, mate, mistletoe, motherwort, parsley, pleurisy root, prickly ash, shepherd's purse, squill and wild carrot. Caution should be exercised while taking these herbs in combination and particularly with allopathic medications used in the treatment of cardiovascular disorders.

EFFECTS OF HERBAL REMEDIES ON CLINICAL LABORATORY TESTS

The following list is based on a literature survey published by Dasgupta and Bernard[7]:

1. Falsely elevated or falsely lowered digoxin levels may be encountered in a patient taking digoxin and the Chinese medicine chan su or dan shen, owing to direct interference of a component of the Chinese medicine with the antibody used in an immunoassay.
2. Abnormally low ciclosporin, digoxin, theophylline or protease inhibitor concentrations may be observed in a patient taking St John's wort due the induced increased clearance of these drugs.
3. Abnormal laboratory results may be encountered owing to altered pathophysiology following the intake of herbs such as kava kava, chaparral and germander which cause liver toxicity. Elevated alanine aminotransferase, aspartate aminotransferase and bilirubin concentrations may be observed in a healthy individual.
4. The presence of an adulterant, most commonly an allopathic medication, would produce an unexpected level of the allopathic medicine despite the subject not receiving the drug following an allopathic prescription (e.g. phenytoin, sibutramine).

REFERENCES

1. Chavez ML, Jordan MA, Chavez PI. Evidence based-drug–herbal interactions. *Life Science* 2006; 78: 2146–2157.
2. Fugh-Berman A, Ernst E. Herb–drug interactions: review and assessment of report reliability. *British Journal of Clinical Pharmacology* 2001; 52: 587–595.
3. Iida R, Otsuka Y, Matsumoto K, Kuriyama S, Hosoya T. Pseudoaldosteronism due to the concurrent use of two herbal medicines containing glycyrrhizin: interaction of glycyrrhizin with angiotensin-converting enzyme inhibitor. *Clinical and Experimental Nephrology* 2006; 10: 131–135.
4. Van den Bout-van den Beukel CJP, Koopmans PP, van der Ven AJAM, De Smet PAGM, Burger DM. Possible drug metabolism interactions of medicinal herbs with antiretroviral agents. *Drug Metabolism Reviews* 2006; 38: 477–514.
5. Mills E, Foster BC, van Heeswijk R, Phillips E, Wilson K, Leonard B, Kosuga K, Kanfer I. Impact of African herbal medicines on antiretroviral metabolism. *AIDS* 2005; 19: 95–97.
6. Beukel CJ, Koopmans PP, van der Ven AJ, De Smet PA, Burger DM. Possible drug metabolism interactions of medicinal herbs with antiretroviral agents. *Drug Metabolism Reviews* 2006; 38: 477–514.
7. Dasgupta A, Bernard DW. Herbal remedies: effects on laboratory tests. *Archives of Pathology and Laboratory Medicine* 2006; 130: 521–528.

BIBLIOGRAPHY

Bressler R. Herb–drug interactions: interactions between saw palmetto and prescription medications. *Geriatrics* 2005; 60 (11): 32,34.

Bressler R. Herb–drug interactions: interactions between *Ginkgo biloba* and prescription medications. *Geriatrics* 2005; 60 (4): 30–33.

Bressler R. Herb–drug interactions: interactions between kava and prescription medications. *Geriatrics* 2005; 60 (9): 24–25.

Bressler R. Herb–drug interactions: interactions between ginseng and prescription medications. *Geriatrics* 2005; 60 (8): 16–17.

Dharmananda S. Director, Institute for Traditional Medicine, Oregon, USA. HIV Drugs and Herb Interactions. Internet www.itmonline.org/arts/hivdrugint.htm

Fugh-Berman A. Herb–drug interactions. *Lancet* 2000; 355: 134–138.

Hu Z, Yang X, Ho PCL, Chan SY, Heng PWS, Chan E, Duan W, Koh HL, Zhou S. Herb–drug interactions. A literature review. *Drugs* 2005; 65: 1239–1262.

Izzo AA, Di Carlo G, Borrelli F, Ernst E. Cardiovascular pharmacotherapy and herbal medicines: the risk of drug interaction. *International Journal of Cardiology* 2005; 98: 1–14.

Kuhn MA. Herbal remedies: herb–drug interactions. *Critical Care Nurse*, 2002: 22; 22–32.

Lambrecht JE, Hamilton W, Rabinovich A. A review of herb–drug interactions: documented and theoretical. US Pharmacist: http://www.uspharmacist.com/oldformat.asp?url

Mayo Cinic. Herb–drug interactions: http:/www.mayohealth.org/mayo/0003/htm/herbdrug.htm

University of New Mexico Employee Health Promotion Program. (EHPP). Interactions with common herbal remedies and prescribed medications: http://www.unm.edu/~ehpp/nutrition%20herb%20interactions.htm

Williamson EM. Interactions between herbal and conventional medicines. *Expert Opinion and Drug Safety* 2005; 4: 355–378.

Glossary

A

Abortifacient – a drug causing abortion (miscarriage)

Acanthosis nigricans – a darkly pigmented skin change around the neck

Acrodynia – a rare disease of infants resulting in weakness, swelling and redness of face, fingers and toes

Acromegaly – a disorder caused by the increased secretion of a hormone (growth hormone) by a tumour (growth) of the pituitary gland

Adaptogen – a term used in traditional medicine indicating an ability to cope with mental and physical stress, and ill health; also sometimes as a 'performance enhancer'

Adenoids – glandular tissue at the back of the throat

Adjuvant – a drug that enhances the effect of other drugs, often without having an effect in its own right

Adrenal glands – two small triangular glands situated on the upper pole of each kidney that secrete hormones vital to life

Aerial – the part of the plant that is above ground

Aglycones – organic compounds (as a phenol or alcohol) combined with the sugar portion of a glycoside

Agonist – a substance that acts in manner similar to another agent/substance that is discussed

Albinism – a group of inherited skin disorders where there is no pigment (melanin) in the skin, hair and eyes

Aldosterone – a hormone secreted by the outside layer (cortex) of the adrenal glands that controls sodium and potassium balance in the body, mainly acting on the kidney

Alkaloids – Natural nitrogen-containing organic (substances that contain a carbon atom) substances which are combined with acids to form crystalline salts. There are numerous alkaloids which are often colourless, complex, and bitter organic bases (as morphine or caffeine) that occur especially in seed plants and are typically physiologically active

Allergens – any substance, usually a protein, which causes the formation of antibodies on entering the human body and reacts with these antibodies to cause mild/moderate/severe allergic (hypersensitivity) reactions

Alopecia – hair loss, either localized or total

Amenorrhoea – absence of the menstrual flow (periods) during the time of life at which it should occur

Amoebic dysentery – a diarrhoea caused by the amoeba *Amoeba histolytica*

Anabolic – a metabolic process by which tissues are built up or strengthened

Anaemia – a condition characterized by inadequate red blood cells and/or haemoglobin in the blood

Analeptic – substances that act as stimulants of the central nervous system

Analgesics – drugs that relieve or abolish pain

Anaphylaxis – an immediate and serious hypersensitivity reaction due to the combination of an allergen with the antibodies in the body

Androgens – a group of hormones that govern the development and characteristics of the sexual organs in males

Aneurysm – a localized swelling or dilation of an artery due to weakening of its wall

Angina pectoris – pain in the centre of the chest, usually behind the sternum (breast bone) due to poor blood supply to the heart muscle, usually a symptom of a heart attack

Angio-oedema – a variant of urticaria (hives) where massive oedema (swelling) involves tissues under the skin (subcutaneous)

Anorexia – loss of appetite

Antacids – drugs traditionally used to reduce the acidity of the stomach and also to treat stomach ulcers

Antibodies – substances which are produced in the body as a form of defence against toxins or bacteria

Anticoagulant – drugs which inhibit the clotting (coagulation) of the blood

Anticonvulsant – drugs which reduce or prevent fits (seizures)

Antiemetic – a drug that prevents or stops vomiting

Antigen – substances which cause the formation of antibodies

Antihelminthic – substances that are effective against worm infestations

Antihistamines – drugs that are used in the treatment of allergic conditions which are due to the production of histamine by the body in response to an allergen

Anti-inflammatory – substances that prevent or treat inflammations

Antimicrobial – substances that are effective against bacterial infections

Anti-neoplastic – substances that are effective against neoplasms (e.g. cancers)

Antioxidant – a compound that can neutralize oxygen-free radicals in the body that could damage cells. Oxidation, or the loss of an electron, can sometimes produce reactive substances known as free radicals that can cause oxidative stress or damage to the cells. Antioxidants are capable of stabilizing free radicals before they can react and cause harm

Antipyretic – substances that reduce body temperature or fever

Antiseptic – substances used to remove disease-causing micro-organisms without damaging living tissues

Antispasmodics – drugs which have the property of preventing spasms, i.e. contractions of muscle in intestine or stomach or ureters of the kidney

Antitussive – prevent or suppress cough

Antivenin – neutralizes the harmful effects of venoms (e.g. snakes, scorpions)

Anxiolytic – drugs for the relief of anxiety

Apthous ulcers – painful ulcers in the mouth usually caused by stress

Aqueous humour – a liquid found in the eye; if the amount is increased it causes an increase in 'intraocular pressure' and eventually the disorder 'glaucoma' (see below)

Arrhythmia – any variation from the normal rhythm of the heart-beat

Arthritis – inflammation of the joints in limbs or spine

Ascites – accumulation of fluid in the abdominal cavity

Asthma – a disorder of breathing characterized by wheezing and shortness of breath due to narrowing of the small tubes (e.g. bronchioles) in the lungs through which air moves in and out

Astringent – prevents the manifestations (signs and symptoms) of an inflammatory reaction

Ataxia – loss of co-ordination, though the power necessary to make the movements is still present

Atherosclerosis – a condition in which there is fatty change in the walls of arteries that usually leads to narrowing of arteries and formation of blood clots (thrombi)

Atony – 'without tone'; absence of tone in muscles and other organs

Atopic – a form of hypersensitivity which usually runs in families

Atrophy – occurs when normal tissue or an organ becomes smaller due to lack of nutrition or inadequate blood supply

Autoimmune – a reaction by an individual's immune system to their own tissues, to which tolerance has been lost, usually causing harm or ill-health

B

Bacteriostatic – substances that stop bacteria increasing in number

Barium enema – an investigation where barium is introduced into the lower bowel via the anus

Biliary colic – severe pain caused contractions of the smooth muscle of the bile duct

Bilirubin – the main pigment in human bile

Borborygmus – flatulence (wind) in the bowels that causes rumbling

Bradycardia – slowing of the heart rate; slow pulse rate

Bronchiectasis – a condition characterized by dilatations of sections of the bronchi (small tubes within the lung that enables movement of air in and out of the lung); which tend to accumulate secretions and get infected.

Bronchitis – inflammation of the bronchial tubes

C

Cachexia – severe weight loss and listlessness produced by serious disease (cancer, tuberculosis or prolonged starvation)

Carbuncles – a cluster of boils

Carcinoma – a progressive growth of cells; cancer, which can spread to other tissues

Carminative – a medicine to relieve flatulence (wind), and any resulting griping

Carotenoids – a class of antioxidant compounds found in many plants

Catecholamines – substances produced in the body, usually by the inner layer (medulla) of the adrenal glands, e.g. adrenaline, which are known to constrict or narrow blood vessels

Cathartics – substances which produce an evacuation of the bowels

Cerebrovascular accidents/stroke – a disease state due to damage to brain tissue caused either by a lack of blood supply (usually a blood clot blocking an artery to the brain) or rupture of a blood vessel within the brain

Chancre – the first local lesion of the sexually transmitted disease syphilis

Chemotherapy – the prevention or treatment, principally of cancers/malignant disease, by chemical substances

Chloretic – stimulates the formation of bile

Cholagogue – a substance which increases the flow of bile by stimulating contraction of the gall bladder

Cholecystectomy – removal of the gall bladder by surgery

Cholesterol – a fat (lipid) that is an important constituent of body cells and is widely distributed throughout the body, present in the blood; increases of blood cholesterol have been associated with an increased risk of heart attack

Chorea – occurrence of short, purposeless involuntary movements of the face, head, hands and feet, as for example in Huntington's chorea

Chronotropic – increases the rate of the heart beat

Claudication – a cramp-like pain that occurs in the muscles of the legs on walking

Climacteric – the menopause

Colic – an attack of spasmodic pain, usually in the abdomen

Conjunctivitis – inflammation of the conjunctiva; that is, the whites of the eye; the most common cause of red eyes

Contusion – bruise; injury to the deeper layers of the skin or underlying tissues, with variable bleeding but without an open wound

Convulsions – commonly called fits, which are rapidly alternating contractions and relaxations of the muscles, causing irregular movements of the limbs or body, which may be associated with loss of consciousness

Cor pulmonale – another name for pulmonary heart disease characterized by failure of the right ventricle of the heart

Corticosteroids – group of hormones produced by the adrenal cortex, also called steroids, which are absolutely essential for life

Cranial nerves – nerves arising from the brain

Crohn's disease – a chronic inflammatory disease of the lower bowel

Crural ulcer – an ulcer connected with the leg

CT or CAT scan – a radiological investigation that produces cross-sectional images of the body

Cyanosis – bluish discolouration of mucous membranes, finger nails, tongue, lips etc due to lack of oxygen

Cyst – a benign hollow tumour containing fluid or soft material

Cystic fibrosis – an inherited disease of the glands of the lungs, pancreas, mouth and gastrointestinal tract, characterized by failure to gain weight, repeated chest infections (bronchitis) and foul smelling stools

Cystitis – inflammation of the bladder

Cytochromes – enzymes (see below) that are found within a cell and are involved in the metabolism of that cell

D

Dementia – an acquired and irreversible deterioration in mental functions, usually seen in old age

Demulcent – a soothing agent

Dermatitis – inflammation of the skin

Diabetes mellitus – a condition where there is an increased amount of glucose (sugar) in the blood due to a deficiency in the production of a hormone which controls blood sugar levels in the body (insulin), that is produced by the pancreas

Diaphoretic – an agent that promotes perspiration (sweating)

Diuretics – substances which increase the flow of urine

Diverticulum – a pouch or pocket of tissue leading off the main cavity of a body organ, or tube, usually in the intestine (gut), which when inflamed causes diverticulitis

Dropsy – retention of fluid within the body; the current medical term is 'oedema'

Dysmenorrhoea – pain during menstruation (periods)

Dyspepsia – another name for indigestion

Dysphonia – altered voice, usually decreased sound

Dysuria – difficulty or pain while passing urine

E

Ectopic pregnancy – pregnancy developing outside the cavity of the uterus, usually in the fallopian tubes (see below)

Eczema – inflammation of the skin with itching and discharge from vesicles (minute swellings in the skin)

Electrocardiograph (ECG) – a record of the variations in electric activity in the heart as it contracts and relaxes

Electroencephalography (EEG) – a graphical record of the brain's electric potentials discharged by nerve cells

Electrolytes – substances whose molecules split into their constituent electrically charged particles when dissolved in water

Emmenagogue – an agent that promotes menstruation (periods)

Emollients – substances which have a softening and soothing effect on the skin

Encephalopathy – conditions in which there are signs of cerebral (brain) irritation without any apparent localized injury/lesion to account for them

Enzymes – a protein which acts as a catalyst for metabolic processes within the body

Epilepsy – a medical disease which is characterized by recurrent fits (seizures)

Epistaxis – bleeding from the nose

Erectile dysfunction – male sexual disorder where erection of the penis is defective

Erysipelas – infection of the skin (caused by the streptococcus bacteria) characterized by fever and a rash on the lower leg or the face

Erythema – redness of the skin due to dilatation of blood vessels

Euphoria – a feeling of well-being. In mental disease there may be an unjustified sense of well-being and this state – unjustified euphoria – can also be brought about by drugs of abuse

Eustachian tube – tubes, one on each side, leading from the middle ear (the chamber of the ear lying immediately behind the ear drum or 'tympanic membrane') to the nasal cavity

Expectorants – drugs that help the removal of secretions from the air passages by promoting coughing

F

Fallopian tubes – tubes, one on each side, which lead from the ovaries to the uterus (womb), having one end attached to the womb and have the other, open end lying close to the ovary, down which eggs travel from the ovaries

Febrifuge – agent used to reduce fever

Fibrinolytic – the way in which blood clots are dissolved within blood vessels

Fibroids – benign tumours arising from the smooth muscle layer of the uterus (womb)

Fibromyalgia – a disease of uncertain causation (aetiology) characterized by many non-specific symptoms, such as pain and fatigue, multiple tender sites in muscles, and disturbed sleep patterns

Flavonoids – a class of antioxidant compounds

Fulminant – a disease developing suddenly

Furuncle/Furunculosis – another term for a boil

G

Galactogogue – promotes production of breast milk

Gall stones – stones found within the gall bladder

Gastritis – inflammation of the stomach lining

Gastrointestinal – pertaining to the stomach and intestines

Gingivitis – inflammation of the gums

Glaucoma – increased pressure within the eye, which over time can lead to blindness

Glomerular nephritis – an inflammatory disease of the kidneys

Glottis – narrow opening at the upper end of the voice box (larynx)

Glycoside – a compound molecule formed of a sugar and a non-sugar unit

Goitre – a swelling in the front of the neck caused by an enlargement of the thyroid gland

Gonorrhoea – a sexually transmitted inflammatory disease affecting the mucous membrane (lining) of the urethra in the male and vagina in the female

Gout – a condition associated with a raised concentration of uric acid in the blood which causes pain in joints, usually the joint of the big toe

H

Haemarthrosis – bleeding into, or the presence of blood in, a joint

Haematemesis – vomiting of blood

Haematoma – a collection of blood within the body forming a definite swelling

Haematuria – passage of blood in the urine

Haemolysis – destruction of red blood cells

Haemolytic anaemia – anaemia which is due to excessive destruction of red blood cells, usually seen in the newborn

Haemophilia – an inherited disorder of blood clotting which results in prolonged bleeding even after minor injury

Haemoptysis – the coughing of blood from the lungs

Haemorrhoids – 'piles'; swollen or dilated veins ('varicose veins') which tend to occur as lumps in the lining of the anus

Halitosis – another term for bad breath

Hepatitis – inflammation of the liver cells

Hernia – the protrusion of an organ, or part of an organ, through the wall of the cavity that normally contains it

Hiatus hernia – a displacement of a portion of the stomach through the opening in the diaphragm through which the oesophagus passes from the chest to the abdominal cavity

Histamines – substances widely distributed in the tissues of plants and animals, including man, which are considered responsible for allergic reactions

Hydrocephaly – an abnormal accumulation of fluid (cerebrospinal fluid) within the skull, which may cause an enlargement of the head

Hypercalcaemia – raised blood calcium concentrations

Hyperhidrosis – excessive sweating

Hyperplasia – usually an abnormal increase in the number of cells in a tissue/organ resulting in organ enlargement

Hypertension – high blood pressure

Hypertrophy – increase in size of cells or organs as a result of on-going increased demand. For example, in body builders the muscles continue to increase in size or hypertrophy owing to regular demands to carry increasing weight

Hyperventilation – an abnormally rapid breathing rate

Hypnotic – a drug that induces sleep

Hypochondria – a delusion of ill health, often severe, by patients

Hypokalaemia – abnormally low concentration of potassium in the blood

Hypothalamus – part of the brain that regulates many body functions

Hypothyroidism – disease due to abnormally low levels of thyroid hormone

I

Ichthyosis – a disorder in which the skin is permanently dry and scaly

Idiopathic – a term applied to diseases to indicate that their cause is unknown

Ileum – the lower part of the small intestine

Immunosuppressants – drugs that suppress the normal immune responses of the body. Usually used to prevent rejection of transplanted organs

Impetigo – an infectious skin disease which causes intense itching rash on the face and elsewhere on the body. Vesicles erupt and may become infected (pustules) and leave yellowing brown scabs

In vitro – a term used in medical research and experimental biology to refer to observations made outside the body, usually in laboratory experiments

Incubation period – the period elapsing between the time when a person becomes infected by some agent and the first appearance of the symptoms of the disease

Infestation – the presence of animal parasites in the intestine, hair or clothing

Inotropic – increase of the force of contraction, usually of heart muscle

Iridoids – constituents of many medicinal plants which may be responsible for the some of their pharmaceutical effects

Ischaemic heart disease – disease of the heart muscle due to poor blood supply to the heart muscle

J

Jaundice – a yellow discoloration of the skin, mucous membranes and eyes due to the deposition of bile pigment

K

Keratitis – inflammation of the cornea (the transparent white lining of the eye which permits light to enter the inner eye) in response to bacterial, chemical, radiation or mechanical trauma

L

Lachrymation – formation of tears by the lachrymal glands, which connect to the eyes via the tear ducts

Lactation – production of milk by the breasts

Laparoscopy – a technique by which the contents of the abdomen may be examined by insertion of a tube with a light, through a small hole made in the abdominal wall

Laparotomy – a surgical operation where the abdominal cavity is opened

Larynx – voice box

Leucorrhoea – whitish discharge from the vagina

Leukaemia – a malignant disease of white blood cells

Leukoplakia – a white plaque on the mucous membranes, usually in the mouth, which may be pre-cancerous

Lichen planus – inflammation of the skin characterized by small shiny papules which may come together to form larger plaques. The cause is unknown but may be due to emotional factors and may also be caused by some drugs, such as chloroquine which is used to treat malaria

Lipoproteins – types of fats bound to proteins found in the blood

Lumbago – pain in the lower region of the back

Lumbar – the lower part of the spinal column

Lymph nodes – collections of cells at various sites in the lymphatic system through which lymph drains

Lymphocytes – a variety of white blood cells produced by lymphoid tissues, which are also involved in the formation of lymph and antibodies

Lymphoma – a malignant proliferation (growth) of lymphoid tissue of which there are two main types Hodgkins and non-Hodgkins; the primary sign is enlarged lymph glands, usually in the neck and armpits (axillae)

M

Malaena – blood in the faeces/stools; passage of dark, tarry masses in the faeces/stools

Mania – a form of mental disorder where an elevated mood is often accompanied by hallucinations and delusions, and often great excitement

Mastitis – inflammation of the breast, most commonly associated with the early days of breast feeding

Megakaryocytes – bone marrow cells which contain large numbers of nuclei and platelet granules from which blood platelets form; that is, precursors of blood platelets, which are essential for the blood clotting process

Melancholia – an old-fashioned term for a form of mental illness characterized by great mental and physical depression

Melanin – pigment which gives colour to the skin, hair and eye

Meningitis – inflammation of the membranes of the brain or spinal cord or, usually, both

Menopause – the term applied to the cessation of menstruation at the end of a woman's reproductive life

Menorrhagia – abnormally heavy blood loss during periods (menstruation)

Metastasis – the process by which malignant disease (e.g. cancers) spreads to distant sites of the body resulting in secondary tumours, also called secondary deposits

Meteorism – the distension of the abdomen by gas produced in the intestines

Methaemoglobinaemia – a condition due to the presence in the blood of a different form of haemoglobin which cannot carry oxygen

MRI scan – a very sensitive and highly developed X-ray technique which is used to examine tissues in a non-invasive manner; unlike standard X-ray it shows soft tissue as well as bone

Mucilage – a viscous substance usually obtained from plant seeds by maceration (softening by soaking)

Mucous membrane – the general name given to the membrane which lines many of the hollow organs of the body (e.g. mouth)

Multiple sclerosis – a progressive disease of the brain and spinal cord which may result in paralysis and tremors and in severe disability

Musculoskeletal – relating to muscle and bones and also tendons

Mutagenic – an agent that causes an alteration in genetic material

Myalgia – pain in muscles

Mydriasis – dilatation of the pupil of the eye

Myeloid – a type of cell in the bone marrow that gives rise to white blood cells

Myeloma – a malignant disease of the blood forming tissues of the bone marrow

Myocardial infarction – heart attack: death of heart muscle due to lack of blood supply, usually due to a blood clot blocking blood flow

Myocarditis – inflammation of the heart muscle
Myocardium – heart muscle

N

Nasal septum – the cartilage that divides the nose into two sections
Nausea – the sensation that vomiting may be about to occur
Necrosis – death of cells, often of a limited part of a tissue, due to disease or damage
Neonatal – pertaining to the first month of life
Nephritis – an inflammatory disease of the kidney
Neuralgia – pain which is the result of damage to or irritation of a nerve
Neurasthenia – fatigue and listlessness attributed to disease of the nerves
Neuritis – inflammation of the nerves
Neurological – pertaining to the nervous system
Neuropathy – a disease affecting the nerves
Neurotransmitters – chemical messengers which transmit impulses from nerve to nerve or nerve to other cells
Neutrophils – type of white blood cells, which usually form the first line of defence in infections
Nociceptive pain – pain attributed to damage of nerves rather than tissues
Nocturia – increased passage of urine at night
Noradrenaline – a chemical messenger (catecholamine) produced by the sympathetic nervous system (part of the autonomic nervous system) and adrenal medulla

O

Occipital – part of the back of the head just above the neck
Oedema – an abnormal accumulation of fluid beneath the skin resulting in swelling
Oesophagus – muscular tube that carries food and drink from the mouth to the stomach
Oestrogen – a female sex hormone
Oliguria – passage of small volumes of urine
Oncology – study of malignant diseases (cancers)
Ophthalmic – associated with the eyes
Opiates – agents like morphine which are derived from the opium plant, commonly referred to as 'the poppy plant' or opium poppy which is *Papaver somniferum*
Optic nerve – the nerve that carries impulses from the eye to the brain
Osteomalacia – softening of bones due to loss of minerals
Osteoporosis – brittleness and increased porosity of bones
Otitis media – inflammation of the middle ear
Ovulation – development and release of an egg or 'ovum' from the ovary

P

Palpitations – being aware of the beating of your heart
Pancreatitis – inflammation of the pancreas
Pancytopenia – a marked reduction in the number of all blood cells
Papules – small solid elevation of the skin or mucous membrane
Paralysis – loss of muscle power due to a lesion in a nerve/s
Parasympathetic – a part of the autonomic nervous system, which controls all the automatic processes in the body, e.g. breathing
Parkinson's – a disease of the nervous system characterized by tremors of the arms and legs and an abnormal way of walking (gait)
Pathology – the study of disease, its causes and development
Pemphigoid – a variant of the autoimmune skin disease pemphigus where blistering occurs as a result of separation of the layers of the skin; it is common in the elderly.
Pemphigus – an autoimmune skin disease where the outer layer of the skin, the 'epidermis', is affected as the cells tend to separate and form blisters.
Peptic ulcer – an ulcer in the stomach or duodenum
Perineum – area of the body between the opening of the bowel and genitalia

Peripheral neuropathy – loss of sensation in the peripheral parts of limbs, principally fingers and toes

Peristalsis – movements or contractions of the muscle in the bowel which propel the intestinal contents towards the rectum and anus

Peritoneal – relating to the lining of the abdominal cavity

Peritonitis – inflammation of the lining of the abdominal cavity, the peritoneum

Petechiae – small red spots or 'macules' due to bleeding in the skin

Pertussis – whooping cough

Pesticides – agents used to kill or control pests

Pharmacology – study of drugs: their actions, adverse effects and uses

Pharyngitis – inflammation of the pharynx (throat)

Phlebitis – inflammation of the veins

Phlegm – secretions (mucus) from the air passages

Photodermatitis – inflammation of the skin caused by sunlight

Photophobia – increased sensitivity to light

Photosensitivity – abnormal sensitivity, usually of the skin, to sunlight

Pigmentation – colour of the skin owing to the amount of melanin in the skin

Pituitary – a gland in the brain which secretes several hormones that in turn control the secretion of hormones from other glands

Placenta – 'after birth' the organ which nourishes the fetus during pregnancy

Plasma – fluid component of the blood without the red and white blood cells

Pneumonia – inflammation of the lung tissue caused by infection

Polyarteritis nodosa – a disease of uncertain causation characterized by pain in muscles, joints, fever and weight loss and skin lesions such as purpurae (see Purpurae below)

Polyarthritis – inflammation of several joints of the body

Polydipsia – excessive thirst

Polymyalgia rheumatica – a disease characterized by pain and tenderness of muscles and joints

Polyp – growth which is attached by a stalk to its site of origin

Polysaccharides – carbohydrates that can be decomposed by hydrolysis into two or more molecules of monosaccharides

Polyuria – increased passage of urine

Post-ictal amnesia – loss of memory for events just prior to a fit

Poultice – soft moist application to the skin usually for infected lesions

Pre-eclampsia – a complication of the latter half of pregnancy characterized by high blood pressure and impairment of kidney function, leading eventually to fits (eclampsia)

Priapism – a prolonged and painful erection of the penis

Proctoscopy – a procedure which enables a health professional to look at the inner lining of the anus and rectum using a short rigid hollow tube that usually contains a light source

Prodromal – symptoms and signs before a disease shows itself fully

Progesterone – a female sex hormone

Prolactin – a hormone produced by the pituitary gland associated with breast-feeding

Prophylaxis – prevention

Prostatectomy – surgical removal of the prostate gland

Protozoa – a single cell animal; for example, an amoeba (see Amoebic dysentery)

Pruritus – another name for itching

Psoriasis – a skin disorder, commonly inherited, which causes scaly skin

Psychosis – a serious psychiatric disorder commonly regarded as a form of insanity, where the brain function is abnormal and the individual loses touch with reality in an extreme way

Purgative – an agent that promotes evacuation of the bowel

Purpurae – a rash caused by bleeding from small blood vessels (capillaries)

Pyelonephritis – inflammation of the kidney, with pus, due to bacteria

R

Radiological – investigations using x-rays

Radiotherapy – treatment using x-rays, usually for cancers

Reflux – fluid flowing in the opposite direction to normal

Remission – a temporary relief of signs and symptoms of diseases

Retina – the layer at the back of the eyeball sensitive to light

Retinopathy – disease of the retina

Rheumatism – a lay term describing pain in muscles and/or joints

Rheumatoid arthritis – inflammation of the lining (synovial) of joints

Rhizome – a root-like stem from which grow both root and shoots

Rickets – a disease of bone (softening) due to a deficiency of vitamin D

Rubefacient – a substance applied to the skin to increase blood flow, which has the effect of causing redness

S

Salicylates – a group of drugs to which aspirin belongs that contain salicylic acid, which is found in many plants and is also synthesized

Saponins – substances found in some plants, which may help lower cholesterol and may have anticancer effects

Scabies – a contagious itching disease caused by mites

Sciatic nerve – the largest nerve in the human body, which runs from the lower end of the spine to the foot, inflammation or compression of which causes sciatica

Scurvy – disease due to lack of vitamin C

Sebaceous glands – glands in the skin that secrete an oily material (sebum)

Sedative – a calming agent/drug, such as Valium

Seizures – fits, convulsions

Sickle cell disease – an inherited disease of the blood due to sickle shape of red blood cells; distortion of the red blood cells occurs when there is, for example, lack of oxygen and this causes the 'sickled cells' to block blood vessels; the red blood cells also have a shortened life-span

Sigmoidoscopy – examination of the lower bowel using an instrument called an endoscope

Sinuses – air-filled passages behind the face through which air flows after being breathed in through the nose; inflammation of the lining of these passages causes sinusitis

Somatic – relating to the body as opposed to the mind

Sphincter – a circular muscle which surrounds an opening in an organ; for example, the muscle at the lower end of the bladder that has to be released in order for urine to pass out of our bodies

Steatorrhoea – passage of fatty stools

Stenosis – an unnatural narrowing of any passage; most commonly narrowing of blood vessels

Syphilis – a sexually transmitted disease. Syphilis is caused by an organism called a spirochaete, *Treponema pallidum* and transmission by kissing, blood transfusion and skin injuries (percutaneous) have been reported. A fetus can become infected through the placenta

Systemic – affecting the whole body

T

Tachycardia – increased heart rate

Tempero-mandibular joint – the joint between the upper part of the jaw and the skull

Teratogenic – the ability to cause physical defects in a fetus during development

Thrombocytopenia – a decrease in the number of blood platelets

Thrombolysis – dissolving of a blood clot

Thrombosis – formation of a blood clot (thrombus) that then blocks the blood vessels

Thrush – an infection caused by the fungus *Candida albicans*

Thyrotoxicosis – a disease due to excess thyroid hormone

Tincture – an alcoholic solution used in pharmacy

Tinnitus – ringing in the ears

Triglycerides – a group of basic substances from which fats are formed

Tuberculosis – a bacterial infectious disease usually of the lungs, but it may affect other structures e.g. bone

Tumours – growths/swellings

Tympanic membrane – the ear drum, that is the membrane between the outer ear and the middle ear

Typhoid – an infectious water-borne disease

U

Ulcerative colitis – an inflammatory disease of the lower bowel

Urethra – passage or tube which carries urine from the bladder to the exterior

Urethritis – inflammation of the urethra

Urticaria/Hives – the rash produced by the sudden release of histamine in the skin; nettle rash

V

Vagal – relating to the vagus nerve, which supplies the pharynx (throat), larynx (voice box), trachea (windpipe), lungs, oesophagus and upper part of the intestinal tract

Vasoconstriction – narrowing of blood vessels

Vasodilatation – dilation of the blood vessels

Ventricular fibrillation – a very dangerous disorder of heart rhythm

Vermifuge – agents that kill and expel parasitic worms

Vertigo – fear of heights and loss of balance

Vitiligo – an acquired skin condition where clearly defined/circumscribed areas are without pigment due to the absence of pigment producing cells or ‘melanocytes’

Volatile oils – oils that vaporize readily

W

Warts – small growths from the outer layer of the skin caused by a viral infection

Index